Caring for Patients
from Different Cultures

Fourth Edition

Caring for Patients from Different Cultures

FOURTH EDITION

Geri-Ann Galanti

PENN

University of Pennsylvania Press

Philadelphia

Published by
University of Pennsylvania Press
Philadelphia, Pennsylvania 19104-4112

Printed in the United States of America on acid-free paper

10 9 8 7 6 5 4 3 2 1

Library of Congress Cataloging-in-Publication Data

Galanti, Geri-Ann.
    Caring for patients from different cultures / Geri-Ann Galanti.—4th ed.
       p.   cm.
    Includes bibliographical references and index.
    ISBN 978-0-8122-2031-5 (alk. paper)
    1. Transcultural nursing—United States—Case studies. 2. Transcultural medical care—United States—Case studies. 3. Hospital care—Psychological aspects—United States—Case studies. 4. Ethnopsychology—United States—Case studies. I. Title.
    [DNLM: 1. Transcultural Nursing—Case Reports. 2. Cultural Competency—Case Reports. 3. Cultural Diversity—Case Reports. WY 107 G146c 2008]
    RT86.54.G35   2008
    610.73—dc22   2008017463

To the many students and clinicians
who generously shared the case studies within this book.
Thank you!

Contents

Preface to the Fourth Edition

As with previous editions, my explicit goal is to help health care professionals achieve greater cultural competence. The path to cultural competence involves learning about, understanding, and respecting the values and beliefs of others, and then being able to apply the knowledge to provide better care for patients of diverse ethnic backgrounds. Thus, I continue to focus on the concepts I think clinicians need to know, and to use the case studies to illustrate them. Although previous editions have emphasized the clash of cultures, this time I have also tried to include many examples that illustrate how potential problems can be avoided when health care providers practice cultural competence. Those cases are marked by having their case number in *italics*. I have also added a chapter called "Making a Difference." It presents some of the changes that various hospitals have made in order to provide more culturally sensitive care. It is certainly not an exhaustive list, but my hope is that it will inspire other health care institutions to make additional changes.

I have also added a list of "key points" in addition to the summary at the end of each chapter. They are addressed to clinicians, and highlight the key practice points I hope they will remember.

Working with patients from a variety of ethnic groups can be challenging, but when health care practitioners make an effort to be sensitive to the cultural needs of their patients it can add an interesting and pleasurable dimension to the work, and often reduce stress and increase patient satisfaction. This in turn can lead to greater adherence and, ultimately, better patient outcomes. Although many clinicians fear that "cultural competence" will just add one more thing to their already overburdened workload, in reality, it overwhelmingly makes for win-win situations.

Once again, I have included an appendix containing profiles of various cultures and religions. Keep in mind that the profiles are merely meant to be a quick guide to broad culture areas; it must always be remembered that the descriptions will never fit individuals perfectly. They are simply intended to give practitioners a place to start to understand the behavior of others. I have not covered all aspects of all cultures; that would be impossible. I also don't believe it's necessary. My hope is to help clinicians shift their thinking to be more open to cultural variations in general. For that reason I also include a few rare cases that most clinicians will probably never run across. Rather than serving as a guide to what to do or avoid, these cases are meant to exemplify the range of human experience. The examples are all based on actual cases, although sometimes I have taken minor liberties in order to make a point.

I have added an appendix on how to use interpreters, as well as a section in Chapter 1 on asking the right questions. The biggest danger of cultural competence training is that, no matter how often you remind people *not* to stereotype (I've just done it twice in two paragraphs), there is a tendency to misuse cultural information. Culturally competent health care is at its core *patient-centered care*. The most important aspect of that is learning to ask the right questions.

I have updated the bibliography. However, rather than including recommended Web sites and media, I refer readers to the appropriate pages on my Web site (www.ggalanti.com). The material there will be far more current.

In earlier editions, I kept nearly all the case studies from the previous edition and added new ones. This time, I have deleted many of the cases from earlier editions, not because they weren't good, but in the interest of space. I have added nearly 100 cases. Most of what is missing is covered in a new case or in one of the other original cases. Those who have earlier editions of my book will now have a larger pool of cases.

I should mention that there is some repetition throughout the book. This is because some ideas are relevant to a number of topics. Because a reader may choose to read a chapter appropriate to his or her specialty rather than the entire book, when I thought it important, I included the same material in more than one chapter. For example, what should you do when the family don't want you to reveal a negative diagnosis to the patient?

The heart of the book is still the case studies. Once again, I must give credit where credit is due, and in this case credit belongs to the thousands of health care professionals who over the years have shared with me the frustration of dealing with the huge variety of ethnic populations in the United States. When I first began teaching nursing classes, I was incredibly idealistic. I thought I could give the students the knowledge they would need to provide culturally appropriate care. I found, however, that most nurses are overworked and have little time to make adjustments for ethnic differences. They work in the "real world," not an academically idealized version of it. Were my classes of no value, then, beyond mere curiosity?

Fortunately, no. I found I could significantly reduce the nurses' stress by explaining why their patients acted as they did. The ethnic populations were not deliberately trying to irritate the staff; they were simply behaving according to what was appropriate within their culture. Now, when people ask me what I do, I explain that I teach health care providers why their patients are *interesting* rather than *annoying*. It makes a difference. Note that throughout the book I make references to "a nurse who was taking a class in cultural diversity"; the class was mine, taught in the School of Nursing at California State University, Dominguez Hills. The class is called Cultural Diversity and Health Care.

This book spends little time on theoretical issues. Over the years, I have found that the most effective way to make a point is to tell a story. People remember anecdotes much better than they do dry facts and theories. Theories that grow out of stories are much easier to grasp and retain than ones presented in a vacuum because they create a sense of empathy and resonate with our emotions. Thus, the emphasis is on case studies and the lessons we can draw from them.

The general organization of the book is identical to that of the previous edition. The first chapter covers basic theoretical concepts. The rest of the book contains the best of the thousands of incidents of conflict and misunderstanding—or cases where conflict has been avoided through the application of cultural competence—that my students experienced. I have tried to give solutions or ways to avoid problems whenever possible, although it is not always possible. In every case, however, I've attempted to explain why people acted the way they did. I hope that the book will help readers to see things through the eyes of people from cultures that are different from theirs. For me, the most important contribution of anthropology is that it can provide us with new perspectives.

My only fear is that people reading this book will feel their ethnic group has been presented in a bad light or that the individual in the case described is a poor representative of his or her ethnic group. Such accusations would not be entirely unjustified. I have chosen cases that created the greatest trouble for the hospital staff, and the individuals involved may not be the best representatives for their ethnic groups. I have tried to choose examples of behavior that reflect cultural values or customs, even if the behavior is an extreme version. It is my intention to promote understanding, not prejudice. (Troublesome members of my own ethnic group are also well represented here.) I will make a blanket apology at the outset, lest I offend anyone. Truly, no offense is meant. I should also add that I intend no disrespect to any members of the health care profession. Some of the nurses and doctors depicted do not come across as very admirable. Individuals should *not* be taken to represent all members of that group. Hopefully, the examples of things clinicians have done right will counterbalance the negative examples.

The book is organized in thirteen chapters. The first introduces the basic relevant anthropological concepts. The following twelve are arranged according to topic: communication; pain; religion and spirituality; activities of daily living and the body; family; men and women; staff relations; birth; end of life; mental health; traditional medicine; and making a difference. I chose a topical organization rather than one by ethnic group, both to be in keeping with standard clinical texts and because I felt it was more suitable for making theoretical points. The chapter divisions, however, are somewhat arbitrary. There may be material in one chapter that could just as easily fit into another. In such cases, I have referred the reader to related material in other chapters. Some material did not fit well into any chapter but did not warrant a separate one. Life does not always fit into neat categories.

Unlike most books, this one can be read in almost any order, a few pages at a time, although the first chapter should be read first. Each case is self-contained and can be understood on its own.

I decided to use names for all the patients and hospital staff in the various case studies; it makes the stories more accessible. I have tried to use ethnically appropriate names whenever possible. All names are fictitious. If I inadvertently use someone's real name, it is accidental. I use first names for the nurses and last names for the doctors to reflect their common usage. For the patients, I generally use first names for individuals under eighteen and last names for those older, consistent with recommended usage.

I should also note that the terms "Hispanic" and "Latino" are interchangeably used throughout the book. Both are in common usage at the time of writing, and each reflects the preferences of different individuals.

The major goal of the book is to help health care professionals recognize the cultural dimensions of problems that occur in hospitals between and among patients, their families, and staff. Obviously, not every possible problem can be documented. There is no easy "recipe" for solving problems; each individual and situation is different. My hope is that this book will give the reader some idea of the range of cultural behaviors and the need to understand others' actions from the perspective of the other person's culture, as well as offer clinicians some alternatives for providing culturally competent care.

The bibliography is intended as a resource guide for those who want to do more research, either out of general interest or to deal with specific problems. It is divided into five sections: journals, books and articles by topic, books and articles by ethnic group, Internet sites, and videos and CD-ROMs. The list is by no means exhaustive, but it should provide a useful starting point.

Acknowledgments

First, second, and third, I want to thank the hundreds of health care practitioners who generously shared with me the cross-cultural misunderstandings they encountered in their work. Without them, there would be no book. Ideally, each case study would include a note stating the name of the student who shared it with me. However, because I didn't keep such records when I first began collecting cases, I'm unable to do that for all of them. And it doesn't seem right to give credit for some and not others. As a result, no one gets credit. But you know who you are . . . and I hope you know that you have my gratitude. This book is dedicated to you.

Next, I am indebted to the School of Nursing at California State University, Dominguez Hills; the Department of Anthropology at California State University, Los Angeles; and at UCLA, both the School of Nursing and the Doctoring program at David Geffen School of Medicine, where I have taught the courses that gave me access to the nurses and medical students who shared their experiences. I would particularly like to acknowledge Carole Shea, who believed in my approach, and Laura Inouye, for always supporting me. Next, I want to thank all those who hired me to conduct workshops on cultural diversity. Lecturing is a two-way street; I always learn from those I teach.

I also want to thank my editors at the University of Pennsylvania Press, Jo Joslyn and Alison Anderson for graciously answering my endless questions. They were a joy to work with. I'm also grateful to Joyce Ippolito for making my writing sound better than it is.

The teachers and mentors whom I acknowledged in the first edition still deserve credit: Robert Edgerton, Allen Johnson, Susan Scrimshaw, and Lowell Sever. Although she doesn't know me, Madeleine Leininger deserves my recognition for creating the field of transcultural nursing. I would also like to thank Jerry Hoffman, Michael Wilkes, Susan Stangl, and Margi Stuber for helping me see the world through the eyes of physicians, and who have been instrumental in training a new generation of caring physicians. Michael Wilkes has been particularly generous in including me on numerous grants to develop training materials for medical students and residents. It has given me an additional entrée into the culture of medicine, as well as the opportunity to organize my thoughts. Jean Gilbert, Robert Like, and Noel Chrisman have earned my eternal gratitude by generously sharing their comprehensive knowledge with me and answering all my many questions. I've been fortunate to have had the opportunity to work with Jean on a number of projects; thank you, Jean. I also want to thank Judy Eighmy, my extremely knowledgeable and helpful resource on hospice.

I'd also like to recognize two people who have helped get my work out into the public arena: Michael Woods and Jackie Brookman. I've collaborated with Michael Woods on a cultural sensitivity booklet, now being published by Joint Commission Resources, and an e-learning course on cultural competence, being used at numerous hospitals and through University HealthSystems Consortium Learning Exchange. Jackie Brookman encouraged me to develop a "tips" booklet for foreign-born nurses working in the United States, as well as a training manual for health educators, orienting foreign-born nurses to work effectively in American hospitals. The reorganization of the chapter on staff relations reflects some of that work. Hopefully, through their efforts, my work will reach more clinicians than ever before.

In researching the material for the last chapter ("Making a Difference"), I was aided by many individuals. In particular, I would like to acknowledge the many members of the CLAS-talk listserv who responded to my request about what hospitals are doing to provide more culturally competent care: Elsa Batica, Cindy Brach, Linda Choi, Martha Davoli, Florentina Dinu, Wendy Friar, Yolanda Gaskins, Vivian Green, Irina Greenchtein, Boris Kalanj, Nataly Kelly, Becky Watt Knight, Susan Martorell, Jacqueline Voigt, and Amy Wilson-Stronks. Special thanks to Julia Puebla Fortier for running the listserv. I am also grateful to Nataly Kelly for providing notes from the National Council in Interpreting in Health Care Open Call on May 25, 2007 on the topic of on-site and remote interpreting.

Without my husband, Donald Sutherland, there would be no book. He originally conceived of the book, as well as made my life easy while I was writing this edition. I am eternally grateful. Thank you, Don, for everything.

I also want to thank my huge Sephardic family. I never realized how different my upbringing was from that of most Americans until I was in college and read the classic article "The Folk Society" by Robert Redfield. My first reaction was: "The folk society? This sounds just like my family." Being raised in my family gave me insight into more traditional cultures as well as surrounding me with the love and security that gave me the courage to make my way in the world.

Finally, I want to thank my friends who, to me, are like family. As always, you make the world a much better place.

Chapter 1
Basic Concepts

If the United States is a melting pot, the cultural stew still has a lot of lumps.

Introduction

What happens when an Iranian doctor and a Filipino nurse treat a Mexican patient? When a Navajo patient calls a medicine man to the hospital? Or when an Anglo nurse refuses to take orders from a Japanese doctor? Generally, the result is confusion and conflict, unless they all have some understanding of cultural differences.

The health care system in the United States has been in a state of crisis for some time. An obvious problem is the cost and apportionment of medical care. Recently, much attention has been paid to the health care disparities that exist in this country. Despite the best intentions of physicians, minority Americans suffer from a greater proportion of diseases, including diabetes, cancer, cardiovascular disease, HIV/AIDS, and asthma. Research has shown that minorities also receive less treatment than whites, including surgical treatment of lung cancer, fewer cardiac diagnostic and therapeutic procedures, and fewer referrals for renal transplants (see Betancourt and Ananeh-Firempong 2004). Although lower socioeconomic status and lack of insurance are major contributors to these disparities, other factors play an important role. A study by Hasnain-Wynia and colleagues (2007) found that minority patients tend to receive care from lower-quality hospitals. The gap was particularly large in terms of patient counseling. This finding underscores the need for better communication, many aspects of which can be influenced by culture.

The goal of the medical system is to provide optimal care for all patients. In a multiethnic society, this goal can be accomplished only if the health care providers understand such things as why Asian patients rarely ask for pain medication whereas patients from Mediterranean countries seem to need it for the slightest discomfort; why Middle Easterners will not allow a male physician to examine their women; and that coin rubbing is an Asian form of medical treatment, not a form of child abuse.

Cultural Competence

This book addresses the cultural differences that create conflicts and misunderstandings and that may result in inferior medical care. The goal is to help the reader achieve *cultural competence*. It begins with understanding your own culture and biases, becoming sensitive to the cultures of others, and appreciating the differences. The next step involves acquiring knowledge and understanding of other cultures, especially their values and beliefs. The final step is to apply that knowledge. Culturally competent health care will lead to greater patient satisfaction, improved clinical outcomes, and greater cost efficiency. Note that throughout the book, I use the terms "cultural competence" and "cultural sensitivity" somewhat interchangeably.

It should be remembered, however, that cultural competence is a journey, not a destination. I was reminded of this recently when I was a speaker at a conference in the South. The setting was lunch in the grand ballroom. There were over 100 people in the room. Salads sat waiting at every plate. My presentation was over; I was hungry. I waited several minutes for people to begin eating. No one did. Finally, I asked one of my hosts if there was some reason no one was eating. He was rather nonresponsive, and I was starving, so I began to eat. No one else followed suit. A few minutes later, a member of the clergy came to the podium and said grace. Then, everyone picked up their fork and began to eat. What I hadn't considered was that people in the South tend to be more religious than those in the West Coast urban center where I live. Apparently, my host hadn't wanted to embarrass me by pointing out my ignorance when I asked about eating. I wish he had. Sometimes we forget that there can be cultural differences even within our own culture. And no matter how much we think we know, we can still make mistakes.

Asking the Right Questions: The 4 C's

Culturally competent care is essentially patient-centered care. Although the case studies used in this book focus on a variety of ethnic cultures, the principles of cultural competence should be applied to *all* patients. The key factor in achieving cultural competence is learning to ask the right questions to elicit an understanding of the patient's point of view. A number of mnemonics have been developed to help practitioners remember what questions to ask. A simple one, developed by myself and physicians Stuart Slavin and Alice Kuo, is called "The 4 C's of Culture." It was inspired by "The 8 Questions" proposed by Arthur Kleinman and his colleagues (1978).

The first C is for "Call," as in *What do you* call *your problem?* This is to remind the clinician to ask, "What do *you* think is wrong?" It's getting at the patient's perception of the problem. This is an important question because the same symptoms may have very different meanings in different cultures and may result in barriers to compliance. For example, among the Hmong, epilepsy is referred to as "the spirit catches you, and you fall down." Seeing epilepsy as spirit possession (which has some positive connotations for the possessed) is very different from seeing it as a disruption of the electrical signals in the brain. This should lead to a very different doctor-patient conversation and might help explain why a Hmong patient may be less anxious than the physician to stop the seizures. For an excellent example of what can happen when caring, competent physicians do not understand the patient's perspective, see Anne Fadiman's 1997 book *The Spirit Catches You and You Fall Down.* Understanding the patient's point of view can help the health care provider deal with potential barriers to adherence and improve the patient-practitioner relationship.

Another medical anthropologist and I were shadowing a pediatric attending on rounds. A young Mexican boy named Pablo Medina presented with cyclic vomiting. His mother reported that the episodes had occurred in conjunction with specific events. The first was when Pablo saw his dog run over in the street and he watched his father carry the dog's bloody body into the house. The second was when a friend of the family was shot while he was standing next to him. Just before his most recent admission his father informed the family that he (dad) was moving back to Mexico. On the day of admission, Pablo's teacher yelled at him for something that he did wrong. His mother was called to pick him up from school for vomiting. My colleague and I both immediately shared a single thought: *susto.* This is a Hispanic folk disease in which a shock—such as the ones the boy experienced—causes the soul to leave the body. (For more on *susto,* see Chapter 12.) No one mentioned *susto*—not the mother, nor the attending, nor the interpreter. My colleague and I wanted to, but as observers we didn't feel it was our place to do so. But we left wondering, what if the attending had said something like, "That sounds like it could be *susto.*" Perhaps the mother didn't see it that way. But what if she did? Would it have changed the clinical management of the boy's condition? Probably not. His symptoms were treated successfully. But what might it have done for the relationship between the patient and the physician?

We tend to think that everyone respects the knowledge of doctors, but that's not always the case. What if you had just moved to a foreign country and were diagnosed with soul loss by the traditional healer who was held in high esteem by all the villagers? Would you be impressed with his diagnostic skill, or would you think he's not very smart and doesn't really understand what's going on? Might some of your patients feel the same way?

No one is expecting physicians or nurses to work within the health model of their patients, but by showing some respect and understanding for it, they can greatly increase patients' trust. Finding out and acknowledging patients' interpretation of what is wrong can aid in that.

The second C is for "Cause." *What do you think* caused *your problem?* This gets at the patient's beliefs regarding the source of the problem. Not everyone believes that disease is caused by germs. In some cultures, it is thought to be caused by upset in body balance, breach of taboo (similar to what is seen in the United States as diseases due to "sin" and punished by God), or spirit possession. Treatment must be appropriate to the cause, or people will not perceive themselves as cured. Doctors thus need to find out what the patient believes caused the problem, and treat that as well. For example, it may sometimes be appropriate to bring in clergy to pray with them if they believe God is punishing them for some transgression.

2   Emma Chapman, a sixty-two-year-old Black woman, was admitted to the coronary care unit because she had continued episodes of acute chest pain after two heart attacks. Her physician recommended an angiogram with a possible cardiac bypass or angioplasty to follow. Mrs. Chapman refused, saying, "If my faith is strong enough and if it is meant to be, God will cure me." When her nurse asked what she thought caused her heart problems, Mrs. Chapman said she had sinned and her illness was a punishment. Her nurse finally got her to agree to the surgery by suggesting she speak with her minister. This case will be discussed again in Chapter 12, with an additional possible solution suggested (see case 254).

The third C is for "Cope." *How do you* cope *with your condition?* This is to remind the practitioner to ask, "What have you done to try to make it better? Who else have you been to for treatment?" This will give the health care provider important information on the use of alternative healers and treatments. As discussed in Chapter 12, most people will try home remedies before coming in to the physician; however, few will share such information due to fear of ridicule or chastisement. It's important that health care providers learn to ask about such remedies in a nonjudgmental way, because the occasional traditional remedy may be dangerous or could lead to a drug interaction with prescribed medications.

3   Olga Salcedo was a seventy-three-year-old Mexican woman who had just had a femoral-popliteal bypass. Anabel, her nurse, observed that Mrs. Salcedo's leg was extremely red and swollen. She often moaned in pain and was too uncomfortable to begin physical therapy. Yet during her shift report, her previous nurse told Anabel that Mrs. Salcedo denied needing pain medication. Later that day, Anabel spoke with the patient through an interpreter and asked what she had done for the pain in her leg prior to surgery. Mrs. Salcedo said that she had sipped herbal teas given to her by a *curandero* (a traditional healer; see Chapter 12); she didn't want to

take the medications prescribed by her physician. Anabel, using cultural competence, asked Mrs. Salcedo's daughter to bring in the tea. Anabel paged the physician about the remedy and brought it to the pharmacist, who researched the ingredients. Because there was nothing contraindicated, the pharmacist contacted Mrs. Salcedo's physician, who told her she could take the tea for her pain. The next day, Mrs. Salcedo was able to go to physical therapy and was much more motivated and positive in demeanor. Although it took some time to coordinate the effort, in the end, it resulted in a better patient outcome. Had Anabel not asked what she had been using to cope with her pain, it is likely Mrs. Salcedo would have delayed physical therapy and thus her recovery.

The fourth and final C is for "Concerns." *What concerns do you have regarding the condition?* This should address questions such as "How serious do you think this is?" "What potential complications do you fear?" "How does it interfere with your life, or your ability to function?" It is important to understand the patient's perception of the course of the illness and the fears they may have about it so you can address their concerns and correct any misconceptions. You also want to know what aspects of the condition pose a problem for the patient; this may help you uncover something very different from what you might have expected. This C also includes *What are your concerns regarding the recommended treatment?* It is also important to know a patient's concerns in order to avoid problems of nonadherence, because some patients may have misplaced concerns based upon their own or others' past experience.

Jorge Valdez, a middle-aged Latino patient, presented with poorly managed diabetes. When Dr. Alegra, his physician, told him that he might have to start taking insulin, he became upset and kept repeating, "No insulin, no insulin." Not until Dr. Alegra asked Mr. Valdez what concerns he had about insulin did he tell her that both his mother and uncle had gone blind after they started taking insulin. He made the logical—though incorrect—assumption that insulin caused blindness. In this case, the patient expressed his fears and because the physician was competent enough to pick up on them and explore them, she was able to allay them. In many cases, however, unless the physician specifically asks about concerns, patients will say nothing and simply not adhere to treatment. By asking, the health care provider can correct any misconceptions that can interfere with treatment.

The remainder of this chapter is devoted to several anthropological concepts that may help the reader understand the source of many of the conflicts and misunderstandings contained within the book. Many will be reviewed in the chapters that follow as well, when additional incidents that illustrate the principles are described.

4

Culture

A basic working definition of culture is that it encompasses beliefs and behaviors that are learned and shared by members of a group.

A man I know removes his shoes when he enters the house. He has indoor shoes and outdoor shoes and will not wear one for the other. Is this a cultural trait or a personal idiosyncrasy? From the information given, it is impossible to tell. One must know his ethnic background. If he were Japanese, it would be a cultural trait. He is not. He is a white Anglo-Saxon Protestant from New York. Thus this trait is a personal idiosyncrasy. For behavior to be cultural, it must be learned and shared by members of a group. New York WASPs do not make a practice of removing their shoes when entering a house. The Japanese do.

Subcultures

Within most cultures, smaller groups of people share certain characteristics not shared by the culture at large. Anthropologists call such groups subcultures. Subcultures may be based upon a variety of things, including ethnicity (Hispanic Americans, Asian Americans), occupation (nurses, physicians), activity (gangs), or sexual orientation (lesbians). When one subculture has more power than another, it is referred to as the "dominant" culture. Those subcultures with less power are called "minority" cultures and are often discriminated against.

Every culture and subculture has its own values, worldview, language ("jargon"), and norms (rules of acceptable behavior). For example, Anglo American culture values independence, a value not shared by many of the other ethnic groups found in the United States. Part of the American worldview is to believe that humans control nature. American social norms include the following rule of behavior: if someone offers you something you want, you may accept it with thanks the first time it is offered. Iranian cultural rules, in contrast, dictate that you wait until it is offered a second time; the first is to be polite; the second is sincere. Chinese cultural rules would have you wait until it is offered a third time. Another American cultural rule is that the needs of your children come before those of your parents, directly opposite to the norm in most Asian cultures. A third American rule of behavior is that you firmly shake hands in greeting someone. This may violate the norm of many Middle Eastern cultures, which prohibit touching between members of the opposite sex.

Nursing and medicine are two examples of subcultures. If you are a health care practitioner, consider what values, worldview, language, and norms describe your subculture. When I was teaching a nursing class several years ago, during a break, several of us were in the restroom. I noticed one of the nurses following an elaborate ritual. After using the toilet, she went to the sink, turned on the water, and scrubbed her hands and arms with much more vigor than I thought necessary for the occasion. She then left the water running while she went to get a paper towel to dry her hands, and finally turned off the faucets using her elbows. I stood there staring. When I brought this up in class, all the students—all nurses—thought her behavior sounded quite normal. From the perspective of an outsider, it was actually quite bizarre. The hand-washing ritual is one of the norms of the nursing subculture; it is based on the worldview belief that germs cause disease.

Stereotype Versus Generalization

I will be making many generalizations in this book. They should not be mistaken for stereotypes. The difference between a stereotype and a generalization lies not in the *content*, but in the *usage* of the information. An example is the assumption that Mexicans have large families. If I meet Rosa, a Mexican woman, and I say to myself, "Rosa is Mexican; she must have a large family," I am stereotyping her. But if I think Mexicans often have large families and then ask Rosa how many people in her family, I am making a generalization.

A *stereotype* is an ending point. No attempt is made to learn whether the individual in question fits the statement. Stereotyping patients can have negative results.

Lily Khalid was a forty-eight-year-old woman from the Middle East. She was in the county hospital to have surgery for gallstones. Sandy, a Mexican American nurse, was caring for her prior to surgery. Sandy cared for Mrs. Khalid for three nights and describes them as a nightmare. Mrs. Khalid did nothing but moan and groan and demand pain medication. She was on the call light continually. Sandy did her job but resented her behavior. She chalked it up to her ethnic background—Middle Easterners are often demanding and express their pain freely and loudly. She looked forward to Mrs. Khalid's surgery; at last, her gallstones would be removed and she could go home.

When Sandy returned to work a week later, she learned that Mrs. Khalid had not had gallstones after all. When the surgeons opened her up, they discovered that cancer had invaded her entire gastrointestinal system. She died on the operating table. Sandy's heart sank. She had stereotyped Mrs. Khalid as just another loud, complaining Middle Easterner. It turned out that she had been moaning and groaning and requesting pain medication not because she was Middle Eastern, but because she was riddled with cancer and in excruciating pain. It was an important lesson for Sandy about the dangers of stereotyping.

6   While taking a course on cultural diversity, Anike Oghogho, a nurse from Nigeria, recognized his tendency to stereotype. He related an example of an African American male patient who presented with a swollen left foot. The patient, Jefferson Bell, kept ringing the call light and asking for more pain medication. Anike said that in the past, he would have assumed Mr. Bell was merely seeking pain meds. This time, however, he reassessed the patient. He discovered that Mr. Bell's fourth and fifth toes were more red and swollen and had pus. Anike summoned the physician, and Mr. Bell was eventually taken to the operating room for incision and drainage of his left foot. Stereotyping could have severely harmed the patient; fortunately, Anike had learned the lesson of *not* stereotyping in his class.

A generalization, in contrast, is a beginning point. It indicates common trends, but further information is needed to ascertain whether the statement is appropriate to a particular individual. Generalizations may be inaccurate when applied to specific individuals, but anthropologists do apply generalizations broadly, looking for common patterns, for beliefs and behaviors that are shared by the group. It is important to remember, however, that there are always differences between individuals; each case must be considered by itself. So why even bother with a generalization? Because it can help us understand and anticipate behavior. Rather than becoming annoyed because my Mexican patient is moaning and groaning in the absence of any serious problems, I might note, "Ah, Mexican culture encourages emotional expressiveness." Or, knowing that Asians value stoicism might help me remember to pay more attention to an Asian patient's pain needs rather than draw conclusions based on the fact that the patient isn't moaning or requesting pain medication. Of course, this should be done with *all* patients.

One of the reasons that stereotyping is so inappropriate is that no one ever belongs to just one culture. We belong to numerous cultures, including those of ethnicity, religion, region of the country, generation, sex, occupation, education, and socioeconomic status. All of them have some varying degree of influence on us. Add to that the degree of assimilation, which includes such factors as the length of time spent in the United States, the age of immigration, desire to assimilate, and residence in an ethnic community or an "American" one. When you also consider the influence of personality factors and individual life experiences, it should be obvious why stereotyping is not just dangerous, but more likely to be incorrect than anything else.

I have purposely chosen examples of individuals who have not assimilated to a great degree and whose beliefs and behaviors deviate from those expressed in the American health care system. It should not be inferred that all or even most members of these groups would act in the manner described. The ones who are most Westernized do not generally present problems. It is those who adhere to traditional ways that are most likely to do so, hence their inclusion in this book. It should be remembered, however, that assimilation occurs in unpredictable stages. Individuals may be quite Westernized in some areas but traditional in others.

I will be making many generalizations throughout this book. I will also be lumping together groups that are actually quite distinct from each other. The term "Hispanic" or "Latino" includes people from such diverse cultures as Mexican, Puerto Rican, Argentinean, and Peruvian. "Asian" refers to people from a variety of countries, including China, Japan, Korea, Vietnam, Cambodia, and the Philippines. It is dangerous and inaccurate to think they are all alike. When I do make such generalizations, it is because there are some traits that are fairly consistent across cultures within the designated group. But never forget individual differences.

Also remember when you come into contact with people from different cultures that it is often highly offensive to them to be labeled by the wrong country. Many are historical enemies. There is also a tremendous amount of prejudice and stereotyping within each larger culture area. A Chinese student shared that many Chinese think that Vietnamese have prominent cheekbones, Koreans have small eyes, and Japanese are short. These are all seen as characteristics that are inferior to those of the more "beautiful" Chinese. A Chinese person would probably be insulted if mistaken for a Korean, and vice versa. Ethnocentrism is universal, and stereotyping occurs even within ethnic groups.

Carla, a half-Mexican nurse, observed that in Mexico those with more European blood often feel superior to those with more Indian heritage. In addition, city people look down somewhat on rural people. It is an insult to call someone "provincial." Those from D.F. (Districto Federal, Mexico City) feel superior to everyone. She, however, prided herself on being immune to all the hierarchical structuring; she firmly believed in the equality of all people.

One day Carla had a patient who was from Mexico. Carla assumed from Mrs. Arroyo's dark skin, black hair, and facial features that she was a Mexican Indian, probably with little education. Carla realized she would have to speak to her rather simply, to make sure that she understood. This was probably her first time in a hospital. She asked the patient which part of Mexico she was from. Mrs. Arroyo looked Carla directly in the eyes and said, "I'm from D.F. And you?"

Carla, who had never realized her own inherent prejudices, was speechless for a moment. She replied, "My father is from Guanajuato." To which Mrs. Arroyo responded, "Yes, I thought as much. I can always spot you provincial people; you are very different."

There are some lessons to be learned from this incident. One is that most of us, even though we may consider ourselves free of prejudice, probably are not. Another is that even within the same culture, people judge and stereotype each other. Finally, it is always a mistake to stereotype people on the basis of appearance.

Generalizations made in this book about large cultural groups such as Asians or Hispanics may be seen as a way of distinguishing broad geographical groupings from each other while recognizing that there are differences within them. Also, on occasion, the only ethnic identity given for a patient is Asian or Hispanic because more detailed information was not known, but the case illustrated a general point common to most cultures within that group.

It is important to recognize that the cases chosen for this book were selected specifically because the misunderstandings were due to cultural differences. Many interactions between individuals of the same two cultures will occur without conflict or misunderstanding, because not every member of an ethnic group adheres to all the traditional beliefs and practices of that group. Alternately, conflicts and misunderstandings will occur between members of different ethnic groups that have nothing to do with culture, but result from individual differences and personality clashes. That is why it is extremely important *not* to stereotype individuals. The generalizations provided in this book are meant to be suggested guideposts, not precise, detailed maps. Ideally, they will help health care providers anticipate possibilities that should be considered, and make sense of behavior that has already occurred.

Prejudice and Discrimination

An important related issue in today's world, given strained inter-ethnic relations, is that of prejudice and discrimination. The long history of slavery in this country, followed by Reconstruction and its aftermath, along with less institutionalized racism, has led many African Americans to distrust the health care system.

8   Mr. Harris, a sixty-eight-year-old African American man, was scheduled to have his cancerous prostate removed at a government hospital. Two days after scheduling the procedure, he called Karen, his nurse, in panic. He had spoken to several friends about his upcoming surgery and now wanted to know about various forms of alternative treatments. Karen spent about an hour on the phone with him and gave him a great deal of information as well as phone numbers he could call to learn about other options. She realized that he was probably overwhelmed and frightened about his diagnosis.

Right before hanging up, Mr. Harris said, "You know I trust *you*, Karen; I just don't know if I trust the hospital to take care of me. I have older friends who were subjected to government studies without knowing it back in the '40s and '50s." Karen suddenly realized it wasn't just the cancer he feared, but what a white institution might do to him, a Black man. The experiments done with syphilitic black men who were left untreated in order to study the course of the disease are infamous.

It is no wonder that many African Americans are distrustful of hospitals—and white institutions in general. Prejudice and discrimination are real. Not surprisingly, if you have been a frequent victim of discrimination, you are likely to come to expect it, even, as in the next two cases, when it is not there.

During a prenatal exam, an obstetrics resident asked the patient whether she had considered having her tubes tied at the time of delivery. The patient, Lotty Parker, was a forty-three-year-old Black woman, pregnant with her twelfth child. Mrs. Parker immediately became angry, saying, "I ain't gonna have no white doctor messin' with my insides!" The resident may have felt that it was his responsibility to explain increased pregnancy risks after forty, but the Black woman apparently viewed his suggestion as a form of racial genocide. Health care personnel must be especially sensitive to this issue when dealing with patients from minority ethnic groups. Rather than directly asking if she wanted her tubes tied, a culturally competent physician might have begun by asking Mrs. Parker if she enjoys having such a large family. If she said she loves it, the doctor wouldn't need to pursue the issue and would avoid asking a racist-sounding question. If, however, she said that it's difficult raising so many children, the physician could then ask if she would like to limit her family size to twelve. If she said yes, the physician could suggest having her tubes tied. In general, health care providers should try to ascertain the *patient*'s attitude, rather than imposing their own.

Another case, which could have ended as badly as the previous one, was rescued by the cultural sensitivity of the clinician. Mrs. Washington, a fifty-year-old African American woman, had had a surgical release for carpal tunnel syndrome—a work-related injury. Linne was assigned to her case. Five months after the surgery, Linne called to see how she was doing. Mrs. Washington replied that she was still having some discomfort when driving and doing household chores. Linne commented that as per their clinical guidelines, she should have been showing improvement after six to eight weeks post op. Linne was concerned that five months later, she was still having problems. Mrs. Washington, however, immediately became defensive and hotly replied, "I'm not in it for the money. I don't want to be in pain."

9

10

Linne felt terrible. She didn't mean to imply that Mrs. Washington was trying to scam the system. She then remembered learning that years of discrimination have led many African Americans to be acutely attuned to signs of prejudice. She realized that Mrs. Washington thought she was implying that rather than return to work, she preferred to stay home and receive worker's compensation. She perceived Linne as being prejudiced and thinking of Blacks as lazy and shiftless.

The situation could have gone very badly from here. Linne could have become defensive and tried to defend her comment. Mrs. Washington might have responded argumentatively, justifying why she was still off work and receiving Worker's Compensation benefits. In fact, several times in the past, that is exactly what had happened to Linne, which resulted in the patients hiring an attorney, which further delayed their release to work and increased the cost of care. This time, however, Linne used cultural competence skills to restore the situation. She immediately apologized for her comment and explained that she only meant to educate her regarding what she could expect following a carpal tunnel release. She wanted to let her know that if she was still having pain, she needed to talk with her physician to see if there were other treatments to help her pain. Linne told her that as her case manager, she would also speak with Mrs. Washington's physician about her ongoing pain. As a result, Mrs. Washington calmed down and became more receptive. A combination of understanding the impact of prejudice and discrimination, followed by a sincere apology, changed a potentially negative outcome to a positive one.

There is good reason for African Americans to be wary of the predominantly white health care institution. Unless one has had the experience of being stopped by the police simply for driving a nice car in a good neighborhood, or been asked by a white salesperson, "Are you sure you can afford it?" when buying a high-ticket item, it is difficult to understand what it is like to be the recipient of racial prejudice. We are all individuals and want to be treated as such, but, unfortunately, minorities are often judged simply by the color of their skin.

At the same time, however, years of discrimination may have led some individuals to be acutely sensitive and to perceive prejudice when it does not exist. Health care providers should be aware of this and do what they can to ensure that their words and actions do not unintentionally hurt their patients. An African American student in one of my classes interviewed 12 elderly African Americans. They all said they preferred African American physicians because they thought they were the only ones who would treat them fairly, without discrimination. Because their "radar" was always up for discriminatory treatment, if something could be interpreted in two ways, they would usually interpret it as a sign of racism—

for example, if the physician was running late, or didn't spend much time with them. Culturally competent physicians will take the time to apologize and explain such situations—to *all* patients.

Values

Values are the things we hold important. Just as each individual holds certain values, so does each culture. U.S. culture (and I use this term loosely because there are literally hundreds of subcultures within the United States) currently values such things as money, freedom, independence, privacy, health and fitness, and physical appearance.

One way to assess a culture's values is to observe how it punishes people. In the United States wrongdoers are punished by being fined (taking away their *money*) or incarcerated (taking away their *freedom*). The Mbuti pygmies of Africa value social support, and they punish people by ignoring them. The kind of health care provided by the American medical system is often influenced by financial considerations, whereas concern for family, low on the list of "American" values, influences much patient behavior in patients from other ethnic groups. Hence conflict may develop between health care providers and patients.

In the United States, *independence* is manifested by the desire to move away from home as soon as one is financially able. In many cultures that value family more than independence, adult children rarely move out before marriage and often not thereafter. The health care culture also supports the values of independence and *autonomy* in its efforts to teach self-care.

Privacy is also very important to most people from the United States, who build fences to separate their houses from each other. The U.S. health care culture tries to provide privacy for patients often giving information only to the patient, excluding other family members, limiting visiting hours, and offering no sleeping accommodations for visitors. Many non-Anglo patients, however, prefer just the opposite.

Health and fitness are popular movements. There are hundreds of food products labeled "low fat" and "low cholesterol." People can be seen jogging on most city streets, and attendance at gyms is high. This obsession with health leads the medical profession to expect patients to comply with suggestions regarding changes in diet and exercise, assuming that health and fitness is a value shared by all. It is not. Furthermore, what is considered "healthy" varies across cultures.

Concern for *physical appearance* is manifested at every magazine stand. There are few women's magazines that do not have articles on the latest diet, makeup, hairdo, and clothing. The incidence of cosmetic surgery for both men and women is at a record high. Surgical techniques are developed to minimize scarring and maintain beauty. What is considered "beautiful," however, is not the same for every culture.

Understanding people's values is the key to understanding their behavior, for our behavior generally reflects our values. A dramatic example occurred in the early 1980s, when a Japanese ship captain was bringing a boatload of cars to the United States. There was a disaster at sea, and the cargo was ruined. The captain had done nothing to cause the disaster, and he could not have prevented it. If an American ship captain had had a similar experience, the first thing he probably would have done when he reached land was call his insurance agent to see who would pay for the damages. The Japanese captain killed himself.

There is obviously a big difference between calling one's insurance agent and killing oneself. The different reactions are dictated by different values. The hypothetical American captain would probably value *money*; his concern would be for the financial loss. The Japanese captain was concerned about his *honor*. As the captain of the ship, he considered himself responsible for the accident. The loss of the cargo meant the loss of his honor. Without honor, he felt he could not live. Committing ritual suicide was the only way for him to regain his honor.

Values influence our everyday behavior as well. Why are you reading this book? Is it because you value knowledge and hope to learn something? Is it because you are required to read it for a course and you value good grades? If so, are you motivated because good grades will get you a better job, and with a better job you will earn more money, and you value money? Nearly everything we do reflects our values on some level.

Values and the American Health Care Culture

One reason for so many conflicts and misunderstandings in hospitals is the great disjunction between the values of the health care culture and that of the patient population.

As mentioned earlier, the health care culture values autonomy and independence. Patients, in contrast, often value the family over the individual. The family may prefer to make decisions as a group and to assist the patient in "self-care" functions the staff thinks the patient should do on his or her own. Furthermore, many patients prefer to have family members with them at all times, leading to chaos and loss of control from the perspective of the nurses.

The health care culture's value of *efficiency* often conflicts with patients' value of *modesty*. Many doctors and nurses find concern about keeping patients covered difficult when their primary focus is performing an appropriate procedure. The health care culture also values *self-control*. Many patients, however, come from cultures in which emotional expressiveness

is the norm. This can lead to resentment toward such patients on the part
of the staff.

Worldview

The second most important concept for understanding people's behavior
is to understand their worldview. Problems can result from a disparity
between the worldview of the health care culture and that of the patient
population. People's worldviews consist of their basic assumptions about
the nature of reality. These become the foundation for all actions and
interpretations. For example, people whose worldview includes the notion
that everything happens for a reason will tend to find meaning in all events.
A childless thirty-five-year-old woman who goes through the emotional
agony of finding a breast lump, only to have the biopsy turn out to be negative, may interpret the experience as a message from the universe reminding her that now is the time to decide whether or not she wants to have
children (breasts metaphorically representing nurturing). As another example, someone who believes that the world is a hostile place and "out to
get them" may perceive a health care provider who is late for an appointment due to a sudden emergency as deliberately displaying prejudice.

An individual's worldview can have an important influence on his or her
health care behavior. For example, someone with a scientific worldview
might perceive birth defects as a mistake in the transcription of DNA during the process of meiosis, while someone whose worldview encompasses
the notion of reincarnation might see it as resulting from improper behavior in a past life, and someone who believes that God rewards good behavior and punishes bad behavior might interpret it as punishment for one's
sins. Thus, one's worldview might affect one's interest in genetic counseling during pregnancy. Again, if part of an individual's worldview is that
the physical body is all there is, that person might want everything possible done to extend their life. A person who believes that this life is but a
precursor to the next, however, might be more willing to "let go." If one's
worldview holds that life begins at conception, abortion will be viewed as
murder; if, however, life is thought to begin at the point that the fetus
becomes viable, a first-trimester abortion is simply a medical procedure.

While we all have our own individual worldview, our culture can influence the way we perceive things. Religion often defines the worldview
of people who are devoutly religious. Belief in the existence of God, for
example, might be part of their worldview. If people believe God confers
both health and illness, it may be very difficult to get them to take certain medications or change their health behavior. They might not share
the health care culture's belief that germs cause disease and that diet and
exercise contribute to one's health. They may see no point in worrying

about high blood pressure or bacteria when moral behavior is the key to good health.

11   Mona had the opportunity to use her understanding of worldview when caring for Ramon Diaz, a Hispanic male who had been admitted to the hospital three times in a single year for uncontrolled diabetes. Despite being given a strict diet and insulin orders to follow, he continued to eat whatever he wanted and refused to monitor his blood sugar. When Mona questioned him about this, he replied, "Okay, I'll start my diabetic diet tomorrow, but it's not going to make any difference. It's in God's hands now." Mona's initial reaction was to become frustrated with him, but instead, noted his fatalistic worldview. She realized that her usual "lecture" and instructions were not going to be enough. So she took the time to explain to him and his wife that if not managed daily, diabetes can have fatal complications. She also went over with them ways to gradually change his diet, which made adherence more likely than would a demand for a complete and sudden change. Mona also used cultural competence skills by including his wife in the teaching, since the family is the primary unit in traditional Hispanic cultures. Since she was also the family cook, it was important to get her on board with the plan. Mona took a further step by talking to her coworkers about a fatalistic world view, hoping this knowledge would keep them from getting frustrated and "giving up" on their patients as they often did. Cultural competence can be contagious; health care practitioners should be encouraged to share their knowledge and experiences with co-workers.

Since people's worldviews consist of their *assumptions* about the nature of reality, they rarely question the veracity of their beliefs. For example, a devout Christian might not be likely to conclude that God does not exist on the basis of the accidental slaughter of innocent children. Rather, the Christian might simply remark, "God works in mysterious ways." No matter how much "evidence" is presented to the contrary, people rarely change or even question their worldview. Instead, they reinterpret events in a manner consistent with their beliefs.

People's Relationship to Nature

Another aspect of worldview involves people's relationship to nature. The culture of the United States, for example, believes people can control nature. If the land is dry, they irrigate. If bacteria cause disease, they destroy them. If the heart does not work, they replace it. This also relates to the health care culture's view of the body as a machine; if it becomes broken, one should simply turn it over to the mechanics (doctors and nurses) to be fixed. To the consternation of many health care professionals, not all cultures share that belief.

Other cultures, such as Asian and Native American, see people as a part of nature. They strive to maintain harmony with the earth and look to the land to provide treatment for disease. Herbal remedies are important in their cultures. Still other cultures, such as Hispanic, believe people have little or no control over natural forces. *Que será, será.* What will be, will be. Preventive health care measures are likely to be ignored; they would do no good anyway. Thus worldview can have important implications for health-related behavior.

Emic and Etic

The terms "emic" and "etic," derived from linguistics and rarely used in ordinary life, are extremely important in anthropology. They refer to perspectives. Emic perspectives are the insiders' perspectives, natives' views of their own behavior. Etic perspectives are those of outsiders. The two simply represent different vantage points, and knowing both helps provide a more complete picture, a fact caregivers would do well to remember when treating patients from different cultures. Try to understand *their* perspective on their condition, as well as your own.

An Etic Perspective on American Medicine

Anne Fadiman, in the now classic book *The Spirit Catches You and You Fall Down* (1998), contrasts biomedicine with traditional Hmong medicine. In doing so, she helps us to see biomedicine from an *etic* perspective, while looking at traditional Hmong medicine from an *emic* perspective. American medicine doesn't come off as well as Hmong medicine.

- A traditional Hmong healer might spend as much as eight hours in a sick person's home, whereas American doctors force their patients, no matter how weak they are, to come to the hospital, and then might spend only twenty minutes at their bedsides.
- Traditional Hmong healers are polite and never need to ask questions; American doctors ask many rude and intimate questions about patients' lives, right down to their sexual and excretory habits.
- Traditional Hmong healers can render an immediate diagnosis; American doctors often demand samples of blood (or even urine or feces, which they like to keep in little bottles), take x-rays, and wait for days for the results to come back from the laboratory—and then, after all that, sometimes they are unable to identify the cause of the problem.
- Traditional Hmong healers never undress their patients; American

doctors ask patients to take off all their clothes, and sometimes dare to put their fingers inside women's vaginas.

- Traditional Hmong healers know that to treat the body without treating the soul is an act of patent folly; American doctors never even mention the soul.

- Traditional Hmong healers preserve unblemished reputations even if their patients don't get well, since the blame is laid on the intransigence of the spirits rather than the competence of the negotiators, whose stock might even rise if they had had to do battle with particularly dangerous opponents; when American doctors fail to heal, it is their own fault.

Ethnocentrism and Cultural Relativism

Two key anthropological concepts are ethnocentrism and cultural relativism. They refer to attitudes. *Ethnocentrism* is the view that one's own culture's way of doing things is the right and natural way. All other ways are inferior, unnatural, and perhaps even barbaric. *Cultural relativism* is the attitude that other ways of doing things are different but equally valid. It tries to understand the behavior in its cultural context. Most humans are ethnocentric. It is natural to think one's own culture's way is best. Anthropologists, however, strive to be culturally relativistic.

If I were to tell most Americans about a group of people in Africa who sometimes kill healthy newborn infants, they would probably take the ethnocentric attitude that these people were barbarians. If I were to explain that they were hunters and gatherers living on the edge of starvation and that if a second child is born too close to the first, chances are close to 100 percent that both will die because the mother does not have enough milk to support both, their attitude might change. They still might not condone infanticide, but they might understand it as the only viable choice in a desperate situation. Rather than seeing the Africans as barbarians, they might realize that the people were forced to extreme measures by difficult circumstances. Their attitude would thus change from ethnocentric to culturally relativistic.

The Western health care system tends to be ethnocentric because practitioners believe that their approaches to healing are superior to all others. There is a lot we can learn, however, from other cultures. Many modern drugs, including quinine, were derived from plants used by native peoples. Westerners are beginning to acknowledge the effectiveness of acupuncture for certain conditions. The goal of all systems of healing is the same; to help people get well. If all cultures could study each other's techniques with a culturally relativistic perspective, the cause of modern medicine would be greatly advanced.

Time Orientation

Time orientation, one's focus regarding time, varies in different cultures. No individual or culture will look exclusively to the past, present, or future, but most will tend to emphasize one over the others. Chinese, British, and Austrian cultures have a past orientation. They are traditional and believe in doing things the way they have always been done. Interestingly, in many cases, countries that emphasize the past are ones that were once more powerful than they are now. This may be their way of recognizing and valuing that time in their history. These cultures usually prefer traditional approaches to healing rather than accepting each new procedure or medication that comes out.

People with a predominantly present time orientation may be less likely to utilize preventive health measures. They reason that there is no point in taking a pill for hypertension when they feel fine, especially if the pill is expensive and causes unpleasant side effects. They do not look ahead in hope of preventing a stroke or heart attack, or they may feel they will deal with it when it happens. Poverty often forces people into a present time orientation. They are not likely to make plans for the future when they are concerned with surviving today.

Middle-class Anglo American culture tends to be future oriented. That is reflected in the medical system's stress on preventive medicine and enthusiasm for each new medical technique or drug. In contrast to past-oriented cultures, progress and change are highly valued. China is also shifting to a future orientation, as evidenced by the long-term plan to reduce the country's population by limiting family size.

Hispanics and African Americans tend to have a present time orientation. This does not mean that they do not recognize the past or the future, but that living in the present is more important to them. Their concept of the future may also be different from the Anglo concept. For example, African Americans are more likely to say "I'll see you" than "I'll see you tomorrow." The former implies the future but is not specific. The future arrives in its own time. From this point of view, one cannot be late. Conflict may occur, however, in interactions with white middle-class people, for whom time is very specific.

As the last statement implies, time orientation can also refer to degree of adherence to clock time versus adherence to activities. From the perspective of one oriented to the clock, someone who arrives at 3:15 for a 2:30 appointment is late. For someone who does not focus on clock time, both represent midafternoon. The time to arrive at the afternoon appointment is after the morning activity is completed.

This type of time orientation appears to be related to subsistence economy. In countries with economies based on agriculture, people tend to be more relaxed about time; as I like to say, "The crops don't care what time they get picked." Many people in traditional agricultural villages do not own clocks; the pace is slower and more attuned to nature's rhythms. They tend to focus more on activities, rather than on the clock. In contrast, industrialized nations must pay attention to clock time. There are large numbers of people to organize, and each must complete his or her task according to schedule in order for the next person to begin. Without clocks, chaos would reign.

Hierarchical Versus Egalitarian Cultures

Just as cultures differ in time orientation, they also vary in social structure. American culture is organized according to an egalitarian model. Theoretically, everyone is equal. Status and power are dependent on an individual's personal qualities rather than characteristics such as age, sex, family, or occupation. In reality, things may operate differently, but we hold equality as our ideal. Many Asian cultures are based on a hierarchical model. Everyone is not equal. Status is based on such characteristics as age, sex, and occupation. Status differences are seen as important, and people of higher status command respect. Hospitals are based on a hierarchical model. Social structure, then, can have an important influence on the way people interact, as will be seen in many of the examples given later in this book.

Family of Orientation Versus Family of Procreation

During the course of their lives, many people are members of two different family groups; the family they are born into and the one they create through marriage and children. Anthropologists distinguish the two as "family of orientation" and "family of procreation." The family of orientation is the one a person is born into, the one to which one first orients oneself. It includes the individual, parents, brothers and sisters, and any other household members. The family of procreation is the one formed through marrying and procreating. It includes the individual, spouse, and children. Some cultures, particularly those in which the married couple continues to reside with the parents of the bride or groom, emphasize the family of orientation. Other cultures emphasize the family of procreation. Americans tend to set up their own nuclear family households, and that family takes precedence over all others. The result is a differing set of loyalties.

Models of Disease

Three primary health belief models have been identified by medical anthropologists. They are the following:

Magico-religious model: The world is an arena in which supernatural forces dominate. One's health depends upon the action of gods or other supernatural forces, which can act on their own or be manipulated by other humans. In some cases, illness is seen as punishment for transgression.

Biomedical model: Life is seen as being controlled by a series of physical and biochemical processes, which can be studied and manipulated.

Holistic model: The forces of nature must be kept in balance or harmony, both within the body and between the individual and the physical and metaphysical universe. Health is a positive state of well-being, and encompasses broader environmental, sociocultural, and behavioral determinants. Healing is aimed at restoring balance.

Note that within any given cultural healing system, elements of more than one paradigm or model may apply. As you read the next section, notice which "causes" of disease belong to which paradigm. Also keep in mind that a common reason for lack of adherence is a conflict between the patient's model of disease and that of the biomedical practitioner. Why adhere to a treatment regime that makes no sense to you?

Disease Etiology

Most Americans believe that germs cause disease. Not all cultures share that belief, however. Other causes of disease include upset in body balance; soul loss, soul theft, and spirit possession; breach of taboo; and object intrusion. Treatment for diseases resulting from such etiologies must vary to be appropriate to the cause.

Upset in body balance is a notion that appears to have originated in China and spread from there to influence beliefs in Asia, India, Spain, and Latin America. It refers to the belief that a healthy body is in a state of balance. When it gets out of balance, illness results. In Asia, the balance is between *yin* and *yang*. All things in the universe are primarily either yin or yang, including diseases, which may result from excess yin, excess yang, deficient yin, or deficient yang. Yin and yang are generally translated as hot (yang) and cold (yin), although these refer to qualities, not temperatures.

The balance between hot and cold can be upset by a number of factors, including an improper balance of foods and strong emotional states. The goal of treatment is to restore balance to the system. This is generally accomplished through the use of foods (for example, cold foods should be eaten to cure a hot illness), herbs, or other treatments. To prevent disease, one should avoid extremes, such as ice water. Diet is exceedingly important. (Dietary staples such as rice are generally thought to be neutral, a fortunate and practical designation.)

Foods that are hot in one culture may be cold in another, so it is difficult to make up a comprehensive list. Patients' beliefs in hot and cold
qualities can generally be ascertained only by observing their behavior.
If they refuse certain foods or medications, it may be that an illness they
perceive as hot is being treated with a hot food or medication. Offering
other foods or liquids to take with the pill to "neutralize" it may solve the
problem. If they will not take the pill with ice water, they might take it with
hot tea, orange juice, or hot chocolate.

Although the importance of maintaining a balance between hot and
cold is not recognized in Western medicine, there is a growing recognition that stress plays an important role in affecting the immune system's
ability to fight disease. Stress represents a kind of imbalance. Recent studies indicate that a person's emotional state may also have a significant influence on the immune system. Thus, though the words we use are different,
body balance is a notion to which we should be able to relate.

Paradoxically, China is moving away from traditional medicine in
favor of Western medicine, while there is increasing interest in the United
States in traditional Chinese healing practices. When I asked several
Chinese nurses how they integrate the concept of yin and yang with germ
theory, they explained that when yin and yang are out of balance, germs
can cause disease. This is nearly identical to the Western notion of the
relationship between stress and disease.

Soul loss, along with *soul theft*, is another category of disease etiology.
The concept is self-explanatory. The soul has either left the body on its
own or been stolen, leaving the body in a weakened and ill state. The goal
of treatment is to return the soul to the body. It usually requires a specialist, such as a shaman, who can "leave" his or her own body to search for
and return the missing soul. Although Western medicine lacks a similar
etiological category, catatonic schizophrenics can be described metaphorically as bodies with "no one home."

Spirit possession involves the taking over of the victim's body by a spirit
being. The victim usually acts in ways that are inappropriate for him or
her. In some cultures, this may give the victim a form of power. It is generally the poor, the oppressed, and minorities who become "possessed."
For example, in Ethiopia, women may become possessed by powerful Zar
spirits. When this occurs, their husbands must treat them with unaccus-
tomed kindness and respect, for they are no longer dealing with their wives
but with powerful Zars. The negative side of possession by a Zar is that
the woman is thought to be crazy and must seek help through a Zar cult.
Exorcism is the treatment for spirit possession.

The next etiological category is *breach of taboo*, which means doing something forbidden—for example, eating food cooked by a menstruating
woman, speaking directly to one's mother-in-law, or, among some Christian

sects, having extramarital or homosexual relations. Disease is the punishment meted out by a supernatural force such as God. Treatment involves penance and atonement.

The final major category is *object intrusion*. It refers to the condition in which a magical foreign object enters the body and causes the individual to become ill. Treatment involves removing the object. In most cases, a shaman will suck it out from the afflicted part of the patient's body. The shaman then produces the offending object. Upon analysis, the object often turns out to be bits of hair, animal parts, teeth, or plant material, mixed with blood from the shaman's mouth. One shaman, accused by an anthropologist of practicing legerdemain, freely admitted to secreting the object in his mouth prior to sucking it out of the patient's body. He explained that the real object he removed was invisible, but that it was important for the patient to see something tangible, so he practiced a bit of sleight of hand (or mouth) for the patient's psychological benefit.

Two important points should be made regarding disease etiology. *First, the treatment must be appropriate to the cause.* If germs cause disease, kill the germs. If the body is out of balance, restore balance. If the soul is gone, retrieve it. If a spirit has taken over the body, exorcise it. If a rule has been violated, do penance. If an object has entered the body, remove it. All these remedies are perfectly logical. Whether these etiologies are the true causes of the disease is irrelevant. A patient who believes he or she is ill because of soul loss will not be cured by any amount of antibiotics. The mind is very powerful, as the placebo effect demonstrates. The patient's beliefs, as well as body, must be treated. Many Americans feel they have not been treated properly if they do not receive an antibiotic for a virus, even though antibiotics are effective only against bacteria. Psychologically, they need the pill to get well. This has unfortunately led to a selection for ever more powerful and antibiotic-resistant bacteria.

Second, we must not let our ethnocentrism blind us to the merits in the beliefs of other cultures. They may be right. It is easy to look down on other systems, citing science to support Western medical beliefs. But all medical systems are based on observed cause-and-effect relationships. The major difference with the scientific approach is that science is falsifiable. A scientific hypothesis can be proven wrong. The beliefs of other systems cannot.

At the level of the individual, however, Americans demand no more proof than do people of any other culture. Most believe germs cause disease because their mothers told them so. Few have ever actually seen a germ, and fewer demand to see proof of viruses or bacteria at work. The experts have done that, and their word, along with our mothers', is enough. The same is true in other cultures. People believe disease is caused by spirit possession or object intrusion because their mothers and cultural experts told them so. They have seen people become ill when that happens and get well when treated. What further proof is necessary?

Theoretical Perspective: Adaptation Theory

As can be inferred from the preceding sections, the underlying theoretical perspective of this book is based on adaptation theory. I believe that, in most cases, people have developed traditions designed to achieve success in the broader environment in which they live. This includes adaptations to both the physical and social environments. Obviously, there are exceptions, and there are other theoretical approaches that are equally fruitful in explaining people's behavior. However, this is the theory that will inform the interpretations given in this book. When cultural conflicts occur, it is often because what is successful under one set of environmental circumstances may be less so under others.

We can better understand the relationship between environment and culture by looking at some examples. These generalizations are very broad, but they should serve to illuminate the underlying principles.

Arabs, for example, developed their culture in a harsh desert environment. Humans can have a limited effect on such an environment without the benefit of advanced technology. It makes sense, then, to have a fatalistic worldview, and to see a supernatural entity (God, or Allah) in control. Many Arabs were traditionally herders. Because men tend to be in charge of the herds, this leads to male authority. Because males are often away from home, tending the herds, female purity becomes important. Otherwise, men would often be raising other men's children. Because it is difficult to keep watch over the herds at all times, they are vulnerable to theft. Without an external policing force, the best way to protect one's animals is through one's reputation. Everyone must know that if your animals are stolen, the consequences will be swift and great. Honor and reputation thus become highly valued. In this way, we can see that the environmental factors of the desert environment and a pastoral (herding) subsistence base led to a fatalistic worldview, a social structure that emphasizes male authority, and the values of female purity and family honor.

These cultural characteristics have important implications with regard to health care. For example, preventive care may be underutilized. Since Allah is in control, what's the point? Wives may defer to husbands when it comes to decision making due to male authority. Women may refuse to be examined by a male physician due to issues about female purity.

Another example is the Japanese. Japan is old and densely populated. Thus the Japanese have had both the time and the need to develop rules that will help avoid chaos. These include the development of a hierarchical social system and the value of emotional control. The Japanese were traditionally agricultural, thus leading to an emphasis on the group over the individual. The combination of an agricultural subsistence base and a hierarchical social structure combined to place great value on the elderly (something which is slowly changing in light of the industrialization of Japan) because they are the ones with the most experience and thus the most useful knowledge.

How do these characteristics influence Japanese health care behavior? Because the Japanese see themselves as a member of a family group, rather than as individuals, families may want to be given patient information themselves, rather than have it be given to the patient. Respect for the hierarchy may lead patients to agree verbally to what the physician requests, even if they have no intention of following through; to disagree would be seen as disrespectful. The emphasis on emotional control may lead them to exhibit little sign of pain, no matter how much discomfort they may be feeling.

Adaptation theory can also help us understand the U.S. health care system. The United States was founded by immigrants who came to avoid religious persecution, and a kind of class system where who you were depended upon the status of your family, so freedom and individualism became highly valued and success was measured by your own worth. One "objective measure" of worth is money, and thus wealth became highly valued. Those who prospered in the early days of this open land were often those who were independent, worked hard, and developed the land, in other words, those who controlled nature. Once the country became industrialized, people had to go where there were jobs available or where jobs could be created, thus family became less important than mobility.

As discussed earlier, these characteristics are closely related to the U.S. health care culture. The view that humans control nature leads to extensive use of life support, fetal monitoring, organ transplants, and so forth. The emphasis on money not only influences the level of health care one receives, but also leads to the notion that with enough money, we can cure any disease. The values of individualism and freedom lead us to give information directly to the patient, rather than the family, and to expect that the patient will make all the decisions concerning his health. The value of independence leads to an emphasis on self-care.

Adaptation theory can help explain many of the similarities between cultures. For example, most agriculturalists, whether from Asia, Latin America, or Africa, will value the family over the individual, because successful small farming requires the combined efforts of all members of the family. Large families will also be desired, because more family members mean more workers, which often translates to greater success.

Cultural Customs

Utilizing adaptation theory, it can be argued that most cultural practices originate for very practical reasons. People, however, do not always act in a practical manner if the benefit to them is not obvious and immediate. They may need a "higher" purpose. Ideological injunctions are much more likely to be followed, as anthropologist Marvin Harris (1974), a leading proponent of the cultural materialism approach, points out.

For example, the Hindu prohibition against killing cows may seem bizarre in a country where many people are starving, but it has a practical basis. Most cows are malnourished and if slaughtered would provide very little food. Living, however, cows are good substitutes for tractors. Their milk provides food. Their dung provides fertilizer, fuel for cooking, and, mixed with water, an excellent household flooring material. Far more use is made of living cows than could ever be gained from dead ones. Hungry individuals might look at a cow and see dinner. Forgetting the animal's other practical uses, they might kill and eat it. But if the animal is made sacred, religious ideology will prevent such killing.

Circumstances sometimes change, obliterating the practical need for a custom. Ideology, however, is enduring and soon becomes tradition. Although many cultural and religious traditions no longer have any practical value, they have an important psychological one—they provide a sense of identity and belonging. They serve as a strong reminder that the individual is not like everyone else; he or she belongs to a special group. Abstaining from meat when everyone else is having hamburgers reminds the Hindu that he is Hindu. Walking to temple instead of driving on the Sabbath reminds the Jew that she is Jewish. In fact, the more difficult or impractical the custom, the stronger the reminder of ethnic or religious identity. Thus the benefits of adhering to seemingly outmoded customs can be enormous in a country like the United States, where feelings of isolation and anomie may be strong.

Key Points

- Culturally competent care is patient-centered care.
- Learn your patient's point of view by asking the right questions.
- One model of the questions to ask is "The 4 C's of Culture":
  - What do you call your problem? (What do you think is wrong?).
  - What do you think caused your problem?
  - What have you done to cope with your problem?
  - What concerns do you have about your problem? About my recommended treatment?

Chapter 2
Communication and Time Orientation

Miscommunication is a frequent problem in hospitals. The most obvious case is when the patient and the hospital personnel do not speak the same language. Interpreters are not always available. When they are, vocabulary may be insufficient. But these problems are obvious. There are more subtle ones that result from cultural differences in verbal and nonverbal communication styles and patterns. This chapter explores these problems in communication as well as another subtle but provocative source of difficulty—cultural differences in time orientation. Patients and staff members may operate on different "time clocks," causing confusion and resentment for all parties.

Language Issues

Idioms

Idioms or other nonliteral expressions can often create misunderstanding. A Chinese-born physician called the night nurse one evening to check on a patient scheduled for surgery the next day. The nurse advised the physician that she noticed a new hesitancy in the patient's attitude. "To tell you the truth, doctor, I think Mrs. Colby is getting cold feet." The physician, not familiar with this idiom, suspected circulation problems and ordered vascular tests.   12

A nervous patient jokingly asked his surgeon if he were going to "kick the bucket." The Korean physician, wanting to reassure the patient that his upcoming surgery would be successful, responded affably, "Oh, yes, you are definitely going to kick the bucket!" The patient was not reassured.   13

In general, it is best to avoid using idioms with people who speak English as a second language, since they may often be misunderstood.

Another English

Language problems can also occur among native English speakers. In England, South Africa, and Australia, the word "fanny" is a derogatory term referring to a woman's vagina. Imagine the shock and horror of a British woman—or the confusion of a British man—when told to prepare for a shot in the fanny. (A South African nurse was appalled when an American aerobics instructor called out to her class, "Tighten your fanny, shake your fanny!")

14 Lynette was educating a patient and her husband on the pain-free method of moving up in bed. Part of her instructions were to "slide your fanny up to the middle of the bed." Both started giggling. They were from England. Fortunately, rather than be offended, the patient called Lynette "a fun nurse."

Similarly, birth control instruction to speakers of the "Queen's English" could be confusing if the instructor referred to a condom as a "rubber." Erasers are not a very effective means of preventing pregnancy.

Same Language, Different Meaning

Words can have different meanings in the same language. In Mexico, the word *horita* means right now. In Puerto Rico, it means in an hour or so. This could cause confusion between two Spanish speakers. Similarly, "just now" in South Africa means "later" in the United States. A South African immigrant reported frequent problems with her boss when she first moved to the United States. At times, when he asked her to do something, she would reply, "I'll get to it just now." He'd come back an hour later, asking for the work, which hadn't been done. He would be angry; she had said she would do it right away, but hadn't. She, on the other hand, would be upset because she told him she would get to it later, and now he was expecting her to have it done immediately.

15 Even American English can have different meanings for hearing and deaf people. While Kelly, a young gay male, was a patient in the hospital, blood was drawn for an HIV test. When the results came back, no interpreters for the deaf were available. Because Kelly was adept at reading lips, he was given the test results directly. He was told that his results were positive, meaning, of course, that he was HIV-positive. In deaf culture, however, "positive" means good and "negative" means bad. Kelly was relieved to hear that his test results were "positive"; that meant he was *not* HIV-positive! He went home and did not return for follow-up. What the nurse should have done was tell him that the results came back negative—that he was, indeed, HIV-positive.

This incident was not unique. Carol Browner and her colleagues discovered that many Mexican-born pregnant women receiving genetic counseling misunderstood the term "positive" when given test results for fetal abnormalities. Rather than understand there was a problem, they thought it meant that everything was good; after all, the counselor said the results were "positive." It is important for health care providers to realize that some terms have a different meaning outside the context of medicine. It is critical to make sure that you give enough explanation to ensure that the patient truly understands the information given. Paying attention to nonverbal reactions is also key; any misunderstanding of test results, for example, will often result in an inappropriate emotional response (such as relief).

The terms "positive" and "negative" as applied to test results can be confusing to anyone. It is important for health care professionals to clarify the significance of "positive" and "negative" findings.

Same Word, Different Language

Sometimes the same word can have different meanings in different languages. Consuela, a Filipino nurse, had for several days been caring for Ramon Ibañez, a Mexican premature baby in intensive care. Everything seemed fine, until the Ibañezes suddenly requested that another nurse be assigned to their baby. Consuela was shocked, particularly since they had not given the social worker any explanation.

Consuela had Graciela, a Spanish-speaking coworker, ask them to explain the problem. They were a bit hesitant, but finally told her that they had overheard Consuela talking to a coworker and mentioning that she had a *puto*. In Spanish, *puto* refers to a male prostitute. Their baby's health had gotten worse; they assumed it was because Consuela had picked up a disease from her male prostitute and passed it on to their child. They were in fact a bit surprised that the hospital would employ such a woman to care for the infants.

Was Consuela really seeing a male prostitute? No. In the Philippines, a *puto* is a rice cake. Consuela had been telling her coworker that she was having a rice cake for lunch. Graciela explained this to the Ibañezes and clarified that babies born severely premature often got worse before getting better; Ramon's condition had nothing to do with Consuela. Fortunately, they understood their misunderstanding. The next week, Consuela brought the Ibañezes some *puto* to eat. Mrs. Ibañez hugged her and again expressed their apologies.

In Dutch, the word for "shower" is *douche*. In English, *douche* is related to a specific form, often offensive, of personal feminine hygiene. A hospitalized American patient might be a bit disconcerted if her Dutch nurse told her it was time for a douche.

Different Connotations in Different Languages

Most Anglo Americans realize that the term "boy" is offensive to African Americans due to its use among white slave owners. Many non-Americans,

16

17

however, are not familiar with the history of slavery in this country and the significance of that word. Colleen, an Anglo nurse from Canada, learned the meaning of "boy" the hard way. Her first job when she moved to the United States was at an inner city hospital. The cafeteria was crowded the first day she was there, but she found an empty place across from two Black men. She went over to them and asked very sweetly, "Do you boys mind if I sit down here?" One answered her by picking up his plate of food and throwing it at her.

Most people would agree that he overreacted, but his response is understandable in the context of race relations in this country. The misunderstanding occurred because Canada has not had the same racial problems as the United States, and in the part of the country Colleen was from, adult men and women commonly refer to each other as boys and girls. No insult is meant or taken. Once someone explained the reason for the man's reaction to Colleen, she did not make that mistake again.

Most people in the United States know that "boy" is highly insulting to an African American man, but fewer are aware that the term "gal" has similar connotations for many African American women in the South. Black slave women were called "gals," which explains why several Anglo nurses reported receiving cold and hostile glares from African American nurses whom they innocently referred to as "gals."

Two other words that can cause problems due to different connotations in different languages are "mama" and "papa." In Filipino culture, these terms convey a sense of respect, and Filipino health care workers will sometimes refer to elderly patients in this way. In other cultures, however, it can be interpreted as a *lack* of respect. Health care professionals from the Philippines should be informed of this cultural difference.

When "Yes" May Mean "No"

18   Cultural values can also create communication problems. Jackie, an Anglo nurse, was explaining the harmful side effects of the medication that Adela Samillan, a Filipino patient, was to take at home after her discharge. Although Mrs. Samillan spoke some English, her husband, who was more fluent, served as interpreter. Throughout Jackie's explanation, the Samillans nodded in agreement and understanding and laughed nervously. When Jackie verbally tested them on the information, however, it was apparent that they understood very little. What had happened?

Dignity and self-esteem are important for all individuals, but particularly so for most Asians. Because the family, rather than the individual, is the primary unit, if you look bad, everyone looks bad. It multiplies the humiliation. Had the Samillans indicated that they did not understand Jackie's instructions, they would have lost their self-esteem for not understanding or they would have caused Jackie to lose hers for not explaining the material well enough. By pretending to understand, Mr. and Mrs. Samillan felt they were preserving everyone's dignity.

Jackie's first clue should have been their nervous laughter. Giggling is often a sign of discomfort and embarrassment. Once Jackie realized they had not understood the material, she went over it until they were able to explain it back to her. It is important not to take smiles and nods of agreement for understanding when dealing with Asian patients. They should be asked to demonstrate their understanding.

A second incident involved Linh Lee, a sixty-four-year-old Chinese woman hospitalized for an acute evolving heart attack. At discharge, her physician suggested that she come back in two weeks for a follow-up examination. She agreed to do so, but never returned. It is likely that she never intended to do so but agreed because he was an authority figure. Chinese people are taught to value accommodation. Rather than refuse to the physician's face and cause him dishonor, Mrs. Lee agreed. She simply did not follow through, sparing everyone embarrassment.

In a similar incident, when Dr. Jacks told Cha Xeng, a Hmong patient, that she needed to have gallbladder surgery, she agreed. Several days later, however, she told the interpreter that she did not plan to have the surgery. The interpreter asked her why she had changed her mind. She hadn't changed her mind, she said; she never intended to have the surgery. But she didn't want to show disrespect to the surgeon by disagreeing with his recommendation. It is not clear that the surgeon could have done anything different in this case, other than present the options to her more objectively, and ask for her feelings rather than simply giving his recommendation.

Grammar

The cases described above involved the use of the word "yes" to avoid the embarrassment of saying "no." "Yes" may also be used inappropriately (from the American perspective) for reasons of grammar. According to common English usage, if someone were asked, "Haven't you taken your medication yet today?" and they had not taken it, they would answer, "No." According to the rules of grammar found in most Asian languages, the accurate response would be "Yes," as in "Yes, it is a true statement that I have not yet taken my medication today." The English speaker would be misled by the Asian patient's affirmative response, thinking that person had already taken the medication when he or she had not. To reduce possible confusion, it is generally best to avoid sentences with negatives.

A related source of misunderstanding involves the phrase, "Do you mind . . . ?" If you ask an Asian, "Do you mind . . . ?" you will probably receive the answer "yes." Americans would generally interpret that to mean

19

20

the other individual *does* mind, but they would be wrong. It is the Asian way of showing agreement or willingness.

Pronouns

Different languages have characteristics that are not directly translatable, as any English speaker who has struggled with remembering the gender of inanimate objects in French or Spanish knows well. English poses a similar problem for many Asians. Mieko, a Japanese nurse, was assigned to care for six patients, two male and four female. During reports, she consistently referred to the female patients as "he." Her supervisor interrupted to point out that there were no male patients in the bed numbers she mentioned. Mieko acknowledged that fact and continued in the same manner. The supervisor became confused. Had four transsexuals slipped in?

The explanation is simple. Many Asian languages do not have pronouns that reflect gender; "he" and "she" do not exist. Thus Asians have no model for using the pronouns "he" or "she" and often mix them up, confusing everyone else in the process. This may seem surprising, given the importance of gender in Asian hierarchical cultures. It might help to think of it in this way—gender is of such importance that it is not diminished by the use of a mere pronoun. An individual would be referred to as "that man" or "that woman." Knowledge of this characteristic of the language can lessen the confusion.

Communication Style

Formal Versus Informal Language

The United States was founded in large part by British settlers who were escaping, among other things, the British system of nobility. The notion of equality became paramount in our national culture, as illustrated in the famous words of the Declaration of Independence: "We hold these truths to be self-evident, that all men are created equal." One manifestation of the importance of equality is the absence of a vocabulary that indicates status differences. At the same time, the westward movement embodied a greater informality, also reflected in our language. In Spanish, for example, different forms of the word "you" are used depending in part on the level of formality of the relationship to the speaker. When addressing one person, the speaker may use *tú* for a young person or for someone with whom he or she has a close relationship. Alternatively, he or she may use *usted* for a stranger or someone occupying a higher social position. The more formal *usted* is used when speaking to someone older or someone you don't know very well. In English, "thee" and "thou" used to serve the same purpose, but these have been replaced by the single word "you," which does not distinguish between formal and informal contexts.

The fact that some languages have formal and informal vocabulary, something that English lacks, can create problems. As you will read in the chapter on staff issues, young Filipino nurses may feel forced to resort to speaking in Tagalog in order to show respect to older Filipino nurses because Tagalog has a formal vocabulary. I have had several Nigerian students tell me they were offended by the "rude" behavior of young people who had the "nerve" to say "hi" to them. Why would they be offended by a friendly greeting? Because they perceived "hi" as rudely informal. Instead, they explained, young people should have the courtesy to say "hello" or "good day."

Directive Versus Nondirective Approaches

Different communication styles can also create misunderstandings. The current emphasis in medicine is on shared decision making. The patient is seen as an equal partner in the health care interaction. However, not all cultures have this expectation, and it can sometimes backfire. Medical anthropologist Carole Browner and her colleagues did research on miscommunication between prenatal genetic service providers and patients born in Mexico.[3] They point out that the nondirective approach taken in genetic counseling was interpreted by many of the patients to reflect a lack of concern about test results. They assumed that if their tests had indicated any serious danger, the clinician would have been more dramatic and directive in recommending amniocentesis. Thus, the standard nondirective style was misinterpreted to indicate that no intervention was necessary.

Personalismo

For many Hispanics, the establishment of personal relationships is extremely important. The health care provider who wants to develop a good relationship with a Hispanic patient will take the time to ask about the patient's family and interests before getting "down to business." Although this may seem to be a "waste of time," in the long run it will save time, as the patient will be more likely to open up more quickly to a trusted health care provider. Furthermore, it will improve the chances of the patient adhering to the health care provider's recommendations, because adherence becomes a matter of a "personal favor."

A middle-aged Hispanic woman had a very bad experience with a physician she saw for the first time. She complained that he didn't care for her as an individual; he wanted only to treat her disease. When asked why she felt this way, she explained that the doctor never bothered even to greet

21

her. Furthermore, he stood in the doorway when taking her history. He was lacking in *personalismo*, and as a result, she felt isolated and did not trust him. Rather than return to him, she went to a *curandero*, a traditional healer.

In contrast, a pediatric nurse who described herself as having "lost touch" over the years with being sensitive and polite in her greetings, changed her approach after learning about the importance of *personalismo*. She began to greet her Hispanic patients and their families with a simple "buenos dias" or "buenas tardes" and would make conversation about family life. For example, she'd ask the ages of the children, or what plans the family had for the holidays. She found that family members exhibited much less reluctance when she had to insert an intravenous line or administer medications to their child. She said the family felt she was on "their side," and doing everything to help improve their child's health and well-being.

22   Stephanie's interaction with Juanita Rios, a forty-nine-year-old Mexican woman, illustrates how *personalismo* can improve patient outcomes through increased adherence to medical recommendations. Mrs. Rios was suffering from both renal failure and diabetes; her condition required her to be on dialysis while waiting for an organ transplant. Stephanie, her nurse, found that as she got to know her better, making several home visits when she could not get a ride to the rural clinic, she began to open up more to her. When Stephanie learned that Mrs. Rios had left several of her children behind in Mexico, a necessity that has caused her great sadness and periodic depression, Stephanie encouraged her to talk about her children and show her their photos. On Mrs. Rios's birthday, she arranged for her to call her sons from the clinic. As a result of Stephanie's display of *personalismo*, Mrs. Rios became much more compliant with diet and fluid restrictions. As Stephanie explained, "She knows we make these requests because we care about her."

Personalismo can sometimes turn difficult patients into cooperative ones, and spare a nurse from a lawsuit, as happened in the following case.

23   Dee was caring for Ramona Medina, a Latina with end-stage renal disease. She was number one on the liver transplant list. When Dee began her shift, the departing nurse warned her that she would be dealing with an extremely difficult family who had already lodged several complaints with the administration. Dee was in the middle of a cultural diversity class, and decided to apply the concepts she had been learning to this apparently difficult case. She obtained permission from the charge nurse to be flexible with the visiting hours. She invited the family to help her with hygiene care for the patient. She *talked* to them and developed a relationship with them. At the end of her shift, they requested that she care for their mother the next night.

When Dee spoke with the oncoming nurse, she tried to convince her to be flexible with visitation, but the nurse insisted on enforcing the re-stricted visiting rules. As a result, the day nurse experienced major con-flicts with the family.

Mrs. Medina never received a liver transplant, and thus died. Afterward, the hospital held a risk management meeting. Mrs. Medina's family was suing the hospital; the lawsuit specifically named staff members the fam-ily felt were unprofessional and uncaring. The only two nurses *not* named in the suit were Dee and another nurse. Management spoke with both of them to see what they had done differently; what they had done right. Both had the same response; they talked with the family and kept them involved in the patient's care. In other words, they demonstrated *personalismo*.

Respeto

An important cultural value in Hispanic cultures can actually lead to poorer communication between patients and providers. I'm referring to the importance of *respeto*, or respect.

When Jesus Chavez, a middle-aged Hispanic male, suffered a severe myocardial infarction, his physician, Dr. Jerome, recommended coronary artery bypass surgery. When the Chavez family came to visit, they would often ask Caron, Mr. Chavez's nurse, many questions regarding his condi-tion and prognosis. Caron finally asked them if they had spoken with the doctor recently. They said they had. When she asked them why they didn't ask *him* all these questions, they said, "The doctor is very busy, and he prob-ably does not have time to answer all of our questions. We don't want to take away from our dad's care." They had too much respect for him to bother him with their questions. Caron then called Dr. Jerome to explain the sit-uation. The physician was surprised. "I just spoke with them last night, and they said that they understand everything, and had no questions."

Caron and Dr. Jerome set up a family conference. Caron gave the fam-ily paper and pen to write down all of their questions. Thus encouraged to ask their questions, they did. Dr. Jerome answered each one of them, which clearly put the family at ease.

Asking Questions

It's important for physicians to remember that doctors are held in very high regard in most cultures. This may make it difficult for patients to feel com-fortable asking questions. However, lack of understanding often results in lack of adherence, so better patient outcomes will often result when ques-tions are encouraged. Culturally competent clinicians will have patients demonstrate their understanding of any patient teaching, as well as ask patients what questions they have. Not "Do you have any questions?"—a question many patients will hesitate to respond to either out of respect for the physician's time, or for fear of appearing stupid—but "What questions do you have?" Their tone should assume that *of course* they will have questions, and it is his or her job to be happy to answer them. In addition, it is always good practice for health care providers to ask patients what they understand about their condition.

Asking Patients Questions About Their Culture or Religion

In order to provide culturally appropriate care, it's necessary to know something about the patient's ethnic and religious background. Some nurses have commented that there are patients who become upset when asked about their religious beliefs. There's the danger of appearing intrusive. The key is in the way it is done. If you explain *why* you're asking such questions, people are more likely to give you answers. For example, "We're making an effort at our hospital to meet the needs of our diverse population. Knowing about your ethnic background, religious preferences, and sexual orientation can help us to provide better care, should you choose to share that information with us."

Names

In the United States, individual names are given first, followed by family names. I would introduce myself as Geri-Ann Galanti. Any native would immediately know that my family name is Galanti, and if they were to address me using a title, such as Ms. or Dr., the title would go before my last name, as in Ms. Galanti. This custom is not the same in all countries, however, and can lead to confusion, especially in the filing of medical records. A few examples are given below.

Egyptian Names

All Egyptian names are essentially first names. The first one listed is yours, the second one is your father's, and the third is your grandfather's (even if you're female). Aziz Mohammad would properly be addressed as "Mr. Aziz" and his wife, Sheida, as "Mrs. Sheida," although in the United States Mrs. Aziz would be acceptable.

Indochinese Names

With the Indochinese, the first name given is generally the family name, followed by the individual name. For example, Ngyuen Thanh's family name is Nguyen; his given name is Thanh. When addressing him, use Mr. with his given name, "Mr. Thanh." Interestingly, this reflects the fact that in many Asian cultures the family is more important than the individual, and thus the family name is given first. The opposite is true in the United States, as reflected by the position and usage of our individual name. Note that for the sake of clarity I generally follow the American conventions for names in this book.

Hispanic Names

It is common for Hispanics to take both their mother's and their father's last names. Typically, the father's name is used first and then the mother's. For example, take a woman named Roberta Canál Santos. Canál is her father's last name; Santos is her mother's last name. If she were to go by only one last name, it would be Canál, her father's name. José, the son of Juan Martinez and Flora Gomez, would go by José Martinez Gomez, or simply José Martinez. While some married women continue to use both the maternal and paternal last names, others drop their maternal last name and add their husbands' last name with "de" between the two. For example, if Roberta married José, she might keep the name Roberta Canál Santos or she might prefer to be called Roberta Canal de Martinez.

First Versus Last Names

Americans tend to address each other by their first names. It is considered a sign of friendliness and equality. To use a first name for anyone other than a close friend, however, is both inappropriate and discourteous in most cultures, including European. In nineteenth-century English novels, even teenage girls referred to each other as Miss until they had been friends for at least a year. Hospital personnel should refer to all adult patients as Mr., Miss, Ms., or Mrs., unless instructed otherwise.

African Americans' sensitivity to perceived slights to their dignity is not surprising given their history in this country. It is therefore especially important to show them respect. Mary Washington, an elderly Black woman, was in the recovery room after surgery. To assess her condition, Cheryl, her nurse, spoke her name, "Mary." The patient slowly opened her eyes and turned her head but made no further sign of acknowledgment. Cheryl became concerned because most patients responded readily and clearly at this point. Shortly afterward Cheryl called the woman Mrs. Washington. She then became alert, pleasant, and cooperative. She had perceived the use of her first name as a lack of respect.

25

Interpreters

In 2001, in an effort to improve access to care, quality of care, and ultimately, health outcomes, the U.S. Department of Health and Human

Services, Office of Minority Health, published national standards for Culturally and Linguistically Appropriate Services in Health Care, commonly known as "CLAS standards" (see National Standards 2001). Three of the fourteen standards focus on culturally competent care, four on language access services, and seven on organizational support. Most of the standards are recommendations; however, those requiring language access services are mandates, required for all recipients of federal funds. Thus, a section on interpreters should no longer be necessary. However, the reality is that there are huge numbers of immigrants from a variety of countries, so it is not feasible to have interpreters in every language on staff 24 hours a day. Often, even if interpreters are on the hospital staff, they are not immediately available. Patients are often accompanied by family members, at least some of whom are usually bilingual. Therefore, the expedient choice often favored by physicians and nurses is to use family members. The case studies in this section illustrate why this is *not* a good idea.

I also want to mention that there are numerous telephonic services available, including some video phones. When used properly, these services work quite well. It is important, however, that speakerphones be used, so that telephone receivers are not handed back and forth, making the process more cumbersome than needed.

First, a case to illustrate the necessity of having interpreters available.

26   Pham Kim, a sixty-five-year-old Vietnamese patient, was diagnosed with poor nutrition and lower abdominal pain. Her refusal to eat was documented by the nurses: "No food intake, but only juice." When the interpreter finally spoke with her, three days post admission, she said she hadn't understood anything the doctor had said to her. When the physician asked through the interpreter why she hadn't been eating, she replied, "I do not like American food." He then asked if she had trouble chewing or swallowing food. "No." When the doctor explained through the interpreter that they were going to put a feeding tube through her nose to feed her, she quickly explained that her daughter (who also did not speak English) brought her rice and hot soup every day at 9:00 P.M. The nurses just hadn't seen her eat. If an interpreter hadn't finally been brought in, Mrs. Kim would have suffered a nasogastric tube, followed by a percutaneous endoscopic gastrostomy tube, all for no reason.

The next set of case studies illustrate the kinds of problems that can occur when family members are used as interpreters. It is particularly dangerous when children are used, yet they are most likely to be bilingual and, therefore, the most expedient choice.

27   Hilda Gomez, a monolingual Spanish-speaking patient, came in to the clinic three days in a row to complain of abdominal pain. The first two times, the staff used her young, bilingual daughter to translate. The staff treated her for the "stomach ache" she described. They didn't understand

why she kept returning with the same problem. Finally, on her third visit, the nurse located a Spanish-speaking interpreter. It turned out that Mrs. Gomez needed treatment for a sexually transmitted disease, but was too embarrassed to talk about her sexual activity with her daughter as interpreter. It taught the staff an important lesson.

At least Mrs. Gomez was finally treated properly. Juan Vega had a less   28
happy outcome when a family member was used to interpret a diagnosis of HIV and a detailed explanation of the disease process and prognosis. The family member left the hospital immediately after interpreting, and never returned. Mr. Vega's family, who had been very supportive of him since he had become ill, abandoned him when they were given the details through the family interpreter. After this unfortunate incident, the staff took time to locate a professional interpreter when the patient did not speak English.

Maria Hidalgo was receiving home hospice care for metastatic breast   29
cancer. She spoke only Spanish, so Patty, her hospice nurse, relied on family members to interpret. Maria was desperately fighting not to let her disease upset normal family routines. She was choosing to compromise her comfort in order to maintain her traditional role in the family as wife and mother; however, her exhaustion was making it increasingly difficult to do so. The rest of the family were having a hard time maintaining the illusion of normalcy, knowing that their lives were changing dramatically. In short, everyone was trying to protect everyone else but collapsing under the strain. It was not until Patty called in a bilingual/bicultural colleague that Maria was able to talk more openly about her needs for pain medication. To discuss this through her family would have let down the pretense of normalcy.

A Hispanic woman, Graciela Mendoza, had to sign an informed con-   30
sent form for a hysterectomy. Her bilingual son served as the interpreter. When he described the procedure to his mother, he appeared to be translating accurately and indicating the appropriate body parts. His mother signed willingly. The next day, however, when she learned that her uterus had been removed and that she could no longer bear children, she became very angry and threatened to sue the hospital. What went wrong?

Because it is inappropriate for a Hispanic male to discuss the private parts of his mother, the embarrassed son explained that a tumor would be removed from her abdomen and pointed to that general area. When Mrs. Garcia learned that her uterus had been removed, she was quite angry and upset because a Hispanic woman's status is derived in large part from the number of children she produces. When dealing with anything remotely sexual, it is best not to use family members; if necessary, at least make every effort to use same-sex family members. However, as the next case illustrates, this may not be sufficient.

31   An Arab woman had just given birth. Her Arab American mother-in-law was asked to translate the health teaching material to the new mother. All went well until the nurse reached the information on contraception. The mother-in-law refused to translate such information. She was part of a culture that valued large families, and she wanted as many grandchildren as possible.

In this case, the woman openly refused to translate. It is just as likely that she might have pretended to convey the information while actually talking about something else. It is important to remember that language is not the only issue involved in translation.

32   Helena became very frustrated while caring for Gwon Chin, a seventy-nine-year-old Korean man who had recently suffered from a stroke. Her frustration and impatience were aimed at Mr. Gwon's wife and daughter. Since Mr. Gwon spoke only Korean, she had asked his bilingual daughter to tell her father not to get out of bed because his gait was unsteady. Helena was afraid he would fall and hurt himself. Throughout the day, however, Mr. Gwon continued to attempt to get out of bed. He became very agitated and his wife and daughter seemed almost afraid of him. When Helena questioned the daughter about it, she would only say that her father was "confused." Eventually Helena called upon a Korean nurse to help her. When the nurse told Mr. Gwon not to get out of bed because he might fall, he asked in a surprised tone, "Why would I fall?" When the nurse explained that he was unsteady from the stroke, the patient was shocked. "I had a stroke?!" Helena was in disbelief. He had been on the unit for two days; how could he not know he had had a stroke? When she questioned Mr. Gwon's daughter about this, she explained that her brother had been out of town. He would be back today and tell him. When Helena, stunned by this, asked the daughter why *she* didn't tell her father, she replied, "I could never tell my father what is wrong with him and what he can or can't do. It would be disrespectful for me to do that when he has always told *me* what to do and what was wrong." Although Helena was angry that Mr. Gwon's daughter preferred having her father possibly fall and hurt himself than tell him why he was in the hospital and that he must stay in bed, Helena remained silent. She asked the Korean nurse to explain to the patient how the numbness on his left side would make walking difficult so he should remain in bed. She also added that his son would be in later that day and explain everything to him. After that, the patient remained calm and stayed in bed.

This case is new to this edition. I had trouble deciding where to place it, because it highlights several important points. It shows the hierarchical nature of communication patterns within many traditional Asian households. Parents tell children what to do, not the reverse. Sons have more status and authority than daughters. It is common for family members to try to protect loved ones from "bad news." And finally, it underscores the need to use professional interpreters rather than family members.

A similar dynamic led Serafin Amador, a Filipino man who had immigrated to the United States fifty years ago, to feel disrespected when the medical staff spoke with his grandchildren, rather than himself, due to the language barrier. He said that if they could not speak with him, at least they should be talking with his eldest son, rather than his grandchildren. Respect for the family hierarchy was important to him. Proper use of a trained interpreter would have avoided the problem.   33

Although professional interpreters are generally a good idea, sometimes they can cause a problem, as in the following case.   34

Susana Ramos, a thirty-six-year-old Latina female, brought her mother to the emergency department for evaluation and treatment. She was her mother's primary caregiver and expected to serve as interpreter. When told that it was hospital policy to use a trained medical interpreter, she became very upset. She was further distressed when told that confidentiality laws also prevented her from serving as her mother's interpreter. (In fact, this is not the case. HIPAA (Health Insurance and Portability and Accountability Act) regulations stipulate that health care providers may share information with others *unless* the patient objects. Confusion over the laws and fear of lawsuits has led many health care providers to be overzealous in the protection of patient privacy; see Gross 2007). Susana felt that she was an ideal interpreter for her mother. As her mother's caretaker, she knew her mother's history. She felt her mother would be more comfortable having her as interpreter. She said the hospital policy made her feel like the staff were hiding something from her, and thus she did not trust them. She did not feel her mother would accurately express her needs or report her family history to a stranger. The nurse who reported this incident said that the rapport and care of this patient suffered as a result of the hospital policy.

What should the staff have done in this case? Under the circumstances, Susana would probably have been an appropriate interpreter. However, an even better approach would have been to explain that her mother's health was their shared priority, and because there might be medical terminology she was not familiar with, they wanted to use a professional medical interpreter. They could also have assured her that they would appreciate having her be part of the interview, once the interpreter ascertained that the patient *wanted* her daughter in the room. If Susana seemed offended by that, they could explain that in the past there had been problems when the patient did not feel comfortable being completely honest with the staff in front of family members, and although it was extremely unlikely in this case, wasn't it best to be sure? Susana would likely have been reassured by their concern that her mother get the best care possible.

One final story about the importance of interpreters, even when you speak the language. It's time for some comic relief.

35   An orthopedic fellow from Latin America had to intervene with a Mexican patient who was screaming that the medical resident was crazy. The resident, who had learned a little Spanish to communicate with his patients, told him that he was going to put a plate in his leg—*un platano.* Unfortunately, although "platano" sounds like a Spanish version of the word "plate," it actually means "banana." The patient was afraid the crazy doctor was going to put a banana in his leg.

Because the Latino population in this country is growing larger each year, many physicians are making an effort to learn some Spanish. Many feel that by talking directly to their patients, they can create greater rapport than they might have using an interpreter. Although that is probably true, it is often best to call for an interpreter anyway. Use the time you are waiting for the interpreter to arrive to develop *personalismo,* and save the medical content for the interpreter.

One final note on interpreters. It is essential that they be utilized properly. See Appendix 4, Tips for Working with Interpreters, developed by medical anthropologist M. Jean Gilbert.

Taking a History

When Someone Else Answers for the Patient

36   Nurses and physicians may sometimes experience difficulty when trying to obtain information from a patient. Jeanie did when trying to get a health history from a young Romany (Gypsy) woman. The patient's mother-in-law insisted upon accompanying her to the examining room. Jeanie assumed she wanted to act as an interpreter, but the woman's English skills were no better than her daughter-in-law's. The patient's reply to every question was the same: "I don't know." She probably knew many of the answers but was respecting a cultural prohibition against giving too much information to Gaje (non-Romany). The patient's mother-in-law may have been there in part to protect her and in part to make sure she did not reveal too much. It is important to try to get some time alone with the patient, especially when asking sensitive questions.

When Silence Is the Response

37   Ramona was trying to get a medical history from Mrs. Cata, a Navajo woman. After each question Ramona asked, there would be a long silence. When Ramona spoke, Mrs. Cata would often stare at the floor. Ramona assumed it meant that Mrs. Cata was shy and had trouble understanding

her, but that was not the case. She was merely indicating in a culturally appropriate manner that she was paying close attention to Ramona. The Navajo value silence. A person who interrupts while someone is speaking is perceived as immature.

Most Americans are uncomfortable with silences and tend to fill them with words, making small talk. The Navajo use silence to formulate their thoughts. Words should have significance. An anthropologist doing field-work among the Navajo commented that it took her a long time to get used to talking with them. She would ask a question and get no response. She assumed they had not heard or understood her. She was wrong. They were trying to give her the most complete answer possible, and that took consideration. Eventually, she became comfortable with long pauses in conversation.

When dealing with Navajo patients, if they seem slow to respond, be patient. Give them time to consider your question before answering. Don't make judgments based on the meaning of your own behavior.

Informed Consent

According to American laws, individuals undergoing surgery must sign a document of informed consent, indicating that they understand the pro-cedure and its intended risks. It is consistent with the American value of autonomy that patients should make their own decisions regarding their health. However, it is not always a simple matter to obtain such consent, because not everyone values autonomy in that way. In addition, some patients may have issues with document signing based upon past experi-ences. Or they may agree to sign without truly understanding what they are signing.

Mr. Fanous was a sixty-five-year-old man from the Middle East who had come to the cardiac cath lab for a heart catheterization. It was Nina's job to get him to sign an informed consent. He read the form, which described the various complications that could result along with the pros and cons of the procedure. After Nina went through everything with him, he did not want to sign the form. He questioned why it was even necessary—why didn't they just go ahead and do the procedure? She explained to him that it was not ethical to talk someone into a procedure, and that it could not be done without his consent. After some discussion, Mr. Fanous finally signed the consent form.

Why had he been so reluctant to sign? Partly, it may have been because he did not want to be at the hospital in the first place; he had come only due to the urging of friends. From a cultural perspective, however, it may be because many Arabs believe that because the doctor is the one with the knowledge and training, the doctor should be the one to make the

38

decision. What did Mr. Fanous know about heart catheterization? Why was the hospital so unwilling to take responsibility for its actions? Although, as Nina suggests, there is probably no way to avoid this kind of cultural misunderstanding, just knowing what to expect might help.

39   Yea Samreth, an elderly Cambodian patient, had been severely burned on her back during a coining treatment when the alcohol being used caught fire. (See Chapter 12 for more information on coining.) This occurred while she was being treated by a traditional healer for diabetes. She spoke very little English. Before she could have a skin graft, she needed to sign informed consent. Rhonda, her nurse, had given Mrs. Samreth the form to sign, but she hadn't done so. Rhonda told Gillian, the nurse coming on shift, to be sure to get the document signed. When Gillian approached Mrs. Samreth with the document, she became agitated, and kept repeating, "Later, I sign later." Because Mrs. Samreth's language skills were minimal, Gillian was unsure as to how much she understood about what she was being asked to sign. There was no interpreter available. Gillian later learned why the patient was likely so reluctant. During the Khmer Rouge war, signed life histories were required from those who were later executed. As a result, many middle-aged and older Cambodians are not comfortable signing written documents. A culturally competent health care provider would have made sure to have a family member available for support, a physician available to answer questions, and an interpreter available to explain the document to her. It would also have been helpful to ask the patient what concerns she had about signing.

40   Andrew Chan, the son of Chan Wen, a seventy-five-year-old Chinese man, was angry with his father's physician. His father was scheduled for an angiogram at noon. The nurse had explained everything to his son the day before, and he intended to come to the hospital that morning, speak to his father's physician, and sign the consent. When he arrived at his father's room at 9:30 A.M., his father handed him the signed consent form. Andrew walked over to the nursing station and furiously demanded to know who had made his father sign a consent form in English when he did not speak the language. After further discussion with Mr. Chan, it was determined that the physician had visited him at 8:00 that morning, and seeing the unsigned consent form on the bedside table, handed it to him to sign. The physician did explain the procedure to him, in English. He had no idea that Mr. Chan did not understand a word, because he was constantly nodding in agreement. Smiling and nodding is a common response in any language, when people do not understand. It is often done in an effort to be polite. Why did Mr. Chan sign a form he could not understand? Out of respect for the authority of the physician. Chinese culture is hierarchical, and physicians are held in high esteem.

    There were a number of mistakes made in this case, beginning with the nurse explaining the procedure to the patient's son rather than using an interpreter to explain it to the patient. In addition, the physician should have taken the time to question the patient about his understanding of the procedure. If he had done that, it would have been clear that the patient did not speak English. Fortunately, there were no adverse effects of the errors.

Nonverbal Communication

Eye Contact

Ellen was trying to teach her Navajo patient, Jim Nez, how to live with his   41
newly diagnosed diabetes. She soon became extremely frustrated because she felt she was not getting through to him. He asked very few questions and never met her eyes. She reasoned from this that he was uninterested and therefore not listening to her.

Rather than signaling disinterest, however, Mr. Nez's behavior demonstrated a respect for the nurse's authority. His lack of eye contact probably reflected the Navajo belief that the eyes are the windows to the soul. To make direct eye contact is disrespectful and can endanger the spirits of both parties. Thus his lack of eye contact actually displayed his concern.

A former student of mine said she automatically rejected job applicants who did not make eye contact on the basis that they could not be trusted. In fact, there may be good cultural reasons why eye contact is purposely avoided.

Many Asians consider it disrespectful to look someone directly in the eye, especially if that person is in a superior position. Most Asian cultures are hierarchical; men are considered superior to women, parents to children, teachers to students, doctors to nurses, and so forth. Looking someone directly in the eye implies equality. An Asian patient may avoid eye contact out of respect for the "superior status" of the doctor or nurse, rather than for reasons of disinterest or dishonesty. A Korean nurse shared that when she scolded her children, she would get angry if they had the nerve to look her in the eye. She instructed them to show respect by looking down.

Angela, a nurse case manager, was doing patient teaching with Cha   42
Xeng, a fourteen-year-old Hmong girl who had just delivered a premature baby. Cha Xeng had been in the United States since she was six years old and spoke English fluently. Angela was disturbed because Cha Xeng avoided making eye contact with her and spoke in a soft, timid voice. She immediately assumed that the young mother was hiding something from her, that she was having trouble bonding with the infant or was not interested in her child's special needs. The nurse even suspected her of using illegal drugs, all because she would not make eye contact.

In reality, Cha Xeng was showing Angela respect by avoiding contact. She kept her voice low to avoid appearing rude. She did not ask for further explanations, not out of lack of interest, but to avoid appearing stupid and/or imply that Angela was doing a poor job of explaining. Hmong culture, like most Asian cultures, is hierarchical. Cha Xeng's respect for the hierarchy led Angela to make many incorrect assumptions.

Direct eye contact is also avoided in Nigeria to show respect. Rather than make eye contact with a physician, the Nigerian patient will probably look down.

Many Middle Easterners regard direct eye contact between a man and a woman as a sexual invitation. Female doctors or nurses dealing with Middle Eastern men must be aware that their eye contact may be interpreted not as directness but as an invitation of a sexual nature. In general, eye contact should be avoided with Middle Easterners of the opposite sex. Medical personnel should be aware of the meaning of eye contact in their patients' cultures and make sure the appropriate communication is both transmitted and received.

Touching

It is considered very poor taste in most Asian countries for people to touch in public. Men and women should not hug, kiss, or hold hands. It is, however, common for individuals of the *same* sex to hold hands or walk arm-in-arm. It merely indicates that they are close friends or relatives.

Juen, a former student from mainland China, told me that when she first came to the United States she was staying in the home of an American family. One evening, a male friend of the family came to visit. When he left, he lightly kissed everyone good-bye, including Juen. She was completely shocked, and said, "When he kissed me, it made me feel so uncomfortable, just like you ate a fly!"

Health care workers should be advised that many Asian coworkers and patients will not be comfortable with the casual touching and hugging that many Latinos and Americans do without even thinking. Observe their behavior (and that of their families) to see what they are comfortable with.

When my mother was hospitalized, a rabbi associated with the hospital came to visit her. My husband and I were in the room at the time. We both introduced ourselves to the rabbi. My husband went first, and offered his hand, which the rabbi immediately shook. When I offered my hand, however, it hung in the air as the rabbi pointedly ignored it. After a moment I realized that he must be Orthodox and was thus forbidden to touch me. I've been told that other Orthodox rabbis *will* shake hands with a woman, rather than cause her embarrassment: this particular rabbi was from Chabad, one of the more ultra-Orthodox sects.

The same rule against touching holds true for Muslims. Whenever possible, same-sex caregivers should be assigned to Orthodox Jews and Muslims, and opposite-sex touching should be avoided.

Gestures

Other forms of nonverbal communication can be equally problematic.   44
An Anglo patient named Jon Smith called out to Maria, a Filipino nurse: "Nurse, nurse." Maria came to Mr. Smith's door and politely asked, "May I help you?" Mr. Smith beckoned for her to come closer by motioning with his right index finger. Maria remained where she was and responded in an angry voice, "What do you want?"

Mr. Smith was confused. Why had Maria's manner suddenly changed? The problem was that the innocent "come here" gesture is used in the Philippines (and in Korea) only to call animals, and in a sense Mr. Smith had called Maria a dog. To summon a person, Filipinos motion with the whole hand, palm in, and fingers down.

Unfortunately, many Americans are confused as to whether this gesture means "come here" or "go away," as Teresa, a Filipino nurse, discovered when she tried to call Nancy, an Anglo American nurse's aide, to assist her with a patient. She motioned to her, palm in, fingers down, to come over. Rather than move nearer to Teresa, Nancy merely smiled and waved back, using the same gesture. At the time, Teresa was confused and a bit hurt over Nancy's refusal to help her. She later learned that Nancy simply thought she was waving goodbye.   45

Problems such as this can best be handled through in-service education classes. If hospital personnel from other cultures are taught the different meanings of gestures, they might not take offense. Maria might have responded to Mr. Smith's request and then politely explained how she felt about the gesture. Mr. Smith would have learned something important about cross-cultural communication and probably refrained from using that gesture with a Filipino again.

Other seemingly innocuous gestures that can create misunderstandings include the "okay" sign (thumb and index fingers together in a circle, other fingers straight up), the "thumbs-up" sign, and the "V" made with the index and middle fingers (used to signify either peace or victory). In Brazil, the "okay" sign is a crude sexual invitation. "Thumbs-up" in Iran and the "V," held palm in, in South Africa, Great Britain, Australia, and New Zealand, are insulting gestures similar to the raised middle finger in U.S. culture.

Body Language

Body language is another form of nonverbal communication fraught with the possibility of unintentional messages. I first learned about this when setting up a demonstration regarding interpreters in one of my classes. I had arranged myself and two other students in a triangle; I was the patient, one of the other students was the physician, and the other was the interpreter. I then asked the class what was wrong with the picture. My intention was to illustrate that the triangle was a poor set-up, since it led to a lack of eye contact between the health care provider and the patient. However, that is not what the first volunteer commented upon.

My student from Ghana noted that I was challenging the physician with my posture. "What posture?" I asked. She indicated the fact that my arms were folded in front of my body, a position I had put them in because I didn't have any pockets and didn't know what to do with my hands. She explained that in Ghana they should be kept behind the body to show respect, "unless," she added, "you're being yelled at, in which case it is okay to keep them in front."

At that point, one of the Vietnamese students joined in the discussion, saying that in Vietnam it is a sign of disrespect to keep your hands in back. The same is true in Korea and the Philippines, according to other students from those countries. The Asian students all agreed that hands should be kept folded in front. In Vietnam, they should be at waist level; in the Philippines, they can be down. Once again, the same gesture can have very different meaning, depending on where you are.

Time Orientation

As explained in the previous chapter, time orientation can refer to two different aspects of how people relate to time. One aspect involves whether they are oriented toward the clock or to activities. Conflicts can occur when someone who is clock oriented interacts with someone who is activity oriented. Another aspect of time orientation is more global, and relates to whether people tend to focus on the past, present, or future. The health care culture, as a subculture of American culture, tends to be future oriented, even though many of the patients are present oriented.

Clock Time Versus Activity Time

Cultural differences in clock time versus activity time become particularly significant in health care clinics, which tend to be run on clock time and are often frequented by people operating on activity time. The following two cases illustrate the problem.

46   Mr. Jacinto, a middle-aged Filipino patient new to the clinic, arrived thirty minutes late for his appointment. The front clerk asked him to reschedule, because he was too late to be seen. Mr. Jacinto was very upset, complaining that in the Philippines his doctor would see him even if he

were an hour late. He didn't realize that there would be a problem. He was adamant that he be seen right away for the physical exam he needed in order to obtain a license from the Department of Motor Vehicles. Araceli, a Filipino nurse, was called over to talk with Mr. Jacinto. Knowing the importance of respect in Filipino culture, she used the words *po* and *opo*, both words of respect in Tagalog. She explained in their mutual native language that according to clinic policy, a patient will be asked to reschedule an appointment if he or she arrives fifteen minutes after the scheduled time to avoid creating a long backup in the clinic. Araceli then found him an appointment for the next day, and emphasized the need to arrive on time. Mr. Jacinto was mollified, and thankful both for the respect he had been given through her use of *po* and *opo*, and for the explanation given to him. Most people will be reasonable if they are treated with respect and are made to understand why things are being done the way they are. Too often patients are simply told the rules, without the reasons behind them, and treated in a curt manner, because health care professionals are often overworked with very little time for the "niceties." However, taking a moment in the first place can often save a lot of time and aggravation later on.

It is possible to work with people's time orientation. Juanita Avelar was   *47* a forty-nine-year-old Mexican woman with kidney failure and diabetes. She relied on her niece and nephew to drive her to the clinic and was often late. In Mexican culture, the needs of the family typically take precedence over those of an individual. The nurses learned to take this into account when scheduling her appointments, and they allowed plenty of time for the family to discuss Mrs. Avelar's condition as a family. When certain tests and medications required specific timing for accuracy and effectiveness, they stressed the importance of time.

People from developing countries often have a present time orientation. These cultures are usually based on agriculture, which does not require adherence to a clock. It is only in industrialized nations that clock time is important because the performance of everyone's job depends on all others doing theirs. It becomes necessary to adhere to a standard of time.

Health care professionals can do little about the present time orientation of patients. It is difficult for people who are not used to running their lives by the clock, who think it is rude to interrupt one activity to start another, or whose poverty makes it difficult for them to adhere to other people's schedules, to change their ways. The best health care professionals can do is to stress how important it is that patients show up on time for scheduled appointments. But they should be prepared for patients to be late, or better yet, design more flexible scheduling if the patient population warrants it. See Chapter 13 for what some clinics are doing to resolve the conflict of time orientations in scheduling.

Past, Present, and Future Time Orientation

As discussed in Chapter 1, a present time orientation can conflict with the future time orientation of the health care profession, often resulting in lack of adherence to medical recommendations.

48   Jaime Ortega, a middle-aged Latino patient, suffered from congestive heart failure and hyperkalemia. He was readmitted to the hospital only two weeks after being discharged. Celia, the admitting nurse, discovered that Mr. Ortega had neglected to take the lasix and potassium the doctor had ordered. Why? Because he felt much better; he no longer had any shortness of breath or swelling in his leg. Because his symptoms had disappeared, he stopped taking the medications. After a few days, fluid began to build in his system, necessitating a return to the hospital. Rather than look ahead to the long-term consequences of his condition and need for medication, Mr. Ortega focused on the present. As soon as he felt well, he discontinued the medication.

Physicians are unlikely to change the time orientation of their patients; however, adherence is often key to positive outcomes. It may be necessary for physicians to spend extra time with patients who have a present time orientation, in order to make sure they clearly understand the reason for following medical advice, and the consequences of lack of adherence. It might be helpful to tie long-term measures or preventive medication to concrete outcomes of values the patient holds, for example, "If you want to see your daughter get married . . ." or "If you want to hold your grandchild. . . ."

Keep in mind that all patients, even those with a future time orientation, are more likely to adhere to medical recommendations if they understand the reasons for it. How many half-full bottles of antibiotics are in medicine cabinets around the country?

Summary

Miscommunication between health care professionals and their patients often has nothing to do with ethnic background. A common problem is the use of medical jargon, for example, "voided" instead of "peed." Patients may lack the technical vocabulary to describe their symptoms in a way that physicians can understand. Some patients may be very forthright, whereas others may need probing; a health care provider must be sensitive to different communication styles. Patients may be too embarrassed to discuss certain problems, particularly those of a sexual nature. A health care provider needs excellent communication skills to be able to handle sensitive issues.

When the health care provider and the patient are of different ethnic backgrounds, there are numerous additional opportunities for misunderstandings. Communication styles and time orientation vary considerably from culture to culture, causing confusion and sometimes annoyance for hospital personnel. As a further complication, people from different cultures may behave in similar ways but for different reasons. Understanding why people communicate (or do not) in the way they do, however, can help relieve the frustration of health care workers and perhaps contribute to better patient care.

Key Points

- Avoid using idioms.
- Avoid using the terms "positive" and "negative" with respect to test results in order to avoid confusion with the lay meaning of those terms.
- Pay attention to patients' nonverbal reactions.
- Avoid asking "yes" or "no" questions with Asian patients; it is generally better to ask open-ended questions with *all* patients.
- Realize that some patients prefer shared decision-making, while others prefer a more directive approach. Be flexible and match your approach to the desires of your patient.
- Some patients expect a more personal relationship with their health care providers.
- Encourage patients to ask questions. Ask, "What questions do you have?" not "Do you have any questions?"
- Ask patients what they know about their condition.
- Ask patients about their ethnic and religious background, and explain why you are asking;
- Use professional, trained interpreters. Use telephone interpreters if live ones are not available. Avoid using family members, especially children, whenever possible.
- Understand that lack of eye contact means different things in different cultures.
- Avoid using gestures; they can mean different things in different cultures.
- People from lower socioeconomic strata often have a present time orientation. They may need additional patient teaching when it comes to preventive medicine, and outcomes should be attached to things they value.

For additional issues related to informed consent, see Chapters 6 and 7.
For additional issues related to language and communication, see Chapter 8.
For additional issues regarding taking a history, see Chapter 7.

Chapter 3
Pain

An important health care issue is the treatment of pain. Untreated pain can interfere with the healing process, both by reducing the amount of movement that is comfortable for the patient and by compromising the immune system. Before it can be treated, however, it must be properly assessed. This can cause confusion for health care providers who are unaware of cultural differences in response to pain, particularly in how it is expressed. Some patients come from cultures that encourage emotional expressiveness. Others come from cultures in which stoicism is valued, thus masking any visual signs of pain that patients might be experiencing, as well as inhibiting requests for pain medication. Also crucial are cultural variations in attitudes toward the use of pain medication.

Expression of Pain

Although the physical experience of pain is universal, there is tremendous variation in the way pain is expressed. Although there are, of course, individual differences, cultures also influence whether or not people will act stoically or expressively in response to pain.

49   Differing responses to pain are well illustrated in the cases of Mr. Wu and Mr. Valdez. Bobbie, the nurse, had two patients who had both had coronary artery bypass grafts. Mr. Valdez, a middle-aged Nicaraguan man, was the first to come up from the recovery room. He was already hooked up to a morphine PCA (patient-controlled analgesia) machine, which allowed him to administer pain medication as needed in controlled doses and at controlled intervals. For the next two hours, he summoned Bobbie every ten minutes to request more pain medication. Bobbie finally called the physician to have his dosage increased and to request additional pain injections every three hours as needed. Every three hours he requested an injection. He continually whimpered in painful agony.

50   Mr. Wu, a Chinese patient, was transferred from the recovery room an hour later. In contrast to Mr. Valdez, he was quiet and passive. He, too, was

in pain, because he used his PCA machine frequently, but he did not show it. When Bobbie offered supplemental pain pills, he refused them. Not once did he use the call light to summon her.

This is an instance of two patients with the same condition, yet vastly different ways of handling the pain. Nurses usually report that "expressive" patients often come from Hispanic, Middle Eastern, and Mediterranean backgrounds, while "stoic" patients often come from Northern European and Asian backgrounds. However, simply knowing a person's ethnicity will not allow you to predict accurately how a patient will respond to pain; in fact, there are great dangers in stereotyping, as the next case demonstrates.

Mrs. Mendez, a sixty-two-year-old Mexican patient, had just had a femoral-popliteal bypass graft on her right leg. She was still under sedation when she entered the recovery room, but an hour later she awoke and began screaming, "Aye! Aye! Aye! Mucho dolor! [Much pain]." Robert, her nurse, immediately administered the dosage of morphine the doctor had prescribed. This did nothing to diminish Mrs. Mendez's cries of pain. He then checked her vital signs and pulse; all were stable. Her dressing had minimal bloody drainage. To all appearances, Mrs. Mendez was in good condition. Robert soon became angry over her outbursts and stereotyped her as a "whining Mexican female who, as usual, was exaggerating her pain."

After another hour, Robert called the physician. The surgical team came on rounds and opened Mrs. Mendez's dressing. Despite a slight swelling in her leg, there was minimal bleeding. However, when the physician inserted a large needle into the incision site, he removed a large amount of blood. The blood had put pressure on the nerves and tissues in the area and caused her excruciating pain.

She was taken back to the operating room. This time, when she returned and awoke in recovery, she was calm and cooperative. She complained only of minimal pain. Had the physician not examined her again and discovered the blood in the incision site, Mrs. Mendez would have probably suffered severe complications.

Despite the fact that Mexicans are generally expressive of their pain, it does not mean that every Mexican patient will be, or that there is not a legitimate basis for their cries. The generalizations in this chapter (and book) are meant to be only generalizations; beware the dangers of stereotyping—it can have disastrous consequences.

One case involving cultural differences in expressing pain had a tragic ending. The Irish mother-in-law of one of my nursing students was in the hospital. She was scheduled for surgery at the end of the week. Her family became very concerned when she suddenly started complaining of pain. They knew Mrs. Carroll was typically Irish in her stoicism. They spoke to

51

52

her doctor, who was from India. He was not worried. In his country, women were usually vocal when in pain. He ignored their requests that the surgery be done sooner, thinking it unnecessary.

When he finally did operate, he discovered that Mrs. Carroll's condition had progressed to the point that she could not be saved. It is possible that if he had recognized her expressions of pain as a sign that something was very wrong and had operated sooner, she might have lived.

53   Serena received Maria Messina, an elderly Italian patient, from triage. The triage nurse warned Sirena that Mrs. Messina was "very dramatic." Fortunately for Mrs. Messina, Serena had been taking a course in cultural diversity. She realized that Italian culture encourages emotional expressiveness. She spoke very calmly to Mrs. Messina and her family and explained what would happen to her while she was in the hospital. She then administered some non-narcotic pain medication. Within ten minutes, Mrs. Messina had calmed down and reported a significant lessening in her pain. She thanked Serena effusively for her wonderful care. It takes so little to turn a difficult patient into a pleasant one.

A classic study done in a New York hospital in the early 1950s sheds some light on Mrs. Messina's behavior. Mark Zborowski's project (1952) focused on three groups: Jews, Italians, and "Old Americans" (White Anglo-Saxon Protestants, or WASPs). These groups were selected because Jews and Italians had a reputation for exaggerating their pain, whereas the behavior of "Old Americans" was consistent with the values of the medical system; they were stoic and undemanding.

Although Jews and Italians reacted similarly to pain—loudly—they did so for different reasons. The Italians complained because the pain hurt. Pain medication usually satisfied them. This remedy was rarely effective with Jewish patients, however. In addition to everything else, they would then worry about becoming addicted. Their primary concern was not the pain sensation but the meaning and significance of the pain. How would it affect them and their families? The next case exemplifies this finding, and the one after typifies the "Old American" response.

54   Jane Stein's pinky finger hurt. Not enough to need an aspirin, but enough to cause her worry for the entire summer of her thirty-fifth year. She was concerned because her grandmother had suffered from bad arthritis. Did the slight pain in her pinky signal oncoming arthritis? Would her hands be gnarled by the time she was forty, and would she be unable to even walk by the time she was fifty? Fortunately, the pain eventually went away, and Jane is fine. But she is a wonderful example of how the concern of many Jewish patients is more for the meaning and significance of the pain than it is for the pain itself.

55   Mimsy Brady took her young daughter Heather to see the doctor. This Anglo American girl was suffering from a very painful condition that

causes her to grow nerve tumors. While the physician poked and prodded Heather, she stiffened, but never cried out. The doctor gave them some bad news about Heather's condition, but both mother and daughter remained stoic. When the physician left the room, Heather burst into tears. When Mrs. Brady asked her why she didn't tell the doctor how much it hurt, she said, "I didn't want to seem like a baby in front of him." Mrs. Brady waited until she was alone to cry.

Zborowski observed that Jews and Italians have a similar socialization process. Children are warned to avoid injury, colds, and fights. Crying elicits sympathy, concern, and aid. The more they complain, the more attention and sympathy they receive. In many Jewish families, even a sneeze is seen as illness, thus predisposing children to become anxious about the meaning and significance of any symptoms. Jewish and Italian children are praised for avoiding physical injury and reprimanded for ignoring bad weather or drafts, or for playing rough games. Although this may not be as true today as it was at the time of the study, the behavior of older patients may still reflect this upbringing.

In contrast, WASP children are encouraged to participate in sports. Boys are taught to "take pain like a man" rather than "cry like a sissy" when injured. The body is seen as a machine, which, when not working (that is, when ill or injured) should be taken to a specialist (a doctor) and treated with as little fuss as possible.

Given their upbringing, it should not be surprising that adult Jews and Italians complain and desire attention when ill, while WASPs tend to be "easy" patients. When they are ill, most people revert to childhood behavior, even if the desired results are not forthcoming. If, like the Jewish patient described earlier, they were rewarded for complaining as children, they will complain as adults. If they were taught to lie quietly and not make a fuss, they will probably do the same when they grow up.

Many nurses find it difficult to care for patients like Mrs. Messina who are expressive of their pain. Nurses often prefer stoicism and compliance. When they do not get it, they tend to do as little as possible, and a new nurse is assigned to such patients each day. However, as many of the examples in this book show, a little patience and understanding can make a difference. The important thing is to figure out the source of the patient's concern, something that can often be learned simply by asking.

Why are people from some cultures generally more expressive of pain than those from others? One theory I would offer is that it has to do in part with the weather and degree of crowding. If it is cold, or heavily populated, such that large numbers of people are forced into close contact for long periods of time, it is generally advantageous to have people control their emotions. Otherwise, fights and general chaos are likely to result. In such cultures, such as those in northern Europe (cold weather) and

Japan (crowding), individuals are socialized to control their emotions. The British (who live on a small island), for example, take pride in having a "stiff upper lip." In warmer and less crowded conditions, if there is conflict, people can leave the scene. There is less inherent danger of chaos and, thus, no cultural "selection" for controlling one's emotions.

Pain Medication

Requesting Pain Medication

There is a general assumption on the part of most health care professionals that if someone is in pain, they will ask for pain medication. Unfortunately, that is not always the case.

56   Some patients tolerate even the most severe pain with little more than a clenched jaw and frequently will refuse pain medication. Osito Seisay, a Nigerian farmer who had been injured by a charging bull, was in the United States for arthroscopic knee surgery. His nurse waited for him to request pain medication, but he never did. Mr. Seisay was Muslim, and he offered his pain to Allah in thanks for the good fortune of being allowed such specialized surgery.

57   Vickie, a research nurse dispensing experimental analgesics, noted that an elderly Filipino patient named Fernando Abatay had not received any pain medication following his shoulder repair. When she asked him how much pain he was experiencing, he replied, "A lot." Vickie then questioned why he had not taken any medication. Mr. Abatay explained, "No one asked me if I wanted a shot and I didn't want to bother the nurses." The regular nurses assigned to him claimed that they could not tell he was in pain, and because he did not request any pain medication, they saw no need to give him any.

    Mr. Abatay's behavior can be explained in part by the Filipino concept of *Bahala na* (God's will). Filipinos may appear stoic because they believe pain is the will of God and thus God will give them the strength to bear it. Besides, one cannot change it. This attitude is reminiscent of the fatalistic Hispanic concept *Qué será, será*. A second explanation relates to Filipinos' respect for authority. Mr. Abatay did not want to bother the nurses. A professional's time is valuable and, unless one's problem is very serious, it is better left unmentioned.

58   Keisha handled a similar situation somewhat differently, applying cultural competence skills. Bjung Hsu, an Asian patient, never requested postoperative pain medication. Keisha, his nurse, realized that he may be practicing stoicism. She therefore looked beyond the absence of complaints and noted his elevated vital signs. She then took the time to educate him on the importance of pain management. She explained that it

would reduce recovery time and the risk of postoperative complications. Mr. Hsu then accepted pain medication and recovered comfortably, without incident.

His attitude is very different from that of most American patients. The Chinese are taught self-restraint. Assertive and individualistic people are considered crude and poorly socialized. The needs of the group are more important than those of the individual. Inconspicuousness is highly valued and in recent history has proved necessary for survival. It is best not to call attention to oneself.

One other factor that may be involved in Asians' refusal of pain medication is courtesy. They generally consider it impolite to accept something the first time it is offered. Several nurses from mainland China said they often went hungry during the first few weeks of their stay in the United States. Whenever someone asked them if they wanted something to eat, they politely refused, awaiting a second offer. It rarely came. They soon learned that in America, if one does not accept something the first time, there might be no second chance. Hospital nurses are so busy that they seldom offer something more than once. They should be aware of Asian rules of etiquette when offering pain medication, food, back rubs, or other services.

The safest approach for the health care professional is to anticipate the needs of an Asian patient for pain medication without waiting for requests. If patients are told that their doctor ordered the medication, they will be less likely to refuse on the grounds of courtesy. Asians tend to respect the authority of the physician. But if patients continue to refuse medication, their wishes should be respected.

Attitudes Toward Pain Medication

Use of pain medication is a somewhat controversial topic due to a widespread and somewhat misplaced fear of drug addiction.

Kari, a nurse from India, recounted the story of her aunt who recently had a total knee replacement. She went to visit her two days after she was discharged from the hospital. Kari noticed that her aunt seemed very tense. She asked her when she had last taken her pain medication. Before her aunt could answer, her son, a physician, responded, "Oh, Mom had her last pain medicine yesterday and she really does not need any more medicine. After all, we don't want her to get too used to taking the pain medication." In this case, reducing the pain medication had a negative impact on her aunt's health. She had stopped using her passive range-of-motion machine because it was too painful. By doing so, she risked not regaining full movement in her knee. It was important that her aunt take her pain medication as prescribed so she could become more mobile as well as more comfortable.

59

The potential problem might have been avoided if the health care provider had explained the rationale behind the use of pain medication. Its purpose is not merely to reduce the pain but also to allow her to do the rehabilitation exercises necessary for recovery.

It is also important for patients and providers to understand the nature of addiction. It is largely a psychological and behavioral disorder rather than a physical dependency. When properly prescribed, patients, unlike addicts, do not need increasingly large doses to treat pain because they do not develop a tolerance for it. If higher dosages are needed, it is usually because an inadequate dosage was prescribed in the first place.

There has been a movement in the past several years to educate health care professionals about pain medication and to combat the general prejudice against using high dosages. This is especially important for dying patients, since many have suffered needless pain due to physicians' fear of overmedication. Perhaps this is part of the legacy of our Puritan forebears, the belief that pain should be stoically borne. But given the advances in pain medication, except under the most unusual circumstances, there is no reason for anyone to die in pain.

The Form of Medication

Medication can be administered in many forms, including orally, intravenously, and intramuscularly via a "shot." Although one might assume that the least painful form would be preferred, that is not always the case.

60   Mr. Hassan was an eighty-one-year-old Egyptian patient suffering from advanced lung cancer with bone metastases. Pain control was achieved with long-acting oral morphine. He was receiving hospice care from a home health agency. According to the hospital discharge planner, his pain was well controlled with two narcotic analgesic tablets twice a day; however, when the hospice nurse did her initial evaluation, she found that the patient was requesting intramuscular or intravenous medications, despite the absence of pain between dosages. She explained to him that oral medications were preferable, but he was not satisfied. Two days later, he was readmitted to the hospital, where he received an intravenous morphine infusion.

Why did he want intravenous medication or even shots when the oral medication was doing its job? Because he is from a culture in which many people believe that the more intrusive the procedure the better it is for them, just as it has been found that many Americans think medicine has to "taste bad" in order for it to be effective. There is a lesson from this example: It is best to ask the patient what type of medication is preferred, rather than assuming it should be the least invasive form.

Instructions on the Use of Pain Medication

It is essential that you carefully explain the use of pain medication, and the reasoning behind it, lest a situation like the following occurs. Jesus Garcia, a middle-aged male Hispanic patient, was admitted to the hospital following an overdose of pain medication. He had no history of depression or suicide attempts. It turned out that the overdose was accidental. He had been told to take up to six tablets of pain medication a day. Since his pain was unbearable, he took all six tablets at once, figuring it would be more effective. 61

It took a meeting with the hospital psychiatrist, who confirmed the facts of the situation with the patient's wife, to understand what had happened. Once it was understood, a nurse then spent time going over the protocol with Mr. Garcia. Had she done that in the first place, she would have prevented a near accidental death.

Terminology

Be careful about the terminology you use with your patients, even if they are English speaking. Hilda, a nurse working at a cancer center, had a patient with unrelated leg pain. Mrs. Patterson, the patient, was referred to the pain team at the center. Hilda was becoming a bit frustrated with Mrs. Patterson because she kept canceling and rescheduling her appointments, while continuing to complain about her pain. When Hilda finally asked her why she wasn't keeping any of her appointments with the pain team, Mrs. Patterson replied that she had already suffered enough pain. She didn't need a team to provide her with more! 62

Once Hilda explained that the pain team would only assess her pain and prescribe pain medication, that there was no pain involved in the process, Mrs. Patterson kept her appointment and stopped calling to complain.

The Influence of the Health Care Provider

It is important for health care providers to be aware of their own cultural and personal biases and how they may affect their response to patients in pain. As Davidhizer and Geiger (2004) point out,

- If they expect patients to be stoic, they might over-react to patients who are expressive, or ignore them because they are "difficult" patients. If they expect patients to be expressive, they might ignore patients who are stoic.
- If they believe that pain is a part of life and to be endured, they may take a less aggressive approach to pain management than someone who believes pain can be managed and should be avoided.

- If they believe that pain is part of the childbirth experience, they may believe it doesn't require as much intervention as the laboring woman does.
- If they are concerned with drug addiction, they may hesitate to provide narcotics.
- If they are fearful of respiratory distress, they may be hesitant to provide a terminally ill patient with enough pain medication to ensure comfort and will thus cause the patient to suffer unnecessary pain.

63   Cecilia was a Filipino nurse in one of my classes. One day we were discussing the tendency of Filipino nurses to undermedicate their pain patients. If the physician prescribes a range of dosages, they will often administer the lowest dose. When asked about this, Filipino students have given a number of explanations: pain medication is scarce in the Philippines, so they are trained not to use too much. One nurse said that in the Philippines families pay for the medicine they get in the hospital. Many can't afford it, which is one reason why nurses use the lowest dosage prescribed. Other reasons mentioned include that addiction is highly feared; stoicism is valued; and, for Catholic Filipinos, there is virtue in suffering. After a few minutes, I noticed tears falling from Cecilia's eyes. When I asked her what was wrong, she explained that a year earlier her mother had died of cancer. The doctor had prescribed high dosages of pain medication in the months before her death. Cecilia administered the medication to her mother, but out of habit had cut each dosage in half before giving it to her mother. She did not want her mother to become addicted, she explained. Now, in class, she realized that she had allowed her mother to suffer needlessly. She was dying; what would it matter if she became addicted to the medication? The important lesson here is that caregivers must examine their own attitudes toward the use of pain medication and not let them affect the way they administer it to patients.

Summary

Pain is an unrelenting fact of human life. Although nearly all people experience pain sensations similarly, there are vast cultural differences in the expression of pain. Some cultures encourage the open expression of pain, while others socialize their members to be stoic. Although it is helpful at times to know these generalizations, inaccurate stereotyping can seriously compromise a patient's life. Treat each patient as an individual. The family can also be helpful in letting you know if the patient's behavior is typical or abnormal.

     With regard to pain medication, it is often best to anticipate a patient's pain needs, since cultural or religious reasons may inhibit a patient from requesting pain medication even when it is medically necessary for recovery. Also realize that not every patient will share a desire for the least intrusive medication possible. When alternatives are available, it is best to check with the patient; which form would he or she prefer?

Key Points

- Culture influences whether a patient will be stoic or expressive in response to pain.
- Do not base your assessment of pain on the patient's expression of pain.
- Anticipate a patient's pain needs; do not wait for him or her to request pain medication, because cultural factors may inhibit them from asking.
- Address the patient's concerns regarding pain; for some it may be the pain sensation, for others, the meaning and significance of the pain.
- When alternate forms of pain medication are available, ask the patient what kind he or she would prefer.
- Address patient concerns about addiction and explain the importance of pain medication to healing.
- Give clear instructions on the use of pain medication and explain the reasoning for it.
- Examine your own biases and make sure they do not affect your response to patients in pain.

For labor pain, see Chapter 9.
For more on medication, see Chapter 12.

Chapter 4
Religion and Spirituality

Religion is rarely a topic of conversation in hospitals, but religious beliefs and spiritual practices are common sources of conflict and misunderstanding. Patients' exercise of their beliefs can result in amusing or even tragic interference with medical care. This chapter examines religious and spiritual beliefs that can create conflicts, misunderstandings, or worse. It also looks at several cases where a culturally competent approach on the part of health care providers made a positive difference for patients.

Religious Practices

Buddhist

64

A twenty-year-old Buddhist monk from Cambodia was in same-day surgery for a hernia repair, accompanied by his mother, aunt, and male cousin. When Lisa, his nurse, entered the room, she greeted him, put her hand on his shoulder, and directed him to a chair across the room. The patient suddenly jumped from her in horror. His mother and aunt lunged at Lisa, shouting at her in Cambodian. Lisa fled the room and called a "code gray," which summoned all male hospital personnel to the area.

When everyone arrived, the cousin was in the corner comforting the patient. Security questioned the patient, but he did not speak enough English to respond. His cousin explained that the patient was a monk and could not be touched by a woman. Should it happen, he was not to look at her, move, or respond in any way. Even a slight tensing of the muscles would be interpreted as showing desire and a breaking of his vows. Because of the incident, he would have to do great penance.

Sadly, this incident could have been avoided. Apparently, the need for strict sexual segregation had been thoroughly discussed with the physician prior to admission. The doctor assured them that there would be no problem. However, he neglected to convey this information to the staff. When questioned, the physician said he thought it would be amusing to see how everyone reacted. It was not. The hospital made arrangements to assure that thereafter the patient would have contact only with males, but the damage had already been done.

Catholic

Hilda Romero, an elderly Spanish-speaking Hispanic patient, was brought into the recovery room following a laparoscopic cholecystectomy. Rita, her nurse, was told Mrs. Romero had requested to be seen by a Catholic priest in the pre-op holding area, but they had been unable to accommodate her request due to time constraints. Rita thought that even though the surgery was over, she should still try to fulfill her patient's request. She called the chaplain's office and asked for a Spanish-speaking priest to come to the recovery room. When the priest arrived, Rita drew her curtains for privacy. Mrs. Romero and the priest spoke a while, and he said a prayer. When Mrs. Romero told her family what Rita had done, they all thanked her profusely. Later that week, Mrs. Romero and her family sent Rita a touching thank-you note and a box of chocolates (which she shared with the staff). Rita then realized the impact that a simple call to a priest had had for the patient.

65

Christian Scientist

Betty Williams, a sixty-five-year-old Anglo American woman, came to see a physician specializing in diseases of the colon and rectum. Although Christian Scientists generally take a spiritual rather than physical approach to healing, utilizing their own practitioners, they are allowed to see a physician, and Mrs. Williams made that choice when she began experiencing rectal pain. She was diagnosed with a rectal tumor. The physician, Dr. James, recommended surgery. She refused, despite the fact that it was a resectable tumor and there was no apparent spread. Dr. James saw her over the next six years. In that time, the tumor grew. Mrs. Williams began to experience bleeding and discomfort. She finally agreed to a colonoscopy, but not to a resection of the tumor. Dr. James operated on her. She was "clean" inside. The tumor had not metastasized. If she had allowed the surgeon to resect the tumor, she would have been cured of colon cancer. But her religious beliefs did not allow her to go that far. She would only allow palliative intervention. She died two years later, after the tumor did metastasize. I spoke with one of Dr. James's partners and asked how the physicians felt about the situation. "Sad," he replied. They could have saved her, but she chose another path. In this case, the physicians acted with cultural competence. Although Mrs. Williams's actions conflicted with their own beliefs, they accepted her decisions, and did what they could to help her while staying within the bounds of her beliefs.

66

This case is also interesting as an illustration of the range of beliefs within a religion. One of the basic tenets of the Christian Science Church is that God's creation of man and the universe is perfect. Disease is thus a "misunderstanding." Further, all reality is thought to be ultimately mental/spiritual, not material/physical. Illness, therefore, is of mental, not physical origin and can be cured through proper mental processes. Treatment consists of prayer and counsel with the sick person, and involves three phases. In the first phase, the practitioner tries to remove the sick person's belief in suffering; in the second, the practitioner tries to convince the patient that he or she is well and knows it; in the final phase, the practitioner focuses on his or her own thoughts to free the afflicted person of his belief in sickness. Due to their beliefs, Christian Scientists will rarely seek out medical care. They have seen the effectiveness of spiritual healing. Yet, as in this case, they are free to choose medical intervention. Mrs. Williams even agreed to a colostomy, but drew the line at surgery to remove her tumor, a decision that ultimately cost her her life but preserved her spiritual integrity. Presumably, Mrs. Williams sought the assistance of a Christian Science practitioner at the same time that she saw Dr. James. Dr. James's associate expressed some small surprise that her tumor went so long without metastasizing. Perhaps spiritual healing kept it at bay.

Indian Orthodox Christian

The following case study is not one that will be experienced frequently, but it contains many interesting aspects.

67   His Holiness, the spiritual leader of an Indian Orthodox Christian church, became a patient in an American hospital when he fell ill during a visit to an American diocese. His condition required cardiac catheterization and open-heart surgery. Because it was determined that despite the extraordinary precautions taken his body had become contaminated during the first procedure, there was a ten-day delay during which he had to undergo a purification ceremony before he could have open-heart surgery.

How had he become contaminated? First of all, the surgical team members had allowed non-Orthodox Christians do the electrocardiogram and blood withdrawal and to shave the groin on His Holiness. Second, priests and bishops within this church must avoid exposing their bodies to any female in order to maintain purity. Although there were no female members directly caring for His Holiness, the director of the catheterization laboratory was a female. Even though she was in the back room, operating the x-ray machines, this was a breach of sexual segregation: His Holiness's private parts had been exposed to a woman.

Although he had not received any food prior to surgery—as is common when anesthesia is used—the medical team allowed him to receive

Holy Communion the morning of his heart catheterization. Unfortunately, this led to a cardinal sin. After surgery, His Holiness vomited and the medical team discarded the emesis. The bread and wine of Holy Communion are the blood and body of Jesus Christ; when he vomited, His Holiness was in essence vomiting Christ. The hospital staff should have saved the emesis to be drunk by the priests and bishops there to take care of His Holiness. Drinking the emesis is considered a very holy act that will wash away one's sins.

The cardiologist in charge of the surgery, himself a member of the church, was held responsible for the breaches of purity. He has been socially isolated from the church as a result. His Holiness's party members, also complicit in the contamination, have probably been banished to remote church monasteries simply because a highly qualified woman was allowed to work the x-ray equipment in the back room and because the hospital staff discarded some vomit.

Although routine sexual segregation is a common practice in many cultures, it is important for health care providers to realize that in some religious contexts it is not just a preference but a mandate. If that rule is to be violated in any way—such as allowing a woman to work the x-ray equipment—this should be discussed beforehand. Had the cardiologist realized the strength of the church's requirements in the matter, he probably would not have had her at that job. Second, it would be a good idea to go over all possible complications (such as vomiting) to discuss any rules in that regard. Recognizing that rules for religious leaders may be much more stringent than those for others, and ascertaining them in advance, will avoid most of the problems.

Muslim

Maggie answered the call light and heard a panic-stricken voice saying, "Please come to my room. My neighbor collapsed on the floor and is lying there, muttering. I think he had a seizure." She ran to the room with the charge nurse and discovered Ali Saeed on the floor behind the curtain, praying. Mr. Saeed did not speak English, and his bilingual son had left the room. When Mr. Saeed knelt on the floor to pray, his neighbor had no idea what he was doing and no way to ask. Concerned, he summoned the nurse with the call light.

Devout Muslims believe they must pray facing toward Mecca, the Holy city, five times a day. They pray on the floor, with their forehead on the ground to show submission to Allah (God). Traditionally, they pray on a prayer rug placed on the floor. Though most Muslims in the United States use prayer rugs only in the privacy of their homes, devout Muslims in the Middle East may take them when they travel. Because Mr. Saeed was scheduled for surgery the next day, he thought it was especially important to pray. Culturally sensitive health care providers will learn upon admission about such practices and arrange for privacy during those times. Some culturally sensitive hospitals provide prayer rugs for their Muslim patients (see Chapter 13).

Jehovah's Witness

Most people are aware of the Jehovah's Witness prohibition about accepting blood transfusions. They believe that blood represents life and is therefore sacred. They base this belief upon several sections of the Bible, including Leviticus 17:10: "Whatsoever man . . . eateth any manner of blood; I will . . . cut him off from among his people"; Leviticus 17:11: "For the life of the flesh is in the blood"; and Acts 15:20: "Abstain from . . . things strangled and from blood." They have no problems accepting any other form of medical treatment, and will use non-blood expanders. Blood is the only medical issue, as in the following case.

69   Susi Givens, a thirty-seven-year-old woman with two children, was horseback riding one day when a snake startled her horse. She was thrown off and landed on a stump, resulting in massive internal injuries. She was rushed to the hospital, where the surgical team discovered that there was a large amount of blood in her abdomen and that she needed to have a kidney removed.

Mrs. Givens had a medical alert card identifying her as a Jehovah's Witness and stating that under no circumstances was she to receive blood. Her physician knew this but felt impelled by his oath to save lives to give her a blood transfusion. The hospital was unable to locate her husband, so the physician decided to transfuse her.

His actions saved her life; however, she was not grateful. She sued her doctor for assault and battery and won a $20,000 settlement. She was a competent adult and had made a decision that her physician chose to ignore. In a study done of Jehovah's Witnesses in the 1980s, two-thirds of those polled said they would sue if transfused against their will. Many feel that this is the only way that others will be protected and have their beliefs taken seriously. A physician in a position like that of Dr. Andrews should realize the possible ramifications (including legal ones) of violating the patient's express wishes in order to fulfill his own beliefs (Hippocratic oath) and make a conscious, fully informed decision.

70   Sometimes a Jehovah's Witness will reconsider at the last minute. For example, a twenty-seven-year-old woman who began bleeding heavily several days after giving birth required a hysterectomy. After the operation, she urgently needed blood but refused it. Two days later, when she developed

acute respiratory distress and had to be placed on a respirator, she agreed to the blood transfusion. It saved her life.

Many health care professionals have strong moral difficulty in respecting the Jehovah's Witness position. The conflict lies in two areas: values and worldview. Jehovah's Witnesses believe that, when Armageddon comes, 144,000 of those who have followed God's laws will rise from the dead to spend eternity in heaven. Those who have followed God's laws but do not go to heaven will spend eternity in a paradise on earth. All those who have violated God's laws (e.g., had a blood transfusion, placed themselves above God by celebrating their own birthdays, or worshipped idols by saluting the American flag) are doomed to spend eternity in nothingness.

Suppose for a moment that they are correct. Choosing to have a blood transfusion can be interpreted as giving up the chance to spend eternity in heaven or paradise in exchange for a few more years on earth. In this scenario, it is not very rational to have a blood transfusion. Few health care professionals are Jehovah's Witnesses. They do not believe that the fate of their soul rests on whether they have a blood transfusion. Thus the worldview of Jehovah's Witness patients comes into direct conflict with that of most health care professionals.

Most health care professionals value the life of the physical body. In refusing blood, the Jehovah's Witness is valuing the life of the soul over that of the physical body. The question is, does any group have the right to impose its values and beliefs on others? Can we be so arrogant and ethnocentric as to be sure we are right and they are wrong?

The issue is most difficult when children are involved. Do their parents have the right to choose for them? This question is not easily answered. In an extreme case, parents abandoned their child after he had been given a blood transfusion under court order.

Finally, there are social issues. If an individual who is a member of a very tightly knit conservative group of Jehovah's Witnesses accepts blood, the act might, for some, lead to rejection by his or her entire social network. A few more years of life may not be worth that price.

Why do some members change their mind and accept blood at the last minute? Obviously, not all members of a religion are equally devout. Many people have doubts about their beliefs. When it is a matter of life and death, faith is often not strong enough to dictate the giving up of life.

Dealing with a Jehovah's Witness patient can be very difficult if the need for a blood transfusion arises. Doctors and nurses often feel helpless and frustrated. They value life so strongly that they find it hard to understand why some people willingly choose to give it up. They should try to see the situation from the emic perspective and consider the possibility that the Jehovah's Witnesses are right. They should also acknowledge the role Jehovah's Witnesses have played in the pioneering of bloodless surgeries.

Jewish

71   Jews also have blood beliefs, in their case with implications for burial, as outlined in the following case study. The incident involved Sarah Weinberg, a four-year-old Jewish girl who was hit by a car and sustained fatal injuries. A paramedic team rushed Sarah to the hospital emergency room, after performing several resuscitation attempts en route. She was still alive when they reached the hospital, but died on the operating table. When Mr. Weinberg was notified of his daughter's death, he approached Robert, one of the nurses who worked on her. Mr. Weinberg accepted Robert's condolences and then asked him for his scrubs. Robert did not understand the request; why would the bereaved father want his clothing? Mr. Weinberg explained that, according to Jewish tradition, the individual must be buried whole. Since Sara's blood was on Robert's scrubs, they had to be buried with her. Although Robert was unfamiliar with this custom, he immediately complied. Fortunately, this case was easily resolved.

72   Another case involving the death of a Jewish patient was also resolved due to the cultural competence of the nurse. Matthew Goldstein, the son of an Orthodox Jewish man, requested that he stay with the body of his deceased father until the mortuary came to pick the body up. According to Reyna, the nurse, hospital policy does not allow that, because it sometimes takes hours for the mortuary service to arrive and hospital beds are in great demand. However, because Reyna was taking a class in cultural competence at the time, she was especially sensitive to meeting Mr. Goldstein's needs. Therefore, she arranged for his father's body to be moved into a little-used and secluded area so he could stay with him until the mortuary arrived the next morning. Reyna reported that she felt very good about being able to accommodate him. "It required very little work on my part and the family was allowed to grieve in the manner they wished."

It is a Jewish custom that the body of the deceased is not to be left unattended. To do so is a sign of disrespect. The custom evolved from early times, in which people went to great lengths to guard the deceased from ghosts and spirits.

73   Every religion has days that are considered holy and on which behavior is often strictly proscribed. Sol Meyers, an Orthodox Jew, created a problem for the nursing staff when he tried to observe the Sabbath. Mr. Meyers brought his wife to the hospital in active labor at 8 P.M. on a Friday. When she gave birth at midnight, the nurses suggested that Mr. Meyers accompany her to the postpartum unit and then return home to rest. He thanked them but explained that he could not drive home because it was the Sabbath. The nurses understood and arranged for him to stay in his wife's room.

In the morning, Mr. Meyers asked the nurses for breakfast. They explained that the hospital provided food only for patients; he would have to buy his breakfast in the dining room. When Mr. Meyers told them he was forbidden to ride in an elevator or handle money, one of the nurses offered to get him food. But Mr. Meyers had no money with him. Frustrated, the nurses finally ordered extra food for his wife to share with him. At lunch, Mr. Meyers once again requested food. This time the nurses suggested that he call a friend or relative to pick him up. Mr. Meyers replied that he could not use the phone on the Sabbath, and even if he made a call, no one would answer because all his friends and relatives were Orthodox. By this time, the nurses were losing patience. If Mr. Meyers could drive to the hospital, why couldn't he drive home? If he knew he would have to stay at the hospital, why had he not brought food with him?

The answers can be found in the Torah. One of the most important laws of the Torah states that Orthodox Jews must observe the Sabbath. It is a time to be with one's family and to worship God. The Sabbath begins at sundown Friday and ends at sundown Saturday. During this time, work of any kind is prohibited, including driving, using the telephone, handling money, and even pushing an elevator button. (A large Jewish hospital in Los Angeles features a few elevators that automatically stop on every floor on Saturday.)

The only law higher than the law of the Sabbath is the law that demands one do everything possible to save a life. Mr. Meyers could drive his wife to the hospital on the Sabbath because her life and that of their child were at stake. He could not drive home, however, because a life was not threatened. Mr. Meyers did not bring food with him because it is forbidden to travel with food on the Sabbath (unless it is milk for a baby). Very little else could have been done in this situation other than to charge extra food to the patient's bill.

Sikh

Raj Singh, a seventy-two-year-old Sikh from India, had been admitted to   74
the hospital after a heart attack. He was scheduled for a heart catheterization to determine the extent of the blockage in his coronary arteries. The procedure involved running a catheter up the femoral artery, located in the groin, and then passing it into his heart where special x-rays could be taken. His son was a cardiologist on staff and had explained the procedure to him in detail.

Susan, his nurse, entered Mr. Singh's room and explained that she had to shave his groin to prevent infection from the catheterization. As she pulled the razor from her pocket, she was suddenly confronted with the sight of shining metal flashing in front of her. Mr. Singh had a short sword in his hand and was waving it at her as he spoke excitedly in his native tongue. Susan got the message. She would not shave his groin.

She put away her "weapon," and he did the same. Susan, thinking the problem was that she was a woman, said she would get a male orderly to shave him. Mr. Singh's eyes lit up again as he angrily yelled, "No shaving of hair by anyone!"

Susan managed to calm him down by agreeing. She then called her supervisor and the attending physician to report the incident. The physician said he would do the procedure on an unshaved groin. At that moment, Mr. Singh's son stopped by. When he heard what had happened, he apologized profusely for not explaining his father's Orthodox Sikh customs.

The Sikh religion forbids cutting or shaving any body hair. Orthodox Sikhs always carry a dagger with them, lest someone try to force them to do something against their religion, as Susan had. The dagger is considered one of the five "outer badges." The others are wearing hair and beard unshorn; wearing a turban; wearing knee-length pants; and wearing a steel bracelet on the right wrist. These badges reflect the Sikhs' military history.

Many of the procedures medical professionals consider necessary are not. Shaving to reduce the risk of serious infection, for example, *may* be valid, but there do not appear to be any good studies to support this. Even if there *is* evidence to support decreased infection risk with shaving, the patient could be presented with the statistics and allowed to decide whether or not to take the additional risk. Evidence-based medicine has become increasingly important in recent years. Physicians should make every effort not to impose their own theoretical concerns (such as the belief that shaving reduces the risk of infection) upon patients, and to let patients make the informed choice to take risks when the medical evidence conflicts with their beliefs.

75   In a similar situation, Griselda avoided a potential problem when she had to shave a Sikh child to prep him for an appendectomy. Knowing that traditional Sikh religion forbids cutting or shaving hair, she took the time to explain to the patient and her mother that only the surgical site would be shaved, and explained that the purpose was to create a sterile field free of germs and microorganisms that could cause an infection. In this case, the family chose to allow the child to be shaved, and any potential problems were avoided.

Sacred Symbols

Catholic

76   Religious and spiritual symbols are not always obvious to members of other religions; this can lead to problems. However, culturally competent

health care personnel can truly make a difference. It was a set of rosary beads that offered Ariadne the opportunity to demonstrate cultural sensitivity and flexibility. Celia Montes, an elderly Latino patient, asked that she be able to wear her rosary beads into surgery. Her request was denied. When Ariadne later spoke to her about it, Celia was distraught. She explained that the beads would bring strength to the surgeons and protect her during the surgery. She was afraid to have the surgery without them. Understanding how important they were to her, Ariadne spoke to the charge nurse in the OR. The charge nurse was hesitant to accommodate her request, explaining that the policy existed because too many things had been lost during surgery; if they didn't allow personal effects into surgery, nothing could get lost. Ariadne assured the OR nurse that she would label the beads, and again, emphasized their importance to the patient. The OR nurse finally relented. When Ariadne told Mrs. Montes that she would be allowed to wear the rosary beads into surgery, her relief and gratitude were palpable. Policies often exist for the convenience of the hospital and staff, but accommodating the needs of the patients should be primary.

Disrespect for the Catholic scapular caused another family to request   77
a transfer to another hospital. Mrs. Arogetti, an elderly Italian woman, was wearing a scapular attached to her hospital gown. When the gown became soiled, it was thrown into the laundry without removing Mrs. Arogetti's scapular, which was then lost. Mrs. Arogetti's relationship with the nurse and hospital might have survived the incident, had the nurse bothered to apologize to Mrs. Arogetti. However, she did not. By discounting the patient's symbol of hope, the nurse caused the family to lose faith in the health care team's ability to help Mrs. Arogetti. Due to this loss of trust, the family requested she be transferred to another hospital. The situation could have been avoided by paying more careful attention to Mrs. Arogetti's religious symbol. It could have later been recovered with a sincere apology that acknowledged the importance of the symbol. Unfortunately, neither was done.

Silvia made a positive difference for a Mexican patient named Juan   78
Robles. Prior to being assigned to him, he was having conflicts with several of the nurses over the religious statues he kept in his room. One of the nurses told him point blank that he had to get rid of the statues because they were in the way and were interfering with his treatment. He was very upset and angry over this. Silvia took the time to sit down with Mr. Robles, and ask him about the importance of the statues to him. He explained that he was Catholic and that the images of the saints would help in his healing. Seeing how important they were to him, Silvia raised the issue at a staff meeting. She suggested that they change their unofficial policy and allow patients to keep statues in the room. The initial response to her

suggestion was quite negative. But Silvia persisted, emphasizing how important they were to patient comfort. She then suggested that the nurses tell the patients that they would have to move them while they were working with the patient, but would return them to their place once they finished. They agreed to this. It made for a little more work for the nurses but greatly increased the comfort of patients like Juan Robles.

79   Sacred symbols for people of one religion can cause problems for people of other religions. Mrs. Rao Chean, a seventy-two-year-old Cambodian woman, was admitted to a Catholic hospital following a motor vehicle accident. Amanda, her nurse, found her unresponsive during the assessment. She noted that Mrs. Rao kept staring at the wall. She assumed it was due to the shock of the accident. Amanda turned to Mrs. Rao's daughter to request that she ask her mother how she was feeling. The daughter then asked Amanda to please remove the crucifix from the wall, because it was bothering her mother. Mrs. Rao was a Buddhist. Amanda quickly removed the crucifix and put the Bible in the bottom drawer. As a result, Mrs. Rao appeared to relax and became more talkative. When Amanda later asked her about the crucifix, she felt it made her feel she was being proselytized to worship a God she does not recognize.

Mormon (Church of Jesus Christ of Latter Day Saints)

80   Grace Kettering, a Mormon woman, was admitted to the hospital for facial surgery. Before entering the operating room, she was told to remove all her clothes except the hospital gown. She refused to remove her long underwear, and the surgeon refused to operate unless she did.

Very devout Mormons who have attained adult religious status in the church wear "the garment." It resembles short-sleeved long underwear and ends just above the knee. Although not exactly magical, it is considered sacred and is generally worn except when it is being cleaned or while one is bathing, swimming, or exercising. Although most Mormon patients will have no trouble removing it for exams or procedures, having to remove the garment associated with God's protection might be very distressing for some, as it was for Mrs. Kettering.

Eventually, Mrs. Kettering's surgeon relented. In such cases, an understanding attitude and a discussion of the options beforehand are advisable. For example, the lower half of the garment could be pulled down to the patient's ankles in the event of abdominal surgery.

Native American

81   Abby, a nurse who worked at a hospital close to the Hoopa Indian reservation in Northern California, told of an elderly Native American man

in intensive care. His granddaughter brought in an object consisting of a circular frame with feathers hanging from it. The object fits the description of a "soul catcher." She asked if she could hang it on the wall. Fortunately, Abby was quite understanding and hung it from the intravenous hook above the patient's bed instead. The granddaughter was both relieved and grateful. It was a small concession on the part of the nurse but provided tremendous psychological comfort for the patient and his family.

Cambodian

A Cambodian infant was brought into the hospital diagnosed with dehydration 5 percent. Mona, the nurse, examined the child's extremities, looking for a vein in which to start an intravenous line. She found one on the baby's arm. At that point, she noticed several strands of dark brown strings, about one-half inch wide, on both wrists. Mona prepared to cut the strings with scissors. Mrs. Tep, the baby's mother, walked in at that moment, looked horrified at what Mona was about to do, and began speaking loudly in her native tongue. Mona assumed she was upset because the infant was crying. But Mrs. Tep kept pointing to the strings; it was obvious that she did not want them cut. Mona did not understand what the problem was, but communicated through gestures that she would not cut the strings.

She then started an intravenous line in the infant's scalp. When the baby's parents saw this, the mother began to cry. While it is distressing for any parent to see intravenous lines put into a sick child's scalp, for many Southeast Asians, it is especially traumatic. As the Teps explained through an interpreter, the head is thought to be the seat of life. By introducing holes into it, the nurse had made an easy exit for the child's soul.

What was the problem with the strings? They are known as *baci*. It is a tradition believed to have originated with the Lao culture, but is practiced by the Mien and Cambodians as well. The strings are tied around a person's wrists at important occasions—birthdays, promotions, weddings, and so forth. They are believed to "tie in the soul" so it doesn't get lost. They should never be cut off; they simply wear off in time. If Mona had cut the strings, she would have jeopardized the infant's life from the Tepses' perspective.

Hindu

Fortunately for Arden Patel, Carrie Ann was taking a course in cultural competence when she he was assigned to her. Mr. Patel, a Hindu patient from India, was dying, and in the process, becoming extremely bloated. His abdomen was distended and he was suffering from severe edema in

82

83

his arms. A Filipino nursing assistant was about to remove a string tied around Mr. Patel's wrist because it was cutting off his circulation. Carrie Ann stopped him, and asked him to wait until the patient's daughter arrived. She knew that Hindus sometimes wore sacred threads around their necks or arms, and felt that since the patient was near death in any case, cutting it off without permission might be more harmful than leaving it on. When Mr. Patel's daughter arrived, Carrie Ann explained her concerns. His daughter agreed to allow the strings to be cut, and thanked Carrie Ann for her sensitivity.

A general rule of thumb is to assume that a patient who is wearing anything that looks unusual may be doing so for religious or spiritual reasons. Hindus may wear sacred threads around their necks or arms; Native Americans may carry medicine bundles; Mexican children may wear a bit of red ribbon; Mediterranean peoples may wear a special charm on a chain, such as a mustard seed in a blue circle or a ram's horn, to ward off the evil eye. If an item must be removed to perform a medical procedure, the reason should be explained to the patient and the family. The item should be removed gently and respectfully and kept in contact with the patient's body if possible.

Spiritual Beliefs and Practices

For many people, spirituality is an integral part of their life. Spiritual needs become even more important when people are ill, but these needs are often either ignored or receive low priority from health care professionals. This can create even greater distress for patients who are already stressed from trying to cope with illness, as the next case illustrates.

84   Marietta Amador, a Filipino woman and nurse, felt she was a "victim of cultural ignorance" when her six-week-old daughter Emilita fell ill with sepsis. Emilita was hospitalized for ten days so she could receive massive doses of antibiotics. Fearing that her child would not survive, Marietta asked the nurse to send a chaplain or other religious person to bless or baptize her daughter. She waited for three days, completely distraught, until the nurse sent someone. Marietta had very strong religious values, and spiritual healing was very important to her. Nurses should make every effort to meet patients' spiritual needs as well as their physical needs in a timely manner.

Prayer

85   A seventy-five-year-old African American woman named Agnes Jones was in the hospital recovering from a heart attack. Mrs. Jones was very religious and spent most of her time praying. Her "brothers and sisters" from

the church visited daily, and she appeared closer to them than to members of her family.

During her hospital stay, Mrs. Jones consented to only the procedures and medications she believed were ordered by God because, according to her worldview, only God could make her well. While the nurses bathed Mrs. Jones, she preached to them about Jesus. Before too long, the hospital staff began to avoid her.

For many African Americans, religion is an essential and integral part of life. God is viewed as the source of both good health and serious illness. God can cure any disease, but to be cured one must pray and have faith. This worldview, like all effective ones, is internally consistent: if a patient is not cured, it is not because God failed but because the patient lacked sufficient faith.

The hospital personnel did not handle Mrs. Jones's case well. Rather than avoiding her, they should have had a team conference to discuss her beliefs and perhaps have invited a minister from her church to attend. The minister might have convinced Mrs. Jones to be more cooperative, and the staff might have learned to be more understanding and tolerant of her beliefs.

An excellent example of how to handle this kind of situation is one involving a diabetic Hispanic woman named Elena Montoya who had stopped taking her medication because she was told by a traditional healer that God had taken away her diabetes. She returned to her physician when her symptoms—excessive thirst and frequent urination—returned, but she was reluctant to go back on her medication. The wise health care practitioner, rather than contradict her, suggested that God might have taken away her diabetes for a while, but that it had returned and perhaps He had brought her to the doctor so that she could treat it with medicine. He encouraged her to continue to pray, but got her to agree to allow him to monitor her condition before stopping her medication again.

Karine's sensitivity and flexibility led to a very positive colonoscopy experience for Laura de la Cruz, an elderly Mexican patient, and her family. When she came in for a pre-procedure assessment, accompanied by13 family members, Mrs. de la Cruz's son commented that the outcome of the procedure "was in God's hands" and requested that they be allowed to pray before their mother's procedure. Although this was not normal procedure, Karine recognized the importance of this family's religious beliefs, and allowed them to pray together in private before the colonoscopy. The family was effusive in their gratitude, and shared that their previous requests to pray had always been denied by health care staff. It took very little to make the experience a much more positive one for both the patient and her family.

86

87

Evil Spirits

88 Lhee Pha, a sixteen-year-old Hmong girl, was brought to the emergency department with abdominal pain. She was diagnosed with appendicitis, and it was determined that surgery was necessary. Her father, however, refused to allow the surgery. Within a few days, her appendix ruptured, and she became septic and died. Linda, her nurse, was very frustrated by the situation. Lhee could have easily been saved had her father allowed her to have surgery. Several days later, Lhee's sister came in to the emergency department on another matter. She thanked Linda for the care she had provided for her sister. Linda asked her if there were anything they could have done differently, or anything they could have said to make Lhee's parents see how serious the situation was, and how necessary the surgery. Lhee's sister explained that her parents knew that Lhee might die without surgery, but they did not want to risk her living with an evil spirit. Linda learned that they believed that not only could an incision create an opening for her soul to leave, but it could also create an opening for an evil spirit to enter. Her parents did not want to risk this, even if it meant their daughter's death. Lhee's sister said her family thought the hospital staff had handled the situation well, and were grateful that they had made an exception to visiting rules and allowed all thirty members of her extended family to be in the room with Lhee as she died. Sometimes, cultural competence involves truly accepting other peoples' beliefs, even when they contradict the highest value of medicine—saving life.

Soul Loss

89 Melissa was working in a busy pediatric intensive care unit the day she inadvertently jeopardized Jimmy Hosea's life. Jimmy was a twelve-year-old Navajo post-op patient. The day he transferred into Melissa's unit, the staff had just been given a new Polaroid camera. She gathered together Jimmy and two other children for a photo. Because her attention was on the two others, who happily mugged for the camera, Melissa never noticed the look of horror on Jimmy's face until she saw the photo. He had disappeared while it was developing.

When Melissa found him, Jimmy was sitting on the edge of his bed, gazing at the floor and looking as though he were ready to die. When she asked him what had happened, he carefully responded, "I've lost my soul." Melissa had no idea what he was talking about. He explained that pictures took the soul out of the face captured on the photograph. Melissa was astounded. How could he believe that?

She told him how sorry she was and offered him the photograph. He took it, saying that his family could help him get his soul back with a "sing," a religious ceremony.

This case is a good example of how important it is to know about the spiritual beliefs of those for whom you are caring. Although it is obviously unrealistic to expect to know everything about every culture, just having an awareness that your patients' beliefs may be different from your own may help you to be more sensitive and aware. Melissa certainly is.

Blood Beliefs

Another case related to the issue of soul loss involves Mien beliefs and attitudes regarding blood. Saelee Mui Chua, a forty-two-year-old Mien man, arrived at the clinic with his twelve-year-old son, who acted as interpreter. The son explained that his father had seen a traditional healer the previous week, but the healer had been unable to cure his father's symptoms: weakness, fatigue, increased urination, and thirst. The symptoms suggested diabetes to the physician, and he ordered a blood glucose test. When Shawnee, the nurse, came to draw the blood, Mr. Saelee fearfully yelled, "No!" His son told Shawnee that his father refused to have his blood drawn. When she asked for an explanation, all he would say is, "My father does not want the test."

The staff assumed that Mr. Saelee was afraid of the needle. However, it is more likely that he was concerned about having his blood drawn. There is a Mien legend about an evil bird that brought bad fortune and death by drinking a person's blood. This is probably connected to the Mien belief that losing blood saps strength (Mr. Saelee was already feeling weak) and may result in the soul leaving the body.

The staff tried to "educate" Mr. Saelee about the procedure of drawing blood, and explained its importance in diagnosing his symptoms, but their efforts were to no avail. He would not give his permission for the procedure and simply left the hospital.

What could have been done? Although there are no guarantees that any intervention could have changed Mr. Saelee's mind, they might have explained that the amount of blood needed was extremely small, and that new blood would be made to replace it. If possible, perhaps the traditional healer could have been involved in the procedure. They might have also spent more time explaining why the tests were so necessary. The connection between his symptoms and his blood is not immediately obvious. The following case study illustrates a more culturally competent approach.

When Leslie admitted a seventy-eight-year-old Cambodian woman who had just suffered a myocardial infarction, she realized that the blood sample she was going to have to draw prior to cardiac catheterization could be traumatic for her patient. She therefore took the time to explain to the woman's daughter why it was necessary to draw blood, and assured her she would take the minimum amount necessary. The daughter then explained it to her mother, and stood by her side while the blood was drawn. The patient remained calm and cooperative. Although Leslie did not find out whether or not her patient shared traditional Cambodian blood beliefs, if she did, the short time it took to explain things may have saved her patient significant distress. And if she didn't, well, it is a good idea to provide patients with explanations in any case.

Blood beliefs are common throughout rural Southeast Asia. Some Hmong may not want blood drawn due to the beliefs that blood is a life force and the body has a limited amount of blood that it cannot replenish. Repeated blood sampling, especially from small children, may thus be thought to be fatal.

Summary

Although conflicting belief systems can be a source of frustration, confusion, and misunderstanding, most can be dealt with successfully. One must understand the patient's beliefs and be willing to respect them. When health care personnel work *with* the patient's beliefs, rather than against them, the outcomes are usually more successful, measured not only in patient satisfaction but also in ease for the medical team in managing the patient and family.

Key Points

- Honor patient requests for same-sex providers whenever possible.
- Provide clergy when requested.
- Respect your patients' religious beliefs, even when they conflict with your own.
- Realize that rules for religious leaders may be much more stringent than those for others. Ascertain them in advance to avoid problems.
- Allow patients privacy for prayer.
- Remember that individuals will vary in their degree of adherence to religious practices.
- Be aware that different religions have different holy days. It is Friday for Muslims, Saturday for Jews, and Sunday for Christians.
- Allow patients to make informed choices regarding risks when medical procedures conflict with their religious beliefs.
- Learn what symbols are sacred to those you treat, and respect them. They can provide tremendous psychological comfort to your patients. Do not cut or remove anything without first discussing it with the patient.
- Recognize that many Southeast Asian patients may have beliefs about blood that will make them reluctant to have it drawn. Ask their concerns and provide clear explanations for the need to draw blood.

Chapter 5
Activities of Daily Living and the Body

There are some basic activities that patients must perform each day, including eating, bathing, using the bathroom, and caring for their hair. Not surprisingly, these activities are influenced by culture and thus a potential source of conflict in the hospital. A second topic concerns the concept of body image. The ideal image varies considerably from culture to culture and may affect patients' attitudes toward specific treatments.

Eating

Dietary practices are an important issue for hospitals. Patients who do not eat are often a cause for concern for physicians and nurses. Is there a gastrointestinal problem? Is the patient suffering from depression? The food is bad, but not bad enough to explain it. The problem may in fact be a religious or cultural one. Issues around diet may also arise when families bring in traditional foods for patients, which may in fact be harmful to their condition. Knowledge of cultural differences in dietary rules and food preferences is essential in terms of both patient satisfaction and health.

Religious Restrictions

Islam prohibits eating from sunrise to sunset during the month of Ramadan. Judaism requires its members to fast from sundown to sundown during Yom Kippur, the Day of Atonement. Both restrict the eating of pork, and Judaism has other restrictions that will be discussed below. Hindus are forbidden to eat meat, as are Seventh Day Adventists. Although alcohol is not generally served in hospitals, dietary departments should be aware that the very devout members of religions that forbid it, including Muslims, Mormons, and Seventh Day Adventists, consider vanilla extract an alcohol. The latter two are also prohibited from caffeine. The body is seen as a gift from God or as a holy temple that should not be polluted by drugs or alcohol. Not every member of these religions will necessarily follow the food prohibitions, but it is important to ask.

Muslim: Ramadan

92   Mona Azula was an older Egyptian Muslim woman who came to Juliana's clinic for management of diabetes and hypertension. It was late November, the time of year when staff and patients brought in sweets and other foods in celebration of the holidays. Juliana said that she often walked around the clinic eating, and offering food to the patients. Because she was taking a class on cultural diversity, seeing Mrs. Azula reminded her it was Ramadan. She immediately apologized for eating in front of her during Ramadan. Juliana reported that this simple statement opened up a line of communication she had been trying to establish with the patient for the past six months. Mrs. Azula then began to talk to her about the spiritual and physical significance of fasting. Juliana learned that during the month of Ramadan, followers of Islam are forbidden to eat from sunrise to sunset in order to detach from material cravings and focus on the spiritual. It is thought to help the rich empathize with the suffering of the poor. Although for many Muslims, illness provides an exemption from the rules, they are obligated to make it up when they are in good health, a time when it will be more difficult because they will be doing it alone.

Through their discussion, Mrs. Azula became much more open about her concerns regarding her medical treatment. Although she was still taking her medications, she was fasting during daylight. She was suffering from cold sweats, fatigue, headaches, lightheadedness, and dizziness, along with anxiety and hand tremors. Juliana and Mrs. Azula then developed a treatment plan for the month of Ramadan that involved taking her diabetes medication only at dinnertime. Juliana went over the symptoms of hypoglycemia with her, and asked Mrs. Azula to let her know if she felt any better after adjusting the medications as they had discussed. Two days later, Mrs. Azula returned to the clinic to thank Juliana and tell her how much better she felt. This is an excellent example of how a little cultural competence—this time, in the form of some knowledge of an important religious holiday—led to greater trust and openness and resulted in the improved health of the patient.

93   It is important to remember that not all Muslim patients are from the Middle East. Juana had a patient from the Philippines who kept getting into conflicts with the Filipino nurses because she refused to eat during the day, would not take her medications at the assigned time, and kept requesting time for prayer. The nurses didn't take the time to ask her *why*; they merely grumbled about her noncompliance. It wasn't until Juana asked Emilita Jacinto why she wasn't eating that she explained she was

Muslim and it was Ramadan. Juana then notified the physician to change her diet and adjust her medications to fit her religious needs. Once Juana's coworkers understood the situation, they realized they had stereotyped Mrs. Jacinto as Catholic because she was from the Philippines, and viewed her simply as noncompliant. This case is instructive as a reminder to (1) avoid stereotyping; (2) ask about patients' religious practices upon admission; and (3) try to understand patients' behavior from their point of view. Noncompliance (or, rather, nonadherence) is often a result of cultural misunderstanding. The case is also a good example of cultural competence on the part of Juana.

Jewish: Kosher Dietary Practices

Why would a fifty-four-year-old man burst into tears when served meat, milk, and butter on the same lunch tray? What would cause an eighty-seven-year-old woman to refuse beef and chicken, even though she was not a vegetarian? Why would the mother of a two-year-old patient refuse to use the flatware provided and instead insist on plastic utensils? All these individuals are Orthodox Jews following the kosher dietary laws. These laws forbid eating pork and shellfish and nonkosher red meat and poultry. They also prohibit mixing meat and dairy products, either in the same meal or by using the same plates, pots, or utensils for both.

As with most cultural and religious laws, there is both a practical and an ideological basis for their origin. The overriding ideology behind the kosher laws is humaneness. The practical reasons are generally associated with health.

Shellfish are to be avoided because they are scavengers. They can pick up diseases and transmit them. Pork, if not properly cooked, can cause trichinosis. Furthermore, pigs require shade, water, and human food. In the desert environment it is not a good idea to raise animals that compete with humans for scarce resources. The last two points might explain why Muslims also forbid eating pork. An alternative explanation suggests that because pork and shellfish were dietary staples in the lands where the Jews lived at different points in their history, the prohibition was designed to prevent the Jews from assimilating. For meat to be considered kosher, animals must be killed with a single blow and not strangled. The pain and suffering an animal experiences between the first and final blows or during the time it takes to die from strangulation can stimulate the release of hormones detrimental to humans. Finally, a common supposition is that if meat and dairy products are combined, bits of meat may lodge in a wooden or pottery bowl, mix with the dairy products, and in the desert sun provide an ideal breeding ground for bacteria.

Again, the notion of humaneness underlies most of the kosher laws. One can get milk from a living cow or goat, eggs from a living chicken, and wool from a living sheep, but pigs are useful only when dead. To raise an animal strictly for slaughter is considered cruel and inhumane, as is mixing the meat of a calf with the milk of its mother. Finally, the most humane death is one that is instantaneous.

The practical reasons for most of the kosher laws no longer exist. Yet Orthodox Jews continue to uphold the traditions. The behavior of the patients described earlier becomes clear in light of these laws. All these situations can easily be avoided through knowledge of these kosher laws and the use of readily available frozen kosher meal trays and nonreusable paper plates and plastic utensils.

Hindu: The Sacred Cow

95   Christy, an Anglo nurse, took pity on an elderly man in the emergency room. He had been there for hours and appeared hungry. She went out of her way to get him a hamburger. When she gave it to him, his son, rather than appear grateful, was angry. His father was Hindu, and therefore forbidden to eat beef. She would have been wise to offer a few alternatives prior to getting him food.

Cultural Restrictions: Hot and Cold

96   Nonreligious food restrictions can also create problems. Mina Asami, a sixty-seven-year-old Pakistani woman, was hospitalized with tuberculosis. When Rachel, her nurse, noticed that Mrs. Asami's appetite was poor, she became concerned. Wanting to make sure her patient received enough protein, she made a concerted effort to feed her meat and potatoes with gravy. Mrs. Asami, however, was uncooperative, eating only fruit and Jello.

When Mrs. Asami's son Davi came to the hospital, he provided information that resolved the problem. Rachel, it appears, was trying to feed Mrs. Asami foods that Pakistanis normally avoid during the summer. Foods are either hot or cold. These are qualities, not temperatures. In the summer, Pakistanis avoid hot foods like beef because they "make our insides hot." In winter, they avoid cold foods that make their insides cold. Beef, pork, potatoes, and whiskey are all considered hot foods and are avoided in summer; in winter, Pakistanis refrain from eating cold foods such as chicken, fish, fruit, and beer. Once Rachel understood this, she ordered the appropriate foods for Mrs. Asami, who suddenly developed a much heartier appetite.

97   It is best to ask about food preferences during the admission interview or to arrange for a family member to bring food in for the patient. The latter approach was taken by the family of Chi-Wa Koo, a Chinese patient

with lung cancer. A complete Chinese kitchen was laid out on a hospital serving cart. Mr. Koo refused to eat anything prepared by the hospital, consuming only those items brought and prepared by his family.

Mr. Koo's family regarded his lung cancer as a *yin*, or cold, condition. To restore balance to his system, it was necessary to give him *yang* or hot foods. Without knowledge of *yin* and *yang*, it would be impossible for the hospital to serve Mr. Koo the appropriate foods. Furthermore, in China, the family traditionally supplies a patient's food. Fortunately, this incident occurred in a national medical center that is used to treating patients from all over the world. The staff willingly accommodated Mr. Koo's needs by allowing his family to bring in his food.

Adhering to the rules of hot and cold was compromising the condition of Juanita Palacio, a forty-nine-year-old Mexican woman with kidney failure and diabetes. She considered her kidney problem to be a "hot" condition that she treated with "cold" food and drinks. Unfortunately, many of the fruits, vegetables, and dairy products that she considered "cold" and thus good for her disease contained large amounts of phosphorus and potassium: dangerous for someone on dialysis. Rather than telling her not to eat these foods, an injunction that would have led to decreased trust and probably be ignored, the nurses emphasized eating large amounts of the "cold" foods that are lower in dangerous minerals, while eating small amounts of the foods that are high in them. They also made adjustments to her dialysis to remove these minerals and waste products from her blood more efficiently. And they frequently monitored her blood chemistry and medications. Although it made more work for the health care providers, the payoff was substantial. Juanita's condition became stable and she was able to follow her cultural traditions. This is an excellent example of cultural compromise.

Food Preferences

Each ethnic group has its own food preferences. Filipinos, for example, like rice with every meal and may feel deprived without it. They sometimes say it is a great comfort to eat rice when they feel ill. Japanese may prefer small amounts of beef or chicken, mixed with vegetables and rice or noodles. Food preferences should be ascertained when a patient is admitted and checked throughout hospitalization because they can have an important psychological effect. Simply discussing the daily menu with the patient can make a significant difference in the patient's attitude and recovery.

Mrs. Vu, a Vietnamese refugee in her late sixties, was brought to the hospital by her sponsor for observation. She was tired and losing weight. Her tests were all negative. The nurses tried to get Mrs. Vu to eat, but without success. Fortunately, a Vietnamese dietitian had recently been

98

99

hired. When consulted, she asked the nurses what kind of food they had offered Mrs. Vu. She had been given beefsteak, mashed potatoes, vegetables, cherry cobbler, milk, and coffee, then considered to be a healthy, well-balanced meal—for an American. Mrs. Vu had never eaten foods prepared in this way. When they gave her rice and vegetables stir-fried with beef, she ate everything on her plate, a simple solution to her dietary problem.

100   Pham Kim, the sixty-five-year-old Vietnamese refugee described in Chapter 2, was dehydrated and malnourished. She was receiving palliative care for cancer. She ate little and did not use the dietitian's recommended liquid supplement.

While interviewing the patient regarding her condition and health care practices, Martha, the home health nurse, learned that she was not taking the dietary supplement the dietitian had recommended. Martha realized that it was in the form of a sweet-tasting shake, agreeable to the Western palate but not to her client. She spoke with the dietitian and obtained a nonsweet substitute, which the client found much more to her liking. She said the taste was similar to that of rice-water. It is important to realize that people of different cultures prefer different "tastes"; nonadherence may simply be a result of unpalatable flavors.

Another kind of dietary problem may result from the intersection of food preferences and belief systems, as illustrated in the following case.

101   An Anglo nurse working in Saudi Arabia encountered a potentially life-threatening dietary problem involving many of her hemodialysis patients. Dates, a favorite food of many Arabs, are very high in potassium, which must be strictly limited in someone suffering from kidney failure. The nurse could not always find an interpreter to explain the situation clearly and convincingly to patients. The situation was further complicated, first, because in Saudi Arabia, food deprivation is considered a precursor to illness. From an Arab's perspective, the nurses were helping to bring on illness by depriving patients of dates. Second, dates are considered a special food by many Muslims. It is the first food generally eaten to break their fast during Ramadan, and was one of the Prophet Mohammad's favorite foods. Finally, Muslims believe that Allah (God) is all-powerful. Neither dates nor potassium would influence their health; rather, it was God's will. If Allah meant them to die, so be it. If not, they would survive. Beyond patient teaching, there is little one can do in such a situation.

Dietary Problems

LACTOSE INTOLERANCE

Some ethnic groups cannot tolerate certain foods. According to some studies, most adult Asians, Africans, African Americans, and Native Americans are lactose intolerant, and milk products give them gas and diarrhea. Calcium needs should be considered, however, in planning meals for pregnant women, whether in the hospital or at home. Calcium supplements may be necessary. Other foods such as tofu, collard greens, bok choy, and sardines, all of which are high in calcium, should be emphasized. Hispanics generally consider pregnancy a hot condition. Protein-rich foods, which are also usually hot, may be avoided during pregnancy to maintain body balance. Physicians should take special care to make sure such women receive adequate protein.

ETHNIC DIETS

Typical ethnic diets must also be taken into account when discharging patients with special dietary requirements. Asian diets are generally very high in sodium but low in fats. Mexican Americans tend to use a lot of salt and fats in their cooking. These cooking styles could prove problematic for hypertensive patients. It may be unrealistic to expect someone to change cooking and eating styles completely. Teaching sessions or adjustment of medications may be necessary. The family cook should be included in all discussions. Fortunately, there are many cookbooks today that adapt traditional recipes to the needs of diabetic and hypertensive patients. Hospitals should keep some of these cookbooks on hand to help with patient teaching.

It is common for nurses to educate patients and family on what foods   *102*
interact with the medications prescribed for them. However, as Libby realized when taking a class on cultural diversity, the kinds of foods she usually covered were probably not the ones her patients were eating. She gave the example of Pepe Acab, a Filipino patient who was being discharged on coumadin, a blood thinner, to prevent clotting. Vitamin K reverses the effect of the drug and must be avoided. Normally, Libby would tell such patients to avoid foods like liver, broccoli, brussels sprouts, spinach, Swiss chard, coriander, collards, cabbage, and any green, leafy vegetables. She suddenly realized, however, that there might be other foods he should avoid. She spoke with Mr. Acab and his wife, and got a list of foods he commonly ate. She then did some research and discovered that two foods on the list—soybeans and fish liver oils—are very high in Vitamin K. She was then able to educate him properly on what to avoid. There is an important lesson here—you must find out what the patient normally eats before you can give appropriate advice on dietary issues.

Bathing

Niki's eyes rolled when she saw her patient, Mr. Johnson. "Another street   103
person," she thought. It wasn't that she had anything against the homeless;

the problem was that they just didn't like to bathe. As a nurse, she thought cleanliness was next to godliness. Sure enough, when she tried to bathe Mr. Johnson, he became visibly upset. "No, no." When she asked him why, he explained that the layer of dirt would help to protect him from illness.

Although this belief is in direct contradiction with Western medicine, it is easy to see why it would be adaptive for people living on the street to develop a belief that is consistent with their circumstances—specifically, greatly reduced access to bathing facilities.

Niki wished she could just force him to bathe, but she knew she couldn't; it was a matter of patients' rights. Only if he had to have surgery could she make him take a shower. She sighed and reminded herself that it was a question of beliefs and values, and she shouldn't impose hers on others.

As an interesting note, not all countries that practice Western medicine share our custom of bathing patients daily. In France, patients are typically bathed on a weekly basis. The difference in frequency can be explained by a difference in cultural beliefs regarding the cause of disease. In the United States, germs are thought to be the primary cause, and great efforts are made to destroy them. Bathing is one way of accomplishing that. Although the French see germs as a source of disease, more important to them is the *terrain*—roughly the equivalent of the immune system. Lynn Payer, in her book *Medicine and Culture* (1988), describes how the French would be more likely to give patients a tonic to build up their immune system, rather than antibiotics to kill germs. I can recall being in France and seeing dogs in restaurants, and going into wonderful pastry shops in which the apple tart they are going to sell you is buzzing with flies. Such violations of "cleanliness" never seem to bother the natives, only the American tourists.

Toileting

The need to eliminate body waste is a human universal. What is not universal, however, are the ways in which it is done. These variations can also create cultural conflicts and misunderstandings, as the following cases illustrate.

Asian Toilets

104   Mr. Abatay, a fifty-eight-year-old Filipino patient, created a problem for the staff with his bathroom habits. The nurses, housekeepers, and his two former hospital "roommates" complained that the lid of the toilet was always dirty, and that there were shoe marks and water all over the toilet seat. Although he was suffering from dizziness and placed on strict bed rest, he refused to use the bedpan or bedside commode. One night the

nurse responded to the emergency call light from Mr. Abatay's room and found him squatting on the toilet seat. He had to be helped back to bed. This explained the mystery of the shoe marks on the toilet seat. But why would he do that, and why was there water all over the seat as well?

Mr. Abatay had been raised in a farming village in the Philippines. His only "bathroom" was a *kasilyas,* or "dig-in-the-pit" toilet. It is necessary to squat over them to use them. Since bathrooms are considered dirty, the *kasilyas* is generally located in the backyard, away from the house. There is no water there; people carry a bucket of water with them. People do not use toilet paper; it is thought to cause irritation and mild bleeding and to be rather ineffective at cleaning the area. Water is used instead to rinse off the area. People do not worry about spills; the water dries on its own. And although homes are meant to be kept spotless, because *kasilyas* are thought to be dirty, no one thinks of cleaning them. Mr. Abatay did not want to use the bedpan and "dirty" his bed.

It is unlikely that hospital staff will be able to "train" patients to use a toilet in a way that is different from the way they have grown accustomed. It is important to realize that not all toilets are designed the way American toilets are. In this case, what could have been done is twofold. The staff could have been educated on the differences in toilets in various parts of the world, and Mr. Abatay could have been provided with clean towels, a wastebasket, and disinfectant spray to use after he went to the bathroom.

In an interesting postscript to this case, I was contacted by the safety director for a small manufacturing company. Employees come from all over the world. He had received numerous complaints about employees' bathroom habits, which result in messy, wet toilet stalls. He was stunned to read the above case study, for it helped explain what was going on. He was feeling frustrated, however, because despite issuing memos on the importance of having their backside as close to the seat as possible, and providing seat covers in all the stalls, the toilets were still a mess. He was hoping that I could direct him to an adult training program on "American" toilet etiquette.

I told him that I was unaware of any such programs, but I suggested that someone from his human resources department should lead small group discussions in which information is presented regarding toilet habits in different countries due to differences in such things as plumbing. In countries where toilets are essentially a hole in the ground, people are used to squatting. In the United States, they may adapt by squatting with their feet on the toilet seat. In other countries, the plumbing cannot handle toilet paper, so it is put into a wastebasket next to the toilet.

A friend of mine was teaching kindergarten in a Mexican neighborhood. She said she was going to have to give her students a lesson in hygiene because they kept throwing their used toilet paper on the floor next to the toilet. I suggested to her that the problem might be one of plumbing rather than hygiene. I suspect that no one has told their parents that the plumbing is better in the United States and can handle the toilet paper. Their parents probably have a wastebasket by the toilet at home. Because there were no wastebaskets in the toilet stalls at school, her students were throwing the toilet paper on the floor.

More than once I have had the experience of going into a public restroom, checking the floor of the stalls for an empty one and, having found it, opened the door to find an Asian woman with her feet on the seat, squatting over the toilet. It is biomechanically easier to move the bowels in this position and is common in many parts of the world where Western plumbing is not found—and, occasionally, where it is. In a museum in southern France several years ago, I went to use the restroom but could not find the toilet. Finally, someone pointed out a hole in the ground. There were depressions on either side in the shape of footprints. I had to overcome a great deal of ethnocentrism before I was able to use it. The experience did, however, help me be more understanding when I open a stall door to discover a woman with her feet on the toilet seat.

Muslims and the Left Hand

106   Conflicts can also occur due to different customs for cleaning oneself after using the toilet. Issam Khattab was an Arab student at an American university. He had a perforated colon and needed a temporary colostomy. Sylvia was the nurse assigned to teach him how to use the pouch applied over the surgical opening on his bowel. Sylvia was surprised to find Issam noncompliant when it came to learning how to perform his self-care with the pouch. The main problem is that he would only use one hand to open and rinse out the pouch; he refused to use both hands. Because this task was extremely difficult to do one-handed, he would always call Sylvia to empty the pouch. Sylvia warned him of the dangers of having the unemptied pouch burst, but he still refused to empty it. Finally, to "teach him a lesson," she let it burst. Issam, now covered with his own feces, was angry and embarrassed, but at last began to care for himself.

Why was he so stubborn? Probably because in the Muslim tradition one uses one's right hand to eat and one's left hand to clean after going to the bathroom. Because food in much of the Middle East is traditionally eaten with one's hand out of a communal bowl, it is an important hygiene measure that people use separate hands for separate tasks. Most likely, Issam was avoiding using his right hand to clean his pouch. It is unfortunate that he did not explain the situation to Sylvia; she could have used disposable pouches that he could change using only one hand. Since that incident, she has done just that with her patients who are reluctant to perform the necessary maintenance of their pouches.

Hair

Many cultures have prohibitions against cutting hair, as was illustrated in the case involving Mr. Singh, the Sikh patient in Chapter 4. The biblical tale of Samson, who lost his strength when his hair was cut, reflects a similar prohibition.

Native Americans

A Native American woman named Estelle Begay brought her fifteen-month-old granddaughter Elena into the emergency room. The child was suffering from severe dehydration and fever. To restore fluids intravenously, the nurse shaved Elena's right temple and inserted an intravenous line. Mrs. Begay was busy completing admitting papers while this was done. When she reached the unit to see her granddaughter, she became very anxious and upset. The nurse tried to reassure her that the intravenous lines were temporary and that as soon as the problem was corrected, the child would be fine. Mrs. Begay responded with sorrow and resignation. "She's going to die." The nurse tried to reassure her, but Mrs. Begay would not leave Elena's bedside.

At one point, Mrs. Begay did leave for a few hours. She returned with two relatives and a "medicine bundle," which she tried to put on Elena's bed. This was against hospital policy and was not permitted. The nurse said she could leave it by the window, if she desired.

Mrs. Begay and the other relatives, who were no longer permitted in the unit except during limited visiting hours, kept a vigil outside the door. The next day, despite Elena's improvement, Mrs. Begay insisted on taking her home against medical advice.

The following day, her mother readmitted Elena. She was still feverish and would not eat. A small bundle was attached to the child's shirt. As the nurse started to remove it, the mother stopped her. "Please let her keep it. It is our custom." She went on to explain why Mrs. Begay had taken the child home against medical advice. She was afraid Elena would die.

"In our culture, it is taboo to cut a child's hair. Long, thick hair is a sign of a healthy child. To cut or shave it means the child will become sick or die." Mrs. Begay had obtained a medicine bundle to counteract the effect of violating the taboo, but was not permitted to put it next to the child. It was useless sitting by the window. Mrs. Begay had no recourse but to take Elena home, where she could use the curative charm. This time, the nurses agreed to let the medicine bundle be placed next to Elena. After four days, her condition improved and she was able to go home.

107

This example illustrates two important points. The first is the same discussed in the previous chapter with respect to religious and spiritual symbols: do not remove them. The second is that hair may have important significance beyond aesthetics for the patient and should not be cut or shaved without prior discussion.

The Body

Scars

108   Most Americans are concerned with their appearance. Surgeons therefore try to leave as small a scar as possible. This effort had a negative effect with forty-one-year-old Nigerian patient Osito Seisay, who was introduced in Chapter 3. He had come to the United States to have his brother operate on his knee, which was injured when a bull charged him.

His nurse was concerned when he did not request pain medication following surgery. She learned the reason when his sister-in-law came to visit and spoke to Mr. Seisay in his native language. He was enduring the pain as an offering to Allah.

The next cultural incident occurred when Mr. Seisay's brother, the surgeon, came to remove the bandages. He was very proud of his work and pointed out how small the surgical scar was. Mr. Seisay, however, did not share his brother's happiness. He was disappointed over the small size of the scar. He felt that without a large scar to mark the surgery, the other members of his tribe would not believe he had suffered very much. What kind of offering to Allah would that be?

His brother had obviously shed most of the old ways. He could not believe Osito still held these beliefs and tried in vain to convince him otherwise. At this point, nothing could be done. One would think that Mr. Seisay's brother, being aware of tribal customs, would have anticipated Osito's response. He did not. He was too Westernized. Surgeons, however, should be aware that all patients do not share the same ideal body image and should discuss such things in advance.

Fat

Mention of body image brings up the subject of fat. American culture values thinness and views obesity as a disease. Many cultures, however, see thinness as a problem and plumpness as the ideal.

109   Jane, a nurse, was about fifty pounds overweight. She was embarrassed about her size and eventually managed to lose most of the excess weight. She related an incident that occurred when she was at her heaviest.

Her Panamanian boyfriend, Mario, brought her home to meet his family. When they saw her, they were delighted that she was so fat. They told her this several times during the evening. Jane was totally humiliated by their remarks. She was already nervous about meeting Mario's family, and now they were insulting her. Yet they seemed so friendly.

Near the end of the evening, Mario, sensing her discomfort, took her aside and explained. In his culture, fat is seen as healthy. A fat woman can have lots of babies. All his other girlfriends had been far too thin to suit his family. At last he was going out with a "real woman." They had not been insulting her by calling her fat; they were bestowing a great compliment. His explanation made Jane feel a little better, though their repeated comments about her size continued to disturb her.

Although this incident did not take place in the hospital, it illustrates a problem that could arise there. Most Latin Americans and Eastern Europeans, among others, share Mario's family's view of body size. Advice that a patient lose weight might not be followed because it would create a negative body image. Imagine a slim American woman being told she should gain twenty-five pounds for the sake of her health. How willing would she be to trade her "attractive" figure for one that she sees as too fat? Health care professionals should be aware of possible resistance and be prepared to deal with it.

An article in the *New York Times* in July 2007 (LaFraniere 2007) focused on the efforts the Mauritanian government has been making in recent years to promote a healthy lifestyle. They are fighting an uphill battle, however, because it is a culture that sees fat as attractive in women, so much so that women go to great lengths to put on as much weight as possible. A 2001 government survey showed that 20 percent of the women between ages fifteen and forty-nine had been deliberately overfed, and nearly 70 percent had no regrets. Obesity is culturally associated with family wealth and epitomizes ideal female beauty. In addition to purposely overeating, many women also take a steroid hormone that can cause weight gain. Others take prescription antihistamines because they make them drowsy, and thus less active and more likely to put on weight. One can only imagine the difficulties a physician might face in trying to convince a woman with such beliefs that it is important to lose weight.

Summary

There are many potential sources of conflict within the hospital. Those that involve activities of daily living have the potential of occurring on a daily basis. Awareness of potential areas of conflict can go a long way toward avoiding them. The most common source of problems is diet. Food is essential to health, yet the traditional diet of many patients may conflict with standard hospital fare. As a result, patients may refuse to eat, which can both compromise their health and confuse their diagnosis. It is advisable for health care personnel to have some knowledge of traditional diets, in terms of both content and preparation, and to involve the patient or family in designing meals. In an era of increasing competition between hospitals for patients, it is the savvy hospital that will make accommodations to the patients' preferred diets.

It is also important to understand that toilets take very different forms in different parts of the world; sitting on a toilet seat may not come naturally for many people in developing countries. Some may prefer washing themselves off to using toilet paper.

Hair is another potentially sensitive issue. Do not expect to cut or shave hair without discussion, especially if the patient is a Sikh or Native American.

Finally, remember that the Anglo American view of the body, where the goal is to be thin and free of scars or other marks, is not necessarily shared by all. In many countries, it is seen as healthier and more attractive to be a bit plump. In others, scars may represent an offering of suffering to God.

Key Points

- Ask about food preferences and religious restrictions on diet during the admission interview.
- Involve the patient and/or family in choosing meals when possible.
- Take ethnic diets into account when discharging patients with special dietary requirements. Heart-healthy ethnic recipes are available online.
- Learn about your patients toilet habits and try to accommodate them.
- If your patient comes from a culture or religion that forbids shaving or cutting hair, do not do so without discussing it first with the patient.
- Realize that not everyone values thinness and unblemished skin.

For more on self-care, see Chapter 6.

Chapter 6
Family

When asked to name their most common problem in dealing with non-Anglo ethnic groups, most nurses respond, "their families." This is understandable, given cultural differences in a number of issues related to family, including decision making and the role of family members when someone is ill. However, the application of cultural sensitivity can make the hospital experience less stressful for patients, family members, *and* health care providers.

Decision Making

Family as Decision Maker

In U.S. culture the individual is the primary unit, and autonomy and independence are highly valued. As such, we expect individuals to make their own decisions regarding health care, as long as they are mentally competent. Many other cultures, however, see the family as the primary unit, and family interdependence is valued over independence. Usually such cultures are agriculturally based, since subsistence farming requires the coordinated efforts of a large family, the larger the better since that means more (unpaid) hands to do the work. What affects one person, affects every member of the family. Health care providers are often ill prepared to deal with patients who refuse to make decisions until they consult with family members.

Mrs. De Luiz was a Latino woman in her late fifties, suffering from diabetes. She and her husband lived with their son and his family. Her physician, Dr. Moustafa, found that the oral medication she had been taking was not doing enough to control her blood sugar levels and wanted to put her on insulin. He expected Mrs. De Luiz to comply; however, she said that she would first have to consult with her family. This both annoyed and confused him. This was her health; why did she need to consult with her family? It is actually somewhat surprising that Dr. Moustafa did not

110

understand, since he was Egyptian and family decision making is common in that culture. However, he was only in his thirties and may have adopted some American attitudes. At the same time, because the physician's authority is paramount in Egypt, he may have been disturbed by the fact that Mrs. De Luiz did not immediately accede to his orders, thus undermining his authority. Somewhat annoyed, he told Mrs. De Luiz to return the next day with her husband or son.

When Mrs. De Luiz returned the next morning with her husband, Dr. Moustafa explained to them the importance of keeping her blood sugar under control. Mr. De Luiz said that he was concerned that if his wife went on insulin, she would be unable to care for their grandson and that if she followed a special diet, she would not cook the foods that he liked.

This case highlights the fact that, in most Hispanic families, the needs of the family take precedence over those of the individual and important decisions are made by the family, not the individual. It also emphasizes the importance of asking the patient what concerns she or he might have in following the physician's recommendations. In this case, the patient's husband was forthcoming, but in others, the likely outcome is that the patient would simply not adhere to the physician's recommendations and the physician would have no clue as to why. At least then the physician can have an opportunity to address the concerns.

Although the nurse who reported this case did not report on the outcome, the clinical implications are clear. When treating Hispanic patients, try to involve the family as much as possible. Understand that what affects one individual affects the entire household. This point is true for all families, not just Hispanic ones. Finally, ask about their concerns regarding treatment. One way to ask is to simply say, "I know that patients sometimes find it hard to follow all my recommendations. What problems do you think you might have in following them?" Compromises can be made, particularly with regard to diet. There are ways to adjust traditional ethnic diets to conform to the needs of patients with diabetes and heart disease; it just takes more time and patient education on the part of the clinician.

111   It is important not to confuse deferred decision making with refusal. Olga Lopez, a twenty-four-year-old Mexican immigrant, was suffering from depression. She was hospitalized after a failed suicide attempt. Her physician wanted to put her on antidepressants. When he told her this, she hesitated. He assumed this meant she did not want to take the medication. It was only later that it came out that she *did* want the drugs, but felt she had to discuss it first with her family. The physician could not understand why she might want to consult anyone before making a decision about her own health.

Health care providers must be aware that making your own decisions about your own health care is very American and reflects our strong value of independence. It is good practice to ask a patient, "Is there anyone you would like to consult with before making a decision?"

Authority Figures

In Chapter 7 you will read about cases in which the husband is the authority figure in the family and responsible for making the major decisions, even those regarding the health of his wife and children. However, in some cases, it may be the grandparents or other family members who are in charge, as with the following case.

Ricardo de Luis was a twenty-two-year-old Mexican patient who needed a kidney biopsy. Carmen, a bilingual nurse, acted as interpreter when Swan, his regular nurse, needed him to sign informed consent. They were both surprised when he refused to sign, since they thought he understood the need for the biopsy. He explained that he could not make the decision; that was the job of his eldest brother, since his father, who would normally make such a decision, was in Mexico. Carmen and Swan insisted that he was old enough to make his own health care decisions. Furthermore, the doctor had advised him to have the procedure as soon as possible. It was Friday, and if he didn't have it done immediately, he would probably have to wait until Monday. But his brother was at work and couldn't make it to the hospital until later that evening.

Fortunately for Ricardo, consent could be obtained over the phone with a doctor's order and two nurses witnessing and signing consent. But the situation could have easily been avoided had staff thought to ask Ricardo upon admission if there was anyone he wanted to consult with before making decisions. He had been in the hospital for two days already, and his brother had been there, signing consents and making medical decisions. This specific consent could have been signed earlier. But everyone involved had made the incorrect assumption that because he was twenty-two years old, he would make his own decisions.

In many cultures, including Romany (Gypsy), Asian, Middle Eastern, and Hispanic, males are traditionally the authority figures. Unless they are very acculturated, it is often best to consider them as the spokespersons for the family. They are often the ones who will make the decisions. This recommendation may be difficult for those with feminist leanings, but it is likely to be the most productive approach. Age is also a sign of authority in Gypsy and Asian cultures, so initial conversations should be addressed to the eldest male.

It is unwise, however, to assume that males are always in charge. In matrilineal cultures such as the Navajo, where descent is traced through the female line, the eldest women may have the greatest authority and decision making power. Even in male-dominated cultures, women may have

112

authority in the home when it comes to children and health issues. I was talking with a pediatrician at a large county hospital that serves a sizeable Mexican population. She said that when a child needs to continue treatment in the home—for example, when a child has asthma—she will ask the mother who gives her advice about child rearing, and if that person lives with them. Often that person will be the grandmother. She said she will then include that person in any teaching, because she has learned through experience that if she can get that authority figure on board with her treatment plan, it has a much greater chance of being successful.

As a general practice, health care providers should *ask* their patients if they would like them to consult with any other family members when decisions need to be made, and expect that the responses will vary along both cultural and individual lines. (It should also be noted that in the case of gay and lesbian patients, the person might not be a "family" member.)

Kinship Structure

Issues regarding who may sign informed consent have the potential for becoming very complicated, due to cultural variations in the way that kinship is structured. For example, the maternal uncle has a very important role in Navajo society. U.S. kinship structure is *bilateral*; we are equally related to members of both sides of our family. Social ties might be closer to one side, but the legal relationship is identical. Many other cultures are *unilineal*; that is, they trace their descent from either a male or a female ancestor. A member of a patrilineal culture (such as many in the Middle East) is considered a member of the father's family, rather than the mother's. In a divorce, the father would usually be granted custody, rather than the mother. In contrast, a member of a matrilineal culture (such as the Navajo or Hopi or some African tribes) is considered more a member of the mother's family than the father's.

Although women tend to have greater power and respect in matrilineal societies than in patrilineal ones, property is usually passed on from male to male, with a boy inheriting from his closest male relative. In this case, it will be his mother's brother, because the boy is not considered a member of his father's family. His father will pass on any property or privileges to his own sister's children. Genetically, this arrangement makes sense. A boy always shares the genes of his mother's brother. It is not so certain that he will carry those of his mother's husband.

Many tribes in Ghana are traditionally matrilineal. Several years ago, one of my Ghanaian students told me that changing circumstances were creating a problem in his country. Traditionally, nephews would work the farms of their maternal uncles, and would later inherit the property. In recent years, however, family members would often move to the city. When a farmer died, the sons, who had grown up working the farm, would expect to inherit it, but often the nephews would suddenly show up from the city, claiming the land. Circumstances had changed, but the kinship structure had not, and the laws had not caught up with the new circumstances. Recently, another student of mine from Ghana shared that when his father died a month earlier, his father's sister called from Ghana, trying to claim inheritance for her sons, despite the fact that her brother— my student's father—had been living with his immediate family in the United States for several years.

The Role of the Family

Another important issue involves the role of the family when a member is ill. The general expectation of the health care system is that families will be there—during visiting hours only—to visit with the patient. Ideally, they will make no demands upon the doctors or nurses but will help out as requested. That is not the way many families behave in reality. Problems with too many visitors is a common nursing complaint. However, a little cultural competence can make a huge difference.

Visitors

Reggie was working in the critical care unit when he was assigned Concepcíon Rios, a fifty-seven-year-old Hispanic female with new-onset chest pain requiring cardiac intervention. The nurse who took the phone report laughed when she warned Reggie that twenty or thirty very emotional family members were accompanying the patient onto the unit. As a precaution, security had already been called.

Fortunately for Mrs. Rios, Reggie used this situation as an opportunity to apply what he had been learning in his cultural competency class. He immediately called for an interpreter and discussed his plan with her before talking with the family, to make sure his ideas were communicated properly.

He and the interpreter greeted the family in the critical care waiting room. The men were huddled together talking while the women were crying loudly. Mrs. Rios had thirteen children, and members of each of their families was in attendance. Reggie told everyone that although hospital policy allowed a maximum of two visitors at a time for up to ten minutes until 9:00 P.M., he understood how important family was to them. Therefore, he would bend the rules and allow one family member to stay at Mrs. Rios's bedside at all times to assist him in caring for her, and that two other family members could rotate visiting throughout the night. The men selected a younger daughter to assist him, and the patient's husband

113

volunteered to be the family spokesperson. Her husband then hugged Reggie and told him that he felt comfortable leaving his wife with their family and "such a nice man."

Reggie included the daughter in as much of the routine care as possible, as she was very eager to assist. Grateful family members visited throughout the night. The daughter kept her father informed of her mother's condition, and in turn, he let the rest of the family know. The daughter expressed her appreciation to Reggie many times.

The entire experience was positive for everyone involved. A potentially hysterical crowd became calm and comfortable during what could have been extremely trying circumstances. Contrary to expectations, security was *not* needed to clear out the room. The patient did well and the family was grateful. It was wonderful PR for the hospital. In order to provide culturally appropriate care, all it took was a little knowledge of the importance of family in Hispanic culture and the willingness to be flexible with the visiting rules. Of course, a private room is essential in such a situation.

114   Terry, a labor and delivery nurse, has found a similar approach to be successful in dealing with large numbers of visitors. She finds that most family members just want to help, so she puts them to work. She'll give the grandmother a rocker at the bedside; her job is to "be there" for the laboring woman. Sisters are given the job of massaging feet, hands, and back. She'll put the husband in charge of applying cool cloths to the forehead, fetching ice chips, and letting her know when the IV bag is down to 100cc. The mother of the patient is put in charge of peri-care. If the father of the patient is there, she puts him in charge of the family—making sure the noise level is kept down, the door kept shut, and the television on the station of the patient's choice. If any children are there, their job is to make sure grandma has everything she needs, from coffee to blankets.

Terry's experience is that big families, rather than creating problems, can actually be helpful if you put them to work. After about an hour or so, she will suggest they take a break or go to lunch, since she'll "be needing them later." Often they take a break on their own. She finds that this approach earns her a lot of positive feedback from her patients.

Asian patients will also often have family at the bedside day and night. The custom in both China and Japan is for the family to take care of the patient's personal needs. The medical staff is there to practice medicine. Both respect and obligation require that children minister to their parents.

The Asian respect for parents can be illustrated by the following hypothetical situation. You are in a boat with your mother and your child when the boat capsizes. You can save only one person. Whom do you save? Most Americans would respond, "My child," reasoning that their mother had lived her life whereas their child's was just beginning. Most Asians perceive the situation differently. They would more likely respond, "My mother," explaining that they can always have another child, but they can have only one mother. (Nigerians ask a similar question, but the boat's occupants are your mother and your *wife*. The culturally "correct" response is the same as that described for Asians.)

The different perspectives also reflect a difference in family relationships. Traditionally, most Asians lived in extended family households and tended to value the family of orientation (the individual, parents, and siblings) above the family of procreation (the individual, spouse, and children). Sons generally lived with their parents until they died, and thus that long-term relationship takes precedence over any other. In contrast, Americans usually live in nuclear family households. Ties to parents are weakened after marriage, while those to spouse and children are strengthened. The choice of whether to save the mother or child reflects the traditionally stronger familial tie.

Roma (commonly known as "Gypsies") cause some of the worst complaints regarding family visitors. For example, when Louis Romano, king of his clan, became ill, thirty to fifty of his relatives, friends, and "elders" literally took over the small hospital where he was a patient in intensive care. They came in the evening and stayed all night, despite the posted notice that visiting hours were limited. Those who were not in the patient's room or lobby roamed the parking lot. Everyone in the hospital—supervisors, security, maintenance, office staff, and nurses—tried in vain to maintain order, politely explaining procedure and protocol, but without effect.

Roma live within a large extended family unit known as a clan. All members are considered immediate family. When any member is ill, it is important to show respect and concern through one's presence. Because the patient in this case was the king, the attendance of the entire clan was almost mandatory. A few elders even came from across the country to be with him.

Roma are commonly nomadic, traveling in groups. When they enter a hospital, that becomes their temporary home. If possible, Rom patients should be put in private rooms at the end of a hall to minimize traffic problems and disturbance to other patients. Other than that, hospital staff must be prepared for a constant stream of people moving into the hospital to be near the patient.

One reason large numbers of ethnic family members who visit patients and often remain twenty-four hours a day create significant difficulties for hospital staff is that hospitals in the United States were built to suit Anglo American culture. Anglo Americans tend to have small families and to live in nuclear family households. Privacy is a major value. Generally few family members live near enough to the hospital to visit very often.

115

When they do, they usually stay for only a short period of time because they feel the patient should be left alone to rest in order to get well. Therefore, hospital rooms rarely have more than one visitor's chair per bed and visiting hours may be extremely limited. In addition, Anglo Americans value money as well as privacy. Hospitals are a business. If there is room for another bed, it should be for a patient, not for a family member who wants to sleep over.

Nurses who have worked in or visited hospitals in other countries describe very different situations from those in the United States. For example, one student of mine reported that at a hospital in Thailand, families would often sleep under the beds (tables with plastic covers), on the floor, or even in the bed with the patient. A nurse who worked at a Thai hospital told her that family members would often provide meals for the patient because it would be embarrassing for the patient if the family didn't "care enough" to bring food. A nurse who visited a hospital in Spain reported that it had rooms situated around a large patio, where family members relaxed and cooked food for the patients. Families were there around the clock and helped bathe and feed patients. The physicians and nurses did only medical care. This arrangement helps make sense of the next case.

116   Betsy Sanders, a former student of mine, broke her leg in a skiing accident in Spain. The doctor at the clinic told Betsy that her ligaments were shredded but that he could correct the condition with surgery. When Betsy awoke from surgery, she was nauseated and in terrible pain but could not vomit. She was too embarrassed. There were ten people in the room waiting to see her. She was in a large private room, and a couch had been turned into a guest bed. All her friends in Spain had gotten together and decided Betsy should never be left alone. They worked out a visiting schedule. One friend even took a leave of absence from work to be with her.

Although Betsy appreciated their concern, their solicitousness made her uncomfortable. All but one of her friends were male. She was in bed with her leg in the air for two weeks, wearing nothing but a little gown. She had to be washed in bed and use a bedpan. She could not wash her hair or even brush her teeth. She looked awful and felt worse. All she wanted was to be left alone.

Her situation was the reverse of the non-Anglo in an American hospital. The hospital staff expected her to have visitors around the clock and provided a bed for that purpose. Her friends assumed she would want company and ignored what they interpreted as her polite protestations that she would be fine if left alone. She did not have any family in Spain, so they were filling in. They would have wanted the same attention had the situation been reversed. In this case, however, what the patient longed for was some privacy.

A young Lebanese nurse changed her attitude toward family visitors   117
when she herself became a patient. The evening she had surgery, eight
relatives came in a group to see her. It made her feel good to be the
object of so much love and support. At the same time, she realized that
had she been the nurse in this case, she would have felt that the large
number of visitors was unacceptable, and would have asked them to leave.
She had done this before with other patients, thinking that it was for the
patients' own good. She realized that, in the past, she might have mistakenly imposed the values of the health care system on her patients.

What she learned from this experience was to talk to her patients about
their feelings regarding visitors before the visitors arrived. Then she could
truly do what was best for her patient. For the patient with a large family
who does want a lot of visitors, you might have them to choose one person to sit with the patient for a specified period (for example, two hours).
That position could be rotated among the family members so that everyone gets a chance to be with the patient. That person could also act as
contact person for the nurse and doctor. This type of plan can serve the
needs of the family, patient, and health care staff.

In summary, then, hospitals are designed with the needs and values of
the culture in mind. Problems arise, as they did with Betsy, when the
patient is of a different ethnic group. In a country like the United States,
with its huge population of non-Anglo residents, this is frequently the case.
It is important to remember that the patient is not just an individual but
also a member of a family. When one member is ill, the entire group is
affected. Ideally, the family can help care for the patient, freeing the staff
for more technical medical care.

Familismo

The concept of *familismo,* or the importance of the extended family sup-   *118*
port system, is essential for understanding Hispanic families. Knowledge
of it can help increase patient satisfaction, as the following case illustrates. Charisse, an RN, worked in the department of the hospital where
patients and families came to express their complaints. One afternoon,
Sonia Sanchez came to her office, accompanied by an older woman and
two children. Normally, Charisse said, she would have greeted Mrs. Sanchez, suggest that she and her family be seated, and then listen to her
concerns. On the surface, this appears to be an appropriate way to deal
with complaints. However, after taking a course in cultural competence,
Charisse had new tools to use in the situation. Applying the concept of
familismo, she first introduced herself to the angry Mrs. Sanchez, and asked
about her companions. As Mrs. Sanchez introduced her to her mother and
children, Charisse greeted each one individually and then proceeded to

inquire after Mrs. Sanchez's concerns. At this point, Mrs. Sanchez visibly relaxed. While Charisse acknowledged that Mrs. Sanchez's change in attitude for the better may have been due to the time she gave her to calm down, it is more likely that it was due to the attention and respect Charisse paid to her family. She reported that the interaction was a positive one, and that she felt Mrs. Sanchez left feeling that her concerns had been heard. It was a small gesture on Charisse's part, but may have made an essential difference in their communication.

Self-Care

Another problem often stems from the fact that in many cultures *interdependence* is valued over *independence*, as can be seen in the following cases.

119   Tome Tanaka, a Japanese man in his sixties, was a patient in the rehabilitation unit. A stroke had left him with significant weakness on his left side. Self-care was an important part of his therapy. He had to relearn to feed himself, dress, shave, use the bathroom, and do other daily activities. Kathy, his nurse, spent a great deal of time carefully explaining to Mr. Tanaka how the staff would work with him on these tasks. The patient and his wife listened passively; his children and grandchildren appeared more interested. Several hours later, when Mr. Tanaka's children and grandchildren left, Kathy came into the room and discovered Mrs. Tanaka waiting on her husband as though he were an invalid.

She was not alone in impeding his progress, however. He refused to do anything for himself and continually barked commands at his wife. Rather than use the toilet, he insisted that she hold the bedpan for him. He refused to brush his teeth, shave, or dress, demanding that his wife do everything for him.

Mr. Tanaka attended physical therapy and occupational therapy sessions each day and did quite well. He learned to walk with a cane. He needed minimal assistance with self-care activities. Despite his progress in therapy, however, as soon as his wife or one of his children arrived, he regressed. He was discharged after four weeks, almost as dependent as when he first came.

Kathy and the other nurses were frustrated over Mr. Tanaka's dependency, especially when they saw that he was capable of taking care of himself. They took his "failure" personally, as though they were not doing their jobs properly. What might the nurses have done differently? First, they needed to understand that patients and their families do not always share the same goals as health care personnel. Second, they might have allowed the family to observe Mr. Tanaka during physical and occupational therapy sessions. Unlike most hospitals, this one barred families from such sessions because of the potential distraction for the patient. In this case, the rule might have been waived.

Juan Martinez, a thirty-six-year-old Mexican man with second-degree burns on his hands and arms, posed a similar problem. The skin grafts had healed, and there was now danger that the area would stiffen and the tissue shorten. The only way to maintain maximum mobility was through regular stretching and exercise. The nurses explained to Mr. Martinez's wife that feeding himself was an essential therapeutic exercise. The act of grasping the utensils and lifting the food to the mouth stretches the necessary areas. Mrs. Martinez seemed to understand the nurses' explanation, yet she continued to cut her husband's food and put it in his mouth.

When Linda, one of his nurses, observed this, she took the fork out of Mrs. Martinez's hand and told Mr. Martinez to feed himself because he needed to exercise his arms and hands. Linda again explained to Mr. Martinez's wife how important it was for him to do it himself. Mrs. Martinez appeared skeptical but did not argue. Mr. Martinez looked at Linda peevishly and made a feeble attempt at eating. His wife watched with pity. Linda knew from seeing Mr. Martinez when his wife was not around that he was perfectly capable of feeding himself. Linda left the room. When she looked in five minutes later, she saw Mrs. Martinez once again cutting her husband's food and putting it in his mouth.

Failure to care for oneself is common in cultures that emphasize the family over the individual—in other words, almost all cultures other than Anglo American. Self-care is important to Americans in part because we value independence so highly. In contrast, Asian and Hispanic cultures emphasize family interdependence over independence. For them, self-care is not an important concept.

In many cases, Americans' ethnocentrism blinds them to the fact that life in a typical Asian or Hispanic household may be different from that in an Anglo home. Self-care may be a practical necessity in the Anglo home, where there may be no one to help the former patient with such tasks. In contrast, many Asians and Hispanics live in large extended family households, where someone is usually at home to care for the patient.

Another significant factor is the difference between egalitarian and hierarchical cultures. In an egalitarian culture such as our own, everyone is theoretically equal. Theoretically, no one in the family is considered subservient to anyone else. In hierarchical Asian cultures, some members of the family are clearly dominant (males and elders) while others are clearly subordinate (females and children). The case study involving the Tanakas illustrates the proper roles of wife and children in hierarchical cultures. It is their duty to obey and care for the dominant family member—the husband and father. An additional element when dealing with elderly Asians is the notion that old age is a time for rest, reflection, and

120

being cared for by loved ones after a lifetime of labor. It is seen as inappropriate to insist on self-care when family members are available to assist.

In the situation with the Martinez couple, duty plays a less prominent role. It is of greater importance that when a family member is ill, love and concern are demonstrated through care and attention. The nurses might have instructed Mrs. Martinez to help her husband in ways that would not hinder his rehabilitation. For example, they could have shown her how to massage lotion onto his hands.

Control may also play a role in the failure to care for oneself. Each of the situations described above involved a man whose culture clearly acknowledged his power and authority. All these men, however, were reduced to a state of physical weakness by their medical condition. Ordering people around and having them wait upon one's every need are ways of demonstrating dominance. It may masquerade as helplessness, but it can be a way of maintaining control.

The wise health care provider will acknowledge the powerful role of family in such cultures. When appropriate, patient teaching should involve all members of the patient's family. They are the ones who will likely be caring for the patient at home.

Demanding Families

The hospital staff often has conflicts with family members over issues other than self-care or too many visitors. In some cultures, part of the "job" of the family is to make sure that the nurses are spending enough time caring for their loved one. Unfortunately, given the huge demands placed on nurses, this is not always possible.

121   Before taking my course in cultural diversity, Jennifer, like all the nurses on her unit, tried to avoid taking care of Naser Assharj, a middle-aged Iranian Muslim patient, because the entire staff found his family to be very "uptight and demanding." The nurses rotated care for this patient, because no one was willing to care for him more than one day at a time. When Jennifer learned a bit about Muslim culture, however, she understood why his family kept demanding a private room and made such a fuss over his meals. It was their way of showing love and care for their family member. He needed a private room so that, as devout Muslims, the family could pray together five times a day as commanded by Allah. It was also important that his food be *halal*, or follow the Muslim laws of what is permissible (see Chapter 5). Once Jennifer realized this, she contacted her supervisor and arranged to have the patient moved to a private room and spoke to the dietician regarding his food. The family members were very grateful for her efforts, and became much easier to deal with.

A speaker at a workshop I attended on cultural diversity told an interesting story that shed some light on why many Iranian patients' families are always on top of the staff and constantly questioning everything and advocating (to use a nice word) for their family member. He said that the medical system in Iran, particularly during the time of transition to the Shah, was pretty poor. Unless family members kept constant watch, patients could die. When his grandmother was in the hospital, his mother kept watch over her. One night around 2 or 3 A.M., his mother noticed that her mother was no longer getting oxygen. She ran down to check on things and discovered that the man in charge of changing the oxygen tanks had fallen asleep. If she hadn't woken him up to do his job, her mother might have died. With experiences like that, how could you *not* be constantly watching for mistakes? Plus given all the bad press about medical errors, it's not surprising that people would be concerned.

A social worker attending the workshop had an excellent strategy for dealing with loud, difficult, demanding family members. She sits down with them to figure out exactly what they want. Then she talks to them about different strategies that can be used to accomplish that: "You've tried yelling and screaming at the nurses, and that hasn't worked out for you so far. The nurses are very overworked, and when they're yelled at, they feel angry and unappreciated. This makes them less likely to do what you want. Why don't you try this strategy . . . ."

As someone who has had family members hospitalized I can well understand the frustration of having someone you care for be seriously ill, yet lacking the medical skills to do anything to help the patient. Staying "on top of" the nurses allows you to feel that you're doing something for your loved one. Although this example focuses on a Middle Eastern family because their culture allows them to be more openly verbally aggressive, families from any ethnic background can be demanding.

What can the staff do? I would suggest that at the beginning of the patient's hospitalization, you spend a few minutes with the family, asking questions about the patient:

- Show that you care.
- Tell them that you will be happy to talk with them on a regular basis (set up a schedule that you feel comfortable with) so you can update them on the patient's condition and they can share their concerns.
- Give the family small, helpful tasks they can do, such as massaging lotion into the patient's hands or feet.
- Let them feel they are doing something for the patient.

Often, families become demanding because they feel helpless and out of control. By following these suggestions, you can help to alleviate some of their frustration.

Protective Families

122   Knowing something about a patient's culture can help health care professionals provide more culturally appropriate care. Doreen was caring for a sixty-two-year-old Korean patient, Su Jo. Doreen had learned that Korean culture is hierarchical, and that negative diagnoses may be withheld from the patient. So, rather than assume that Mr. Jo was aware of his cancer diagnosis, she asked his son what his father knew about his medical condition. She also asked the son whether he was the family spokesperson. The son then told her that his father *was* aware of his condition, but asked that she not tell his mother. He also asked that any questions be directed toward him. Things went much more smoothly than they might have, due to Doreen's cultural competence skills. She said that she now asks this question (how much does the patient know about his or her condition?) with all her patients.

A nurse who worked in a hospital in Africa for a few years said that they rarely gave detailed information to patients about their diagnosis or treatment. Such information was usually given to the family. It was felt that having the family relay such news would help to prevent a severe emotional breakdown.

123   An extreme example of the lengths people will go to protect family members was the case of a Pakistani woman. Her son, who was living in the United States, had died of cancer at the age of fifty. She was old and in ill health, and her family were afraid the news would kill her. They even went to the extent of having her son-in-law call her in Pakistan, pretending to be her son. She died not knowing that her son had predeceased her.

Because you cannot know how much a patient truly wants to know about their condition, it is wise to ask. (For more on this subject, see Chapter 10.)

Gifts

124   A more pleasant problem arose during a Korean woman's discharge. Mrs. Choo had been cared for during her week in the hospital by a nurse named Florine. Florine frequently stopped in to see Mrs. Choo, offering to help in any way she could to make her patient more comfortable. Mrs. Choo's family was often there and observed Florine's kindness. When Mrs. Choo was being discharged, her twenty-five-year-old son, Jim, took Florine aside and gave her some money. Florine thanked him but refused it, explaining that she could not accept money for doing her job. Furthermore, it was against hospital policy. He insisted that she take it and put it in her pocket. "My mother wants you to have this. She wants to thank you." Florine took the money from her pocket, this time more adamant in her refusal. Jim in turn became extremely embarrassed.

In Korea, it is common for the family to give a patient's nurse food, money, or a special gift to show gratitude for the care she is giving. For Florine to refuse the gift was both insulting and improper. Reciprocity is important in many Asian cultures. When someone does something for another, something is owed in exchange. If the exchange is not completed, the person receiving the kindness is in the other's debt. Because this is an uncomfortable position to be in, it is extremely important not to let such indebtedness occur. A gift to the nurses satisfies the reciprocal obligation.

The stalemate ended when Florine told Jim to take the money and buy some candy for all the nurses to share. This suggestion took care of the Choo family's need to show their appreciation and allowed Florine to adhere to her own values and hospital policy.

The families of Jewish patients also often give nurses gifts while the patient is in the hospital. It is not done so much through a feeling of obligation and reciprocity, however, but as a way of ensuring good care.

In Japan, it is traditional for families to give gifts to those who have helped them during the year, including physicians, and gifts may also be given in advance of surgery. A Japanese physician, John Takayama (2001), reports that many Japanese patients in San Francisco carry on the tradition. He states that while it makes him uncomfortable to think that these gifts may unconsciously affect the way he treats his patients, he also fears that refusing them would be considered impolite and would damage his relationship with them, because gift giving may reinforce a sense of community.

Whatever the reason for gift giving, when a family member presents a gift to the nurse or doctor, refusing it will likely create a great deal of awkwardness. The solution most commonly practiced is for the health care provider to share the gift with the other staff members. If the gift is inappropriate (e.g., too expensive or too personal), then the physician or nurse should do his or her best to refuse it graciously.

Summary

Family structure and relationships are not the same in every culture. In many cases accommodation will be difficult, if not impossible, given hospital architecture, American medical values, and the American legal system. At the very least, however, greater understanding of the ways of other cultures may have a positive effect on the attitudes of those providing patient care. Culturally competent practices will include involving the family in patient care, both in the hospital and at home.

Key Points

- In cultures where the family, rather than the individual, is the primary unit, decisions are often made by the family. In such cultures, interdependence is usually valued over independence.

- When medical decisions need to be made, ask patients if there is any-one they would like to consult with before making a decision. Ideally, they should be asked before the need arises. Expect that the responses will vary along both cultural and individual lines.
- Be sure to ask patients if they have any concerns regarding your recommendations.
- Males are traditionally the authority figure in most cultures and often act as spokespersons for the family and make decisions for the family.
- In many cultures, it is expected that family members will remain with the hospitalized patient. Try to be flexible regarding visiting rules.
- Involve the family in patient care when they so desire. Emphasize self-care only when it is desired by the patient or necessary for physical recovery; do not impose the value of independence upon those who do not share it.
- When appropriate, patient teaching should involve all members of the patient's family. They are the ones who will likely be caring for the patient at home.
- Show family members that you care about their loved one.
- Set up a schedule for updates on the patient's condition.
- Ask your patients how much they know about their condition. Family members may try to protect them from a negative diagnosis/prognosis.
- When a patient gives you an inappropriate gift, try to refuse it graciously. If possible, accept gifts and share them with the staff.

Chapter 7
Men and Women

Sex and gender are frequent sources of conflict and misunderstanding. Not every culture has been affected by the women's movement. Few share the American ideal of equality between the sexes.

Sex Roles

Since the advent of the women's movement in the 1970s, a concerted effort has been made to eliminate restrictive sex roles. Rather than having opportunities limited by one's sex, the emphasis is on treating each person as an individual and allowing free expression of their abilities. Admittedly, that is an idealized version of what is happening, but it reflects our cultural ideology and the direction in which we are trying to move. Not all cultures, however, share this notion of gender equality, as the following case illustrates.

Women as Wives, Mothers, and Housekeepers

The contrast of both age and sex roles was the source of conflict in the following case, which almost involved filing a child abuse report on a Maria, a fifteen-year-old young Mexican woman who was married and living in California. Karen, her public health nurse, was concerned that her in-laws were possibly holding her as a captive housekeeper and sex slave. She based this on the fact that Maria was pregnant and spent most of her day doing housework. When Karen confronted her, she appeared quiet and unresponsive. Karen arranged to have Ramona, an Anglo American public health nurse who had spent much of her youth in Latin America, check out the situation.

After talking with Maria, it became clear to Ramona that this was a case of ethnocentrism on the part of Karen, who could not understand why a fifteen-year-old girl would voluntarily get pregnant and spend her time keeping house for her in-laws. What Karen didn't understand was that in rural Mexico, where Maria was born, it is expected that a woman's role in life is to be a wife and mother. The Quinceanera, the traditional Hispanic rite of passage for fifteen-year-old girls (*quince* means fifteen) was originally a kind of "coming-out" party designed to announce to the community that the young woman was now eligible for marriage. The ceremony itself, replete with male and female attendants much like "bridesmaids" and "groomsmen," mirrors a wedding ceremony. Given the twin circumstances of high infant mortality rates and the fact that children are highly valued, childbearing is often begun early. Ramona found that Maria took much pride in her pregnancy and in the way she kept the home of her in-laws, with whom she and her husband lived. In fact, her mother-in-law often tried to help with the housekeeping, but was unable to meet Maria's high standards.

Karen's concern about Maria's demeanor also reflected a difference in cultural values. What Karen saw as unassertive and indecisive, needing protection, Maria experienced as the behavior of someone who had been "well brought up." She was showing respect and deference to the public health nurse. It would be wrong, from her point of view, to challenge Karen's values, even though they were not her own.

Had Ramona been the original public health nurse caring for Maria, she probably would have understood the situation and not seen it as a potential case for child protective services. Fortunately, she was brought into the situation before it went that far. One additional note: although it is unknown how old Maria's husband was, it would not be surprising if he were significantly older. It is very common in rural areas of Mexico for parents to marry off their daughters to older men as a way of trying to ensure their economic security.

Men as Decision Makers

Part of the ideology of gender equality extends to decision making. The mainstream Anglo American ideal that husbands and wives should share equally in the decision making is not shared by all Americans and is often not the case for people from other cultures.

126   A twenty-six-year-old Mexican woman named Rosa Gutierrez brought her two-month-old son to the emergency department. She was concerned because he had diarrhea and had not been nursing. The staff discovered that he was also suffering from sepsis, dehydration, and high fever. The physician wanted to perform a routine spinal tap, but Mrs. Gutierrez refused to allow it. When asked why, she said she needed her husband's permission before anything could be done to the baby. The staff tried to convince her that this was a routine procedure, but she was adamant. Nothing could be done until her husband arrived.

Although legally she could have signed the consent, culturally she lacked the authority. In the traditional Mexican household, the man is the head of the family and makes all major decisions. Rosa was unwilling to violate that norm. Fortunately, her husband soon arrived and signed the informed consent.

A pediatrician who encountered a similar problem found a solution that proved effective. A female resident could not get a Hispanic mother to sign consent for a procedure for her child; she, too, insisted on waiting for her husband. In this case, however, it was urgent that the procedure be done as soon as possible. The resident asked an older male physician to speak to the mother. Apparently, the combination of his age and gender were enough to convince her to sign consent without speaking first to her husband.

In another example, Trin Binh and her children were involved in a motor vehicle accident; both she and two of her children sustained serious injuries. Mr. Trin was at work, and did not yet know about the accident. Mrs. Binh and her family were brought by ambulance to the nearest emergency department, where it was determined they would need immediate surgery. Mrs. Binh had emigrated from Vietnam in 1975 and spoke fluent English. She was alert and oriented. However, she refused to sign any consents for herself or her children. She insisted that she must wait until her husband arrived and everything was explained to him. Although the staff explained why there was no time to wait for her husband, who was at least an hour's drive away, Mrs. Binh was adamant.

The situation was resolved when the staff called her husband on the telephone. A physician gave him a detailed explanation of his wife's and children's injuries, as well as what needed to be done. He then spoke with his wife. When she hung up the phone, she agreed to sign consent for the surgical procedures.

Amiya Nidhi was a young woman in her twenties who had recently emigrated to the United States from India. She was in the hospital to give birth. Her support person was her sister, Marala. Marala kept telling her to get an epidural, but Amiya said that even though she would like one, she could not get one; her husband would not allow it. Cindy, her nurse, overheard the conversation. Having learned that husbands are the authority figure in the traditional Indian household, she went to speak with Mr. Nidhi. She explained why an epidural would be advisable. She said that he seemed pleased that she came to him about it. He said he would think about it, and let her know. About thirty minutes later, he came to Cindy and told her that he would like his wife to have an epidural. Everyone was pleased. By using cultural competence, Cindy helped her patient get the care she wanted, while still respecting the authority structure within the family.

As a professional woman and wife who has always shared decision making with my husband, I have to admit that it was hard for me to understand the position of women from other cultures who allow their husbands to make decisions. Although I understand it intellectually, it was something I never understood in my gut until one of my Filipino students shared her point of view. Rosaria was in her early twenties, and had lived in the United States all of her life. Her parents, however, were very traditional, and her father made all the important household decisions. She had recently married a Filipino man who, she was a bit dismayed to learn, wanted her to share equally in the decision making. "It was so much easier having my father make all the decisions. There's so much responsibility involved in decision making. I really hate it." That was something I *could* understand.

I should also point out that sex roles are changing as young women, growing up in the United States, become Americanized and educated. We were discussing this subject in one of my undergraduate anthropology classes that was populated largely by Mexican American students. The women told me that their grandmothers (living in Mexico) taught them that their husband was the boss and that their job was to make their husband's life easier. Their mothers (born in Mexico, but living in the United States) advised them to let their husbands *think* they're the boss, but to manipulate them to do what *they* wanted. The attitude of my students, all of whom planned to get jobs after college, was that there was no way they were going to let their husband be the boss; they would share that job equally. The Mexican male students were rather quiet on the topic, although a few expressed some regret over the changing norms.

Men as Authority Figures

Male dominance is the norm in most cultures, a fact that can create problems for female health care providers, as in the following cases.

130   Anandi Kothari, a middle-aged Indian woman, was being discharged following an angioplasty. Her husband was at her bedside. Her physician wrote out discharge orders and left them at the nurse's station. The nurse, Athula, a female from Sri Lanka, entered Mrs. Kothari's room to remove her IV and give her discharge instructions. Unfortunately, Mr. Kothari refused to accept instructions from Athula. Zakia, a female nurse practitioner on the unit, got the same response. In the end, the male physician had to give the instructions to both Mr. and Mrs. Kothari. Mr. Kothari simply refused to take orders from a nurse, and a female one at that.

131   An Iranian mother and father admitted their thirteen-month-old child, Ali, to the pediatrics unit. After three days of rigorous testing and examination, it was discovered that Ali had Wilms tumor, a type of childhood cancer. Fortunately, the survival rate is 70 to 80 percent with proper treatment.

Before meeting with the pediatric oncologist to discuss Ali's treatment, Mr. and Mrs. Mohar were concerned and frightened, yet cooperative. Afterward, however, they became completely uncooperative. They refused permission for even the most routine procedures. Mr. Mohar would not even talk with the physician or the nurses. Instead, he called other specialists to discuss Ali's case.

After several frustrating days, the oncologist decided to turn the case over to a colleague. He met with the Mohars and found them extremely cooperative. What caused their sudden reversal in behavior? The fact that the original oncologist was a woman.

Even though the Mohars had described themselves as "Americanized," the Iranian tradition of male authority was still strong. They could not accept a woman making life-and-death decisions for their son. Ali's treatment was too important to be decided by a woman.

Several weeks later, it became necessary to insert a permanent line into Ali to administer his medication. The nurse attempted to show Mrs. Mohar how to care for the intravenous line, but Mr. Mohar stopped her. "It is my responsibility only. You should never expect my wife to care for it." Throughout each encounter with the hospital staff, Mrs. Mohar remained silent and deferred to her husband.

Interestingly enough, the nurses had few problems with the Mohars. They were treated with respect because, as Mr. Mohar stated, they were functioning under the direction of the physician. Their only problem was in understanding why the Mohars initially refused treatment for Ali. They had assumed that because both parents were educated in American universities and had described themselves as Americanized, they would accept the American ideal of equality. The stress of their son's illness, however, had made them revert to traditional ways.

The dual role of father and male is evident in the following case study. Magdi Bal was a twenty-seven-year-old woman from Saudi Arabia. Her father was at her bedside when Danielle was doing her preoperative assessment. The surgery Ms. Bal was about to undergo could result in sterilization. Danielle wanted to make sure that she understood before signing the consent. The problem was that her father refused to allow her to sign. Mr. Bal was insistent that she not have a hysterectomy under any circumstances.

The staff was outraged. If the surgeon found uterine cancer, as he expected, a hysterectomy might be the only thing that could save Ms. Bal's life. The physician, Dr. Allen, spoke with her. She said that she wanted to leave all decisions to her father. Dr. Allen spoke next with Mr. Bal. He was adamant—no hysterectomy, no matter what. The physician had no choice but to proceed without compromising her reproductive system.

Danielle spoke with Mr. Bal while Ms. Bal was in surgery. He explained that if she could not bear children, she would not get married. If she could not marry, her worth would be greatly diminished in the eyes of their culture.

Saudi culture is strongly male dominant. It was entirely consistent that an unmarried daughter, even a twenty-seven-year-old one, allowed her father to make all the decisions. Once she married, her husband would take over that job. Furthermore, it is common in Saudi Arabia for a woman to live with her husband's family after marriage. If Magdi Bal could not marry, she would be a burden to her family for the rest of her life.

The doctors and nurses involved in the case later met to discuss it. All were angry with the father for his apparent lack of concern regarding his daughter's health. The women were particularly angry with Magdi for not being more independent. They were further incensed when Danielle told them what Mr. Bal had said. "We are not baby-making machines and our ability to have a productive life is not dependent on having children!"

Once they had vented their anger, they realized that it was not their place to judge. The patient had maintained her rights—in this case, the right to choose someone else to make the decision. They recognized that their values were different from that of the patient's; in other words, they achieved a measure of cultural relativism.

Men as Spokespersons

133   A nineteen-year-old Saudi Arabian woman named Sheida Nazih had just given birth. Her husband, Abdul, had been away on business during most of their ten-month marriage but brought her to the United States to have their baby. He moved into the hospital room with Sheida immediately after she gave birth. He kept the door to their room shut and questioned everyone who entered, including the nurses. The nurses were not happy with this procedure but felt they had no choice except to comply.

Although Sheida could speak some English, the only time she would speak directly to the nurses was when Abdul was out of the room. Otherwise, he answered all questions addressed to her. He also decided when she would eat and bathe. As leader of the family, Abdul felt it was his role to act as intermediary between his wife and the world. This behavior is often interpreted as a sign of domestic violence, and can create additional confusion for Western health care providers (see case study #145 below).

Gender Preferences

134   The gender of a child can influence the treatment it receives from the family. A fifteen-year-old Taiwanese boy named Henry Ting was dying of liver cancer. His parents spent as much time with him as possible during the year he was a patient at the hospital. One of them always spent the

night with Henry, even though they had two daughters, aged eleven and thirteen, at home. Henry's mother prepared most of his meals. His father often drove to Chinatown to obtain Chinese herbs they hoped would help his condition. Mr. and Mrs. Ting were extremely devoted parents—at least to their son. The nurses were shocked to hear the Tings state on several occasions that it would have been better if one of their daughters had cancer instead. Did they value their daughters so little?

As discussed in the previous chapter, sons play an important role in traditional Chinese culture. Henry was their only son. He would be the one to carry on the family name and care for them in their old age. If he died, whom could they rely on? Who would carry on the Ting name? Henry had always been given preferential treatment. The daughters understood their parents' attitude and did not seem to mind. It was the way things were. They, too, spent all their free time with Henry, catering to his frequent demands.

The nurses had difficulty accepting this situation. They understood the Tings' position intellectually but not emotionally. They responded by frequently pointing out how kind and sweet their daughters were. They also recommended that a psychologist meet with the family. The session was a waste of time. Although polite, the Tings refused to speak openly with the psychologist. In Asian culture, psychotherapy is reserved for the hopelessly mentally insane and carries a great deal of stigma. It is not surprising that they would not speak with him.

After a year in the hospital, Henry died. Two years later, his parents had still not recovered. They visited the cemetery daily. The elder daughter did volunteer work at the hospital to help "pay" for the care Henry received, and the younger daughter planned to join her when she became sixteen.

In a situation such as that involving the Tings, nothing can be done to change the parents' attitudes. Although it may be difficult, nurses should try to understand their point of view. Preference for sons is so strong in some cultures that, according to reports from countries such as China and India, there are many fewer females than would be statistically expected. This is thought to be due to differential care of sick children (i.e., ill sons are taken to the doctor right away; when daughters are sick, parents "wait and see") as well as selective abortion and infanticide.

Female Purity

Sexual Segregation

In the Muslim world, female purity is a major concern. This can have important repercussions in a health care setting.

Parey Assadian, a first-generation Iranian American, was admitted to the hospital with heart problems. Her condition was serious; the monitors

135

showed that heart rate was greatly elevated. She needed to be seen by a physician immediately, but her husband vehemently refused to allow the doctor entrance to the room. Why? Simply because the physician was male. As a result, Mrs. Assadian's treatment was delayed and her life endangered.

136   In a similar case, a twenty-eight-year-old Arab man named Abdul Nazih refused to let a male lab technician enter his wife's room to draw blood. She had just given birth. When the nurse finally convinced Abdul of the need, he reluctantly allowed the technician in the room. He took the precaution, however, of making sure Sheida was completely covered. Only her arm stuck out from beneath the blankets. Abdul watched the technician intently throughout the procedure.

Another time, the toilet in Sheida's room overflowed. Abdul flew into a rage when three men from engineering and housekeeping were about to enter the room after knocking. He refused to allow them in. The toilet went unrepaired until the couple left the next day.

Both incidents stem from the fact that among Arabs and Muslims, family honor is one of the highest values. Because family honor is tied to female purity, extreme modesty and sexual segregation must be maintained at all times. According to Geraldine Brooks, author of *Nine Parts of Desire* (1995), Mohammed, who did much to improve the condition of women in the Arab world, began the segregation of women in order to protect his wives from scandal. Others, wanting to emulate the great prophet, followed suit. No matter what the origin, however, it is a tradition that has become firmly ensconced in the Muslim world. Hospitals that do not have female physicians on staff should have a referral system so one can be found when needed. Female housekeepers should clean the rooms of Middle Eastern females. Male nurses definitely should not be assigned to female Muslim patients. Same-sex staff should be used whenever possible. For an example of a culturally competent approach to treating observant Muslim women, see the next case study.

137   Leila Habib was a sixty-seven-year-old Lebanese women with a high-risk mitral and tricuspid valve replacement. She was intubated and sedated, and doing poorly. She required a great deal of inotropic support. Maron, the nurse caring for her, said that with patients requiring as much care as Mrs. Habib did, cultural sensitivity and family support tend to get ignored. When Maron was introduced to Mrs. Habib's son, she noticed that he refused to shake her hand. She said that normally she would have taken this as a sign of rudeness, but because she had taken a diversity course, she decided to investigate it instead. She engaged the son in conversation, and learned that they had moved to the United States fifteen years earlier. He wanted to make sure that his family did not lose their cultural roots, so he made sure that his children learned both Arabic and English. He didn't want them to lose the ability to communicate with their relatives

in Lebanon, where they visited often. Maron asked how she could support him and his mother in a culturally appropriate manner. He explained that it was inappropriate to touch members of the opposite sex (thus explaining his lack of handshake), and requested that she safeguard his mother's modesty as much a possible. Maron said that it was easy to comply, and told Mr. Habib that she would request female nurses when possible. As a result, Mr. Habib expressed great gratitude and Maron was able to build a trusting and rewarding relationship with the family.

Female Genital Cutting

One of the more controversial traditional practices is that of *female circumcision* (as it is seen from an emic perspective) or *female genital mutilation* (FGM in the human and women's rights literature). The origins of this tradition are ancient and largely unknown, but it is consistent with Islamic beliefs regarding sexual desire. As Brooks explains, it is believed that Allah (God) created sexual desire in ten parts; he gave nine to women and only one to men (hence the title of Brooks's book cited above), which is why female sexuality must be kept under control. One way it is done is by keeping the woman covered, veiled, and segregated. Another method, used in some remote regions of Egypt, and particularly in other parts of Africa, is through FGM. It is believed that the practice reduces women's sexual desire, and that without it, women might be unable to control their exceptionally strong libido, and family honor might be lost. Although there has been a great deal of press coverage in the West of this tradition, nurses tell me that it is still extremely shocking to see.

In one instance, a twelve-year-old Somalian girl was admitted to the hospital with a temperature of 102 degrees. When the physician examined her, he discovered that her labia minora and labia majora had been sewn together so tightly that he could not insert a foley catheter. He had to call in a urologist to place the foley. The fever resulted from a severe urinary tract infection, likely caused by the infibulation. 138

In another case, an Egyptian woman in labor presented an unusual problem for the nursing staff. Her vagina was severely deformed, and they were unable to find any of the appropriate "landmarks." The entire area appeared to have been badly burned, yet no other parts of her body showed evidence of fire. The doctor and nurses were mystified. They did not realize that the woman had been "circumcised." 139

The procedure is generally performed when a girl is seven or eight years old. Older women will come in the night, hold her down, and then start cutting. The most minor form involves cutting off the tip of the clitoris. The most severe, known as infibulation, is the removal of the entire clitoris, labia minora, and parts of the labia majora. The outer lips of the vagina are then held together with thorns, sutures, or a paste like material. A small opening is left for urine and menstrual blood. The girl's legs are tied together for several weeks until she heals. As can be imagined, this practice often leads to myriad urinary, menstrual, and intrapartum problems, apart from the risk of infection and death at the time.

In 1985, a world congress was held in Africa in an effort to reduce or eradicate the practice. Surprisingly, the greatest opposition to the elimination of the custom came not from men but from older women and young girls. The older women wanted to maintain tradition. The young girls were afraid that if they were not circumcised, they would be unable to find husbands. Circumcision is seen as the ultimate proof of purity; why would any man marry a woman without a guarantee of her virginity?

In the years since that world congress, little if any progress has been made toward eradication of the custom. In fact, newspaper and magazine reports indicate that it is spreading, as African women move out of Africa. Anthropologists recognize that it is difficult, if not impossible, to merely eliminate a traditional cultural ritual; efforts would be better aimed at trying to promote the *sunna* form, which involves cutting only the tip of the clitoris, over infibulation. Complicating the issue is that opposition to the practice has been associated with the Western world, and there is much anti-American feeling in parts of the world where FGM is practiced. For some, continuing the practice is an anti-American statement.

When the topic of female circumcision came up in one of my nursing classes, a student from Sierra Leone, where most (if not all) women are circumcised, shared something of the experience. She explained that they only cut off the clitoris there; they don't do the full infibulation. She felt the loss of the clitoris was no big deal. Her attitude was that sex is for procreation, not fun, and since African men generally do not perform oral sex on the woman, the clitoris was superfluous. She added that women there still have orgasms, since orgasms are more psychological than physiological. She had no negative feelings toward female circumcision, although she did not plan to have her daughter circumcised because it generally isn't done there. She would not hesitate to do it if they were living in Africa. To help us understand her perspective, she explained that there are a year's worth of festivities associated with the circumcision. It is a very big time in a girl's life. It is followed by an arranged marriage and "devirginization" (her term). This is the ceremony in which the girl is "deflowered" by her husband while all the relatives wait outside for the bloody sheet and listen for the appropriate moans of pain.

In another class, I happened to have two Nigerian students, both of whom were circumcised. But they were from different tribes, and had very different experiences, despite the fact that both had the more minor *sunna* form, where only the tip of the clitoris was removed. The Igbo student had been circumcised as an infant and has no memory of it. She's had no problems resulting from it, and says if she had daughters and moved back to Nigeria, she would definitely have it done to them; it's their tradition. The Izon student had it done when she was twelve. Her parents did *not* want to have her circumcised, but she was the daughter of a prince, and the first-born girl of his first wife (he had three wives), so they had no choice. She remembers being taken by women from the village, who held her down and performed the surgery with a sharp razor. No anesthesia was used, nothing to stop the pain. At the same time, because she was a princess, they also "tattooed" her stomach, creating a geometric pattern of keloid scars across her entire belly. This woman was completely traumatized by the circumcision and tattooing. She said that when she gave birth to her child here in the United States, the midwife delivering the baby didn't realize she was circumcised. When she saw her vagina, she reacted in horror. This led my student to believe that something was wrong with her baby and she was very distressed and embarrassed. Her son is autistic, and despite her training in biomedical nursing, she attributes his condition to her circumcision. She is adamantly opposed to circumcision and said she would never have it done to her daughter. It was particularly interesting to note the differences between two women from the same country due to the fact that they are of different tribes.

Doctors and nurses caring for circumcised women should be especially sensitive to their needs and feelings. Female providers should be used whenever possible, and the patient should be kept draped for privacy. Physicians need to know how to handle labor and delivery, because the episiotomy must be done at an earlier stage. Above all, do not express any ridicule or judgment. You might, however, gently discuss the relationship between their infibulation and any health problems they may have experienced, so that they can make an informed choice for their own daughters. It might also be appropriate to let them know that the practice raises issues of illegality and child abuse in the United States.

Female Virginity

The importance of female virginity and purity are unfortunately well illustrated in the following case. Fatima, an eighteen-year-old Bedouin girl from a remote, conservative village, was brought into an American air force hospital in Saudi Arabia after she received a gunshot wound to her pelvis. Her cousin Hamid had shot her. Her family had arranged for her to marry him, as was local custom, but she wanted nothing to do with him. She was in love with someone else. An argument ensued, and Hamid left. He returned several hours later, drunk, and shot Fatima, leaving her paralyzed from the waist down.

140

Fatima's parents cared for her for several weeks after the incident but finally brought her to the hospital, looking for a "magic" cure. The physician took a series of x-rays to determine the extent of Fatima's injuries. To his surprise, they revealed that she was pregnant. Sarah, the American nurse on duty, was asked to give her a pelvic exam. She confirmed the report on the x-rays. Fatima, however, had no idea that she was carrying a child. Bedouin girls are not given any sex education.

Three physicians were involved in the case: an American neurosurgeon who had worked in the region for two years; a European obstetrics and gynecology specialist who had lived in the Middle East for ten years; and a young American internist who had recently arrived. No Muslims were involved. The x-ray technician was sworn to secrecy. They all realized they had a potentially explosive situation on their hands. Tribal law punished out-of-wedlock pregnancies with death.

The obstetrician arranged to have Fatima flown to London for a secret abortion. He told the family that the bullet wound was complicated and required the technical skill available in a British hospital.

The only opposition came from the American internist. He felt the family should be told about the girl's condition. The other two physicians explained the seriousness of the situation to him. Girls in Fatima's condition were commonly stoned to death. An out-of-wedlock pregnancy is seen as a direct slur upon the males of the family, particularly the father and brothers, who are charged with protecting her honor. Her misconduct implies that the males did not do their duty. The only way for the family to regain honor is to punish the girl by death.

Finally, the internist acquiesced and agreed to say nothing. At the last minute, however, he decided he could not live with his conscience. As Fatima was being wheeled to the waiting airplane, he told her father about her pregnancy.

The father did not say a word. He simply grabbed his daughter off the gurney, threw her into the car, and drove away. Two weeks later, the obstetrician saw one of Fatima's brothers. He asked him how Fatima was. The boy looked down at the ground and mumbled, "She died." Family honor had been restored. The ethnocentric internist had a nervous breakdown and had to be sent back to the United States.

Female Modesty

Female modesty is valued in many cultures. A Nigerian student shared that it may be difficult for a Nigerian woman to undress in front of a male health care provider, or to open her legs for a gynecologist. It would be best to assign female practitioners to such women. At the very least, they should be asked if they have a preference.

While at an imaging center for a mammogram, I overheard Clara, the   141
receptionist from El Salvador, closing the curtain where one of the patients
was changing her clothes. The patient must have said something about it
not being necessary, because I heard Clara say, "I don't want patients to
have to expose themselves, even though we're all women here." I spoke
to her about it afterward and she said that modesty is very important to
her. Like her own mother, she will not wear low-cut dresses or short skirts.
I was not at all surprised to find a Hispanic woman more concerned about
the modesty of her Anglo patients than they were. A Guatemalan student
once told me that her grandmother used to tell her that modesty is an
asset, and not to let anyone other than her husband see her body. It shows
that you have respect for yourself and gives you a sense of pride.

Southeast Asians consider the area between the waist and knees particularly private. Traditional Asian physicians did not touch a woman's
body except to take her pulse. Instead, the woman pointed to the corre-
sponding area of a doll to indicate the site of her problem. It was believed
that only a woman's husband should see her genitals. Knowing this, Erin
handled a potentially difficult situation with cultural competence.

Erin was caring for Hoang Van Chau, a sixty-seven-year-old-Vietnamese   *142*
patient with an irregular cardiac rhythm. As the nursing assistant began
to do the EKG, she exposed the patient's chest. Erin noticed that Mrs.
Hoang appeared embarrassed and tried to cover herself. The nursing assistant ignored her discomfort, and told her to keep her hands down. Erin
moved to the head of the bed and pulled the covers over Mrs. Hoang, but
kept them up so the nursing assistant could place the leads correctly. Mrs.
Hoang relaxed a bit. When she completed her task, Erin let down the blanket and made sure her patient was completely covered. Erin removed the
leads after the procedure and made sure the blanket stayed in place. Afterward, Mrs. Hoang took Erin's hand, bowed her head, and said "Thank
you." The satisfaction Erin felt at making her patient more comfortable
greatly outweighed the extra effort involved in keeping her covered.

Sofia Toledo, a sixty-five-year-old upper class Mexican woman, refused   143
to be dialyzed when she learned that her usual dialysis station was unavailable. She said she would wait until her next treatment, when she could
have her customary place. Unfortunately, this was not a viable alternative.
Missing a treatment could result in serious complications or even death.
When Julia, the nurse, asked her why the new station was unacceptable,
Mrs. Toledo was very vague.

Julia finally called Mrs. Toledo's daughter, and together they solved the
problem. Mrs. Toledo's usual station was unusual in that neither the nurses
nor the patients at the other dialysis stations could see it very well. The rest
of the stations were very open, designed for high visibility by the nurses.
To be dialyzed, the patient had to remove her pants and don a patient

gown. Her underwear was exposed during the process. Mrs. Toledo's sense of modesty, a quality very strong in Hispanic women, made the more open station intolerable.

Julia said that at the time she found Mrs. Toledo's behavior annoying. She and the other nurses saw it as a delay that would prevent them from leaving early. They did not want to have the extra work of moving machinery or remixing the dialysate. She did not understand the importance of modesty in Hispanic culture, but she did realize that it was important to Mrs. Toledo, a normally compliant patient. In this case, a screen or curtain might have alleviated the problem.

144   Farishta Amanullah, a female Afghani patient with open reduction and internal fixation of her left hip, was labeled as "difficult," along with the rest of her family. When Harold, her nurse, went to change her dressing, Mrs. Amanullah's family refused to allow him to do the procedure. When it was time for her physical therapy, her relatives were reluctant to allow her to get out of bed. Tammy, the charge nurse, was taking a course in cultural diversity and decided to explore the situation. She realized that, "difficult" patients are often patients with cultural issues. Tammy approached the family and asked if they had any concerns about Farishta's care. They told her that they preferred to have a female nurse care for her. They were also concerned about Farishta exposing her body in the open and revealing patient gown when she went to physical therapy. Tammy made sure to assign a female nurse to Mrs. Amanullah, and the director of the physical therapy department came to the room and told her that she would be given a second gown to cover her back and protect her modesty and dignity. Once these needs were addressed, Farishta and her family lost their status as "difficult" patients and in fact became quite cooperative. The beauty of cultural competence is not only that it makes medical care more pleasant for the patient, but that it also makes things much easier for the health care providers. All it takes is asking the right questions and making simple accommodations.

Domestic Violence

145   The next case both illustrates the value of modesty and raises the issue of domestic violence. It began when Betty, an RN, looked over the chart given to her by the triage nurse. Betty's first reaction was irritation over the paucity of information. The chart noted only that the patient, an Iranian woman, had multiple injuries resulting from a fall. No description of the injuries was given, and only limited vital signs were noted. When Betty entered the room to meet the patient, she saw a woman completely covered in the dark, heavy cloth known as a *chador*, accompanied by her husband. The patient, Noor Esfahani, looked up at Betty for an instant, and then put

her head down as her husband spoke. Mr. Esfahani explained that his wife was very clumsy and had fallen down the stairs in their apartment. Betty turned her attention to Mrs. Esfahani, asking simple, noninvasive questions. Before Mrs. Esfahani would answer in halting English, she would quickly look over to her husband for approval. When Betty asked her how she had sustained the injuries, Mr. Esfahani stopped her from responding with a quick shake of his head. He then repeated his original explanation.

Betty decided it was time to examine the patient, and asked her to put on a gown while she drew the curtain. Mr. Esfahani stepped outside the curtained area while she changed. Betty noticed that many of the bruises were on Mrs. Esfahani's stomach and inner thighs, locations inconsistent with the story of a fall down the stairs. At this point, Michael, the physician assistant on duty at the time, poked his head in the curtained area. Mr. Esfahani reacted to this intrusion by loudly yelling and pushing Michael, while his wife grabbed sheets and blankets to cover herself. Betty tried to calm the situation, but Mrs. Esfahani quickly dressed and left with her enraged husband against all Betty's protests.

This case raises two issues. The first has to do with sexual segregation. The most obvious sign of cultural conflict occurred when the male physician assistant entered the room and saw Mrs. Esfahani without her *chador*. Although it was acceptable for Betty, a woman, to see Mrs. Esfahani undressed, it violated cultural norms for Michael, a man, to do so. The larger issue, however, has to do with domestic violence. Medical students are taught that one of the first signs of spouse abuse is when the husband speaks for the wife. In cultures in which males are dominant, including many of those in the Middle East, Asia, and Latin America, it is common for the husband to answer questions put to his wife. It is a way of "protecting" her from the outside world. Health care providers should not jump to unwarranted conclusions based on that evidence alone.

In this particular case, however, given the inconsistency of the location of the injuries with the explanation provided, spousal abuse was likely. What should have been done, aside from keeping male health care providers out of the room? Betty might have been more amenable to allowing Mr. Esfahani to answer her questions; this may help gain his trust. When she was ready to examine Mrs. Esfahani, however, she might have asked an assistant to get Mr. Esfahani something to eat or drink in another room, thus leaving her alone with the patient. She might then have said to Mrs. Esfahani something along the lines of, "Most couples fight at home and men sometimes lose their temper and hit their wives. Has that ever happened to you?" It is important that the health care provider make the patient/victim feel respected and supported, that she is being taken seriously, that she doesn't deserve the abuse, and that the health care provider is her ally.

Several nurses who work in an emergency room commented that they frequently see cases of domestic violence among Mexican immigrants. One said that she has had to testify against the husband for spousal abuse in two separate cases. One case involved a twenty-seven-year-old man who beat his fifteen-year-old wife badly enough that she suffered head injuries and required sutures to her face and mouth. She was holding their five-month-old son at the time. In the second case, the wife was not as badly injured, but the state pressed charges, even though the wife refused to do so.

Another nurse reported that she has been asked on two separate occasions by Mexican employees not to report their husbands for abuse.

146   In one instance, Marta Villegas, a thirty-seven-year-old Mexican woman, had come into the emergency department after being beaten by her husband. The attending physician reported it to the police. Mrs. Villegas begged Rowena, her nursing supervisor, to tell the police that it was an accident; her husband didn't really mean to hurt her. Rowena told her that she could not do as she requested; she was concerned for her welfare. She offered some alternatives to returning home, but Mrs. Villega refused them. She knew that her husband would be even angrier now that the police were involved, and she feared reprisals.

Is spouse abuse a part of Mexican culture? No. However, aspects of Mexican culture and the living conditions of Mexicans in the United States may make it likely. Traditional Mexican women are taught that a good wife should be submissive and take orders from her husband. She should not question him, but rather stand behind whatever he decides, even if she disagrees. She must also be tolerant of his behavior. The traditional male role emphasizes the concept of *machismo*. While a man with *machismo* is one who works hard, is a good provider, and lives up to his responsibilities, the term can also refer to a man who is a heavy drinker and can hold his alcohol, traits that are both socially acceptable and proof of manhood. There is a strong correlation between alcohol and spousal abuse. In addition, increased exposure of Mexican Americans to urban violence and poverty lead to feelings of alienation, powerlessness, and hopelessness—all conditions known to be associated with domestic violence. There is also a high degree of violence toward women in rural Mexico by husbands who migrate back and forth between the United States and Mexico. Many women feel that they must be subservient and obey their husbands, and accept violent treatment. "He works so hard for us. If he beats me when he's home, that's okay. It's only for a few weeks. It's a very small sacrifice for all he does for us."

It should be noted that as difficult as it is for physicians to get American women to admit to being victims of domestic violence, women from Middle Eastern, Asian, and Latin American cultures might be even more reluctant to discuss the issue. In these male-dominated cultures women may be both less likely to see domestic violence as a problem issue and less likely to report it. In addition, immigrant women from these cultures are generally dependent upon men for support, and there is greater stigma attached to divorce. It will take an extraordinary amount of sensitivity on the part of the health care provider to get a woman to open up about her situation. It is important to explore options with the victim, especially resources within her own family.

Summary

What conclusions can be drawn from these cases? In general, same-sex physicians and nurses should be assigned if possible when dealing with non-Anglo ethnic groups. Try to keep patients' genitals covered whenever possible. Be alert for cases of domestic violence, but don't assume that simply because a man speaks for his wife he is abusing her. Recognize that sex roles and authority figures vary, though males generally hold the dominant position. Use that knowledge when dealing with patients or families from other ethnic groups. This advice may rankle many women, who may interpret it as reinforcing male domination. Perhaps it does, but if the goals are patient compliance, smooth working relationships, and the best possible patient care, this will be the most expedient way of achieving those goals.

Key Points

- In many cultures, males are the decision makers. Respect family dynamics.
- If your patient comes from a culture which practices sexual segregation, do your best to assign female caregivers to female patients.
- Be especially sensitive to the needs and feelings of circumcised women.
- Try to maintain the modesty of women whenever possible.
- Inquire about the needs and concerns of your patients.
- Realize that domestic violence is an extremely complicated issue for women from many other countries.

Chapter 8
Staff Relations

Not only is the patient population culturally diverse, the staff population is as well. In addition to Anglo staff, hospitals frequently have large populations of doctors from Asia and the Middle East, nurses from the Philippines and Mexico, and orderlies from a variety of countries. This chapter addresses some of the problems and misunderstandings that can occur when hospital staff members from diverse cultural backgrounds interact, as well as some of the problems that occur as a result of differences in training.

Nurses and Doctors

A frequent source of problems stems from the differing status of both women and nurses in the United States and in other countries. In many other countries, particularly those of the Middle East and Asia, men have much higher status than women. In general, women are to obey men. Further, physicians often have very high status. Even in the United States, doctors have always had much higher status than nurses; they have many more years of education, and use their skills to "cure" patients; nurses merely "care" for patients. In recent years, however, nurses as a group have moved toward greater professionalism. Many are obtaining advanced degrees. In many hospitals physicians and nurses are taking more of a team approach, rather than the traditional hierarchical one. Younger nurses have grown up with the influence of the women's movement. More men are going into the profession. For these and other reasons many nurses, particularly the younger ones, are refusing to be subservient to physicians. This is not the case in many other societies, where traditional sex roles combined with the hierarchical nature of the health care profession create an even larger gap between nurses and doctors. This can lead to conflict between traditional foreign-born and American-trained health care providers.

The Role of the Nurse

The role of the nurse varies from country to country as do expectations of appropriate behavior. In the United States, nurses are seen as an essential part of the health care team. They use critical thinking skills and the nursing process to assess, plan, and evaluate each and every aspect of patient care. They

- provide professional technical care;
- provide nonspecialized care (e.g., bathe patients, assist with bedpans, take vital signs);
- serve as patient advocates;
- provide psychosocial care;
- educate the patients about self-care.

Critical thinking is an essential skill for nurses. It involves openness to questioning and the ability to reflect on the reasoning process. The goal is to ensure safe nursing practice and quality care. Nurses must be able to look at the entire situation—the tasks, staffing, patient load, and acuity—in order to organize and prioritize their workload. RNs are expected to analyze the entire situation and think critically before delegating any tasks, especially to unlicensed staff such as nursing aides.

Managers at many hospitals say they have had numerous problems with nurses trained in other countries. Their technical skills are often excellent, but they often fall short in areas of patient advocacy and psychosocial care. They may not demonstrate the level of critical thinking skills required for the job. It's not that they are incapable of doing these aspects of the job, but in many cases, they simply may not know that it's expected.

For example, a nurse trained in the Philippines said when she came to the United States, she had trouble clarifying doctor's orders and decisions. Because physicians are in a position of authority, she didn't feel she could question them. In the Philippines, such behavior would be seen as "deviant and rude." Patient education was also difficult for her, because it was not emphasized in the Philippines; nor was psychosocial care. The family took care of any emotional needs.

A nurse working on a unit where many nurses were brought over from India to work in the intensive care unit (ICU) and telemetry floor said they had a lot of problems getting the Indian nurses to advocate for patients, answer questions for patients and family members, and use critical thinking skills in anticipating the needs of the patients. She learned that in India, a nurse is more of an assistant to the physician. The physician is always nearby, and is the one who talks with the patient. In India, nurses never discussed the disease or care plan with the patient or family members.

An American nurse working in Egypt reported that Egyptian nurses have little autonomy. They are essentially "handmaidens" to the doctors. The medical residents perform many of the tasks done by nurses in American hospitals while the nurses merely serve as aides to the physicians. Critical thinking is not part of the job requirement.

A nurse trained in Vietnam said that RNs there usually perform the duties done here by LVNs—monitoring blood pressure, changing dressings, and administering medication. They were not expected to do patient education, discuss the patient's condition, do personal care for the patient, or provide psychosocial support. They were trained to listen to physicians and *follow* their orders, not *question* them.

Duties of the Nurse

147   Vuong Hue disliked her job as a nurse when she first arrived in America from Vietnam. Before fleeing her native country for her life, she had been happy in her nursing position. However, she soon learned, nursing in America was far different from that in Vietnam. In Vietnam, she had but one function: to provide professional technical care. Nurses were responsible only for giving medications, taking vital signs, and changing dressings per doctors' orders. They were not required to attend to the patient or family's emotional needs. Nor did they have to bathe, feed, or turn the patient, or make the patient's bed. Her coworkers thought she was stuck-up because she acted as if bathing patients and cleaning bedpans were beneath her dignity. It wasn't that, exactly; she just wasn't used to having to do it. As any American-trained nurse will admit, that is not the most pleasant part of the job! Psychosocial nursing was unnecessary as well; more than that, Hue viewed it as improper. The patient's family took care of personal issues; it was rude for her to pry into their personal lives.

It took Hue several years, but she eventually became accustomed to the different roles that American nurses must take. Her coworkers no longer saw her as stuck-up. It might be helpful for American hospitals to have special in-service programs for foreign nurses to discuss explicitly the differences in nursing roles in various cultures. It would go a long way toward avoiding misunderstanding.

Patient Advocacy

148   Before he left the hospital for the evening, Dr. Akram wrote orders for Mr. Harriman, a patient with emphysema, indicating not to use oxygen greater than one and a half liters, and not to do pulse oximeter checks or arterial blood gases. Tula, Mr. Harriman's nurse, was concerned because too much oxygen can shut down the patient's respiratory drive, while not enough

can provide less-than-optimal care to the patient. Without those diagnostic aids, there is no way to know how the patient is doing and what treatment would be most appropriate. Tula suspected that Dr. Akram didn't want these things done because he didn't want to be disturbed in the night with problematic values that he would then be obligated to treat. Mr. Harriman was acutely ill, and complaining that he felt like he needed "more air." The problem, however, was that Tula didn't feel that she could question Dr. Akram's authority. Not only was he chief of internal medicine, but he was from Pakistan and had very traditional ideas regarding the authority of the physician and subservience of the nurse. And, in fact, Tula shared his notion of the authority of the physician, so she said nothing (this case is taken from Galanti 2007).

In fact, as a nurse working in the United States, it is Tula's *job* to question the physician's authority if she feels it is in the best interests of the patient. It is part of being a patient advocate. There are ways in which this can be done, however, that minimize the potentially confrontational nature of advocacy. Tula might have said something along the lines of, "Dr. Akram, I feel like I need some direction. I know you've ordered no more than one and a half liters of oxygen, and I know it's important not to give COPD patients too much. However, Mr. Harriman is complaining that he feels like he needs more air, and I'm not comfortable *not* doing an ABG to see what his oxygenation is like, and not monitoring him with a pulse oximeter. I can see you have a plan, but I'm worried about my inability to assess him properly. Would you be able to take a moment and help me understand what your plan is, and how you'd like me to respond to his needs?" After the physician clarifies his expectations, this often opens a chance for more dialogue. A last statement might be along the line of, "If he gets more symptomatic, what would you like me to do for him before I call you, so you can have the information you need?" This kind of approach maintains respect for the physician while still accomplishing the advocacy role of the nurse.

When American-trained nurses do their job as patient advocates, they can come into conflict with foreign-trained physicians who do not expect such assertive behavior from nurses, based on physician-nurse relationships in their native country.

Annie, an American female nurse, had an unpleasant encounter with Dr. Rao, an East Indian male physician. He had ordered her to restrain a patient whom she felt did not need restraining. When she confronted him with her opinion, he became angry and accused her of questioning his authority. When she asked him why he felt the patient needed to be restrained, his only response was, "Because I'm the doctor and I feel that the patient needs to be restrained." Annie was angry at this obvious non-answer. As a nurse, part of her job was to be a patient advocate, and she did not feel that the patient's needs were being met. As their argument continued, an East Indian nurse who had observed the encounter told the physician that this was America and the rules were different here. "This is not India where you can do whatever you want because you men are the only ones who have rights. You need to explain to her why you want the patient restrained, because the patient has rights and the nurse has the right to know why she's restraining the patient."

Upset by the support given Annie, Dr. Rao left the room. The East Indian nurse explained to Annie that his ego was hurt; in India, it is considered highly disrespectful for a nurse to question a doctor. Does this mean that nurses should never question Indian physicians? Obviously not. Perhaps the most effective solution would be to have all foreign health care personnel participate in an in-service seminar on the culture of the American health care system. However, until that happens, because such physicians are not as likely to change their behavior, nurses who want to communicate more effectively with such coworkers might utilize a less confrontational approach.

150   Dr. Fukushima, a Japanese physician, ordered Lisa to give a patient a certain dosage of a medication. Lisa refused on the grounds that the dosage might be harmful to the patient. Dr. Fukushima insisted, but she was adamant. The interesting twist to this situation is that when Dr. Fukushima reported Lisa to her supervisor, the physician suggested that she should have *agreed* to give the medication, but simply not have done it.

Asians generally believe it is important both to avoid conflict and to show respect for authority. Rather than refuse directly, it is more appropriate to agree to the supervisor's face and then not follow through. Americans, in contrast, feel it is important to be direct and honest. Disagreement is not avoided. Assertiveness is valued, as is an egalitarian ideal. Dr. Fukushima's major complaint was not that the nurse disobeyed him but that she disagreed to his face, thereby denying him proper respect.

It would be easy to suggest that nurses dealing with Asian physicians take that advice, but it is not that simple. Laws require nurses to follow through on orders they agree to. Nurses would be well advised, however, to remember that Asian men are very concerned about their dignity and self-esteem. And, once again, hospitals should consider offering foreign-born physicians training in the role of nurses in American hospitals.

151   Jackie, a thirty-five-year-old Anglo American nurse, and Dr. Hussein, a sixty-seven-year-old Iraqi physician, got into a conflict over the timing of the discharge of a female cardiac patient. Dr. Hussein called in his order to discharge the patient. Jackie did not think the patient was ready to be discharged and refused, saying that she would not discharge her until the physician examined her and read her chart. Jackie had noted several problems on the chart the previous day. Dr. Hussein was furious that she would

not follow his orders, and insisted that she do so. Her response was to threaten to call the unit medical director, a threat that she carried out. When Dr. Hussein came into the hospital, he became enraged over what he saw as her failure to "respect his word." He demanded to know why she was questioning his judgment. She replied, "Because your decision was not the right thing for the patient." They ended up taking the case to administration.

What went wrong? From the nurse's perspective, she was merely doing her job as patient advocate, since in her best clinical judgment the patient was not well enough to be discharged. From the physician's perspective, a subordinate and a female was questioning his authority and abilities. She was operating along American rules, he along Iraqi ones. Jackie also felt that he valued the patient in question less than he did some of his other patients because she was a woman. She also felt that he might have been prejudiced against the patient because he had made a notation in her chart that she had a reputation for promiscuity. What could have been done to avoid the problem? This is a tricky situation. Most Americans, particularly but not exclusively women, would probably take the side of the nurse. However, if the goal is to achieve a smooth-running workplace, compromises must be made. When the physician first called, Jackie might have respectfully asked if she could review the events of the weekend with regard to the patient. For example, she could say, "I'd like your medical opinion on the events that have occurred since you last saw the patient. I think you'll understand why I'm worried about her." By showing respect for his opinion, he might have been more willing to listen to her. Instead, by demanding that he come in to see the patient before she would discharge her, she forced him into a position of having to defend his honor and clinical skills. Often, people feel compelled to maintain their position simply because someone has challenged it. Even if he had refused, she then might have suggested that he choose another physician to review the patient's chart and status. This would protect the nurse from a legal standpoint and the physician might have been more comfortable with the opinion of a professional equal. At the point when he asked why she was questioning his judgment, rather than acknowledge that she was doing so, she might have said that she was not questioning his judgment, but rather doing her job as patient advocate. Pleading that "the system" caused her to do this might have helped him save face. Because nurses are legally and ethically responsible for acting as patient advocate, he might see that by checking on the patient, he would be helping her out. He could later have explained to her the importance of respect to him and explain that her lack of it made him feel defensive.

The comments of an American nurse who worked for several years in Egypt may shed some light on the attitudes of physicians from Middle

Eastern countries. Nursing is a highly stigmatized occupation for women. Wages are very low and, as a result, nurses expect tips or *baksheesh* for patient care tasks, further contributing to the lack of professional status.

Note that the suggestions for handling the situation put most of the burden on the nurse, despite the fact that her behavior was more in line with American cultural values. The truth is, it is more realistic to expect the nurse to make accommodations than the physician. However, I would once again urge all hospitals to have an orientation for foreign-born staff on American cultural values in the workplace.

In case you're wondering how the incident was resolved: the patient remained in the hospital and had open-heart surgery the following week. The relationship between the doctor and nurse was permanently destroyed.

152   The following interaction between an authoritarian Asian physician and an Anglo nurse illustrates how understanding culture can help improve working relationships. Kayla was a staff nurse on a medical-surgical floor when she first met Dr. Ling, an Asian physician. They got along well until Kayla transferred to the diabetes clinic. Clinic protocols allow nurses to order new medications, adjust medications, and order lab work as needed, as long as they get a physician to sign the order. When Kayla would ask Dr. Ling for his signature, he would rudely question her as to why she felt the medication was necessary, and on a few occasions refused to sign, stating that he disagreed with the medication she had ordered. After learning more about Asian culture in a cultural competence course, she realized he probably perceived her approach as showing a lack of respect, despite the fact that she was following clinic protocols. She then changed her approach. Rather than just asking him to sign the medication start, she would go to him, explain the situation with the patient, tell him what she was considering, and ask him what he would like done. Kayla reported that Dr. Ling is much more receptive to this approach, probably because it allows him to feel respected and in control. Taking the extra time to do this has repaired the lines of communication between them. Although it could be argued that Dr. Ling is the one who should change his behavior, that is probably less realistic than having Kayla apply her cultural knowledge to achieve the results that she wants.

Patient advocacy also involves asking questions, something foreign-born nurses may have a problem doing.

153   Dr. Kim, a Korean physician, ordered Isra Srisai, a Thai nurse, to give Digoxin to a patient. Isra, however, thought he had said Dilantin. When she repeated the order to Rowena, the charge nurse, Rowena corrected her. She had been in the room at the time Dr. Kim gave the order. Rowena told Isra that she would have to clarify the order with Dr. Kim. Isra, however, clearly did not want to do that. Rowena, concerned with the safety of the patient, went ahead and clarified the order with Dr. Kim and

presented the information to Isra. Fortunately, nothing bad happened in this situation.

However, nurse managers often report that Asian-trained nurses are hesitant to question physicians, either when they disagree with their orders or when they don't understand an order. Asian respect for authority often conflicts with the patient advocate aspect of the nurse's job in the United States. If the physician is male and the nurse female, respect plays an even bigger role. It is important that foreign-trained nurses be taught that patient advocacy is an important aspect of their job; that it is okay to challenge a physician if they think it is in the best interests of the patient. Suggestions for how to do that in a diplomatic manner can be found in some of the previous cases. Nurses are expected to think critically.

Many Asian-trained nurses also find it challenging to ask questions when they don't understand something, for fear of seeming incompetent. Again, hospital orientation for foreign-trained nurses should emphasize that it is expected they will ask questions.

Critical Thinking

Susan, an Anglo American nurse, asked Marietta, a nurse trained in the 154 Philippines, to cover for her while she took a lunch break. Susan told her that one of her patients, Mrs. Smith, would probably want her pain medication while she was at lunch, since it would be exactly four hours since her last dose. Mrs. Smith had severe chronic back pain and was in for some tests. As predicted, Mrs. Smith called for the nurse while Susan was on her lunch break. Marietta brought her the pain medication. Mrs. Smith told Marietta that her pain was much worse and that she now also had a terrible headache. Marietta told her to see if the medication also helped her headache, and to tell Susan if it didn't. When Susan returned, Marietta reported to her that she gave Mrs. Smith the pain medication. When Susan made rounds after returning from her break an hour later, she ended in Mrs. Smith's room. Susan didn't start with her because she was (supposedly) recently assessed by Marietta. She found Mrs. Smith slumped over and slurring her words; she was having a stroke. Her physician ordered procedures and medications to treat and manage the severity of the stroke, but unfortunately, it was too late to prevent lasting affects. Mrs. Smith could no longer speak and was paralyzed on her dominant side. Marietta asked Susan whether Mrs. Smith had ever told her about her headache. She hadn't, because she was having a stroke when Susan first saw her (this case is taken from Galanti 2007).

This tragedy occurred because the role of the nurse is different in different countries. *In many other countries, nurses are primarily seen as aides to the physician. They are not expected to think on their own.* They are expected to carry out physicians' orders, but not to analyze and assess patients on their own. Nursing in the United States has a much broader scope. Nurses are expected to apply critical thinking skills in the performance of their job. In this case, Marietta should have done several things beyond simply giving Mrs. Smith her pain medication. She should have also:

- assessed Mrs. Smith and found out that the headache was a new symptom, and assessed for pain level;
- documented the complaint of headache and pain level;
- checked the chart for other diagnoses that would trigger a need to call the doctor (such as severe headache in a patient with hypertension);
- checked on Mrs. Smith or assigned an aide to sit with her;
- reported the headache to Susan when she first returned.

Whatever happens to the patients during Susan's break is Marietta's responsibility. Just because the only thing Susan told Marietta about this patient is that she would need pain medication doesn't mean that that is all Marietta has to do for her or Susan's other patients. As an RN in this country, Marietta is expected to assess any situation she walks into and handle it appropriately. The sudden severe headache was a signal that a stroke was occurring. This was essentially ignored by Marietta, an RN who had been trained to assess symptoms. It was her duty to report any significant change in the patient's condition to the physician. Unfortunately, Marietta didn't do her job, and the patient suffered permanent damage because of it.

In the United States, nurses are accountable for everything they do or don't do. RNs are responsible for people's lives in the same way that physicians are responsible for lives. Marietta was too task oriented and took her "assignment" too literally. She merely gave out the pain medication as requested, and neglected the more important aspect of her job—to use critical thinking skills to assess and care for *all* the patients she sees. It is essential that hospitals realize that the scope of nursing is different in different countries, and that they provide orientation and training on the specific expectations for nurses working in the United States.

Psychosocial Care

I often hear the same complaint from Anglo Americans who have been hospitalized. They criticize what they perceive as the "coldness" of Filipino nurses. I brought this up in one of my classes that was populated largely by Filipino nurses. I was curious as to how they would respond to the charge. They explained to me that what is perceived as "coldness" is intended to be a display of "professionalism." It is a sign of respect to show distance. Further adding to the Anglo perspective is the fact that Filipinos are trained not to be physically affectionate, so they may not touch as much as other nurses. I think that another contributing factor is the lack of training in psychosocial care. In the Philippines, as in many parts of the world, family members remain with the patient day and night. They take care of any psychosocial needs the patient might have. In fact, it would be considered rude for a stranger to involve herself in the personal life of a patient. In the United States, the situation is different. Family members often live in different cities, often in different states. Thus, they may not be available to take care of the patient's psychosocial needs. Nurses are expected to take on that function. While, of course, there will be much individual variation, it is important for all foreign-born health care professionals to receive training in American culture, so that they understand that distance is perceived not as professionalism but rather as a lack of warmth and caring and that psychosocial care is not only appropriate, but expected.

Cultural Influences on Nursing

In addition to differences in role expectations, cultural differences also impact the relationships between nurses on the job and lead to misunderstandings and conflicts between nurses of different cultures.

Gender Role Conflict

Traditional dominant and subordinate roles can be a source of friction among hospital staff. For example, Ikem Nwoye, a Nigerian male nurse assistant, would have what one nurse described as a temper tantrum whenever a female registered nurse asked him to do something. At other times he would sulk and simply leave the room. What he would not do was take instructions from a woman. In Nigeria, men are considered superior to women. Men tell women what to do, not the reverse.

Nursing is a hierarchical profession in which orders are followed according to rank, not sex. The nurses thus expected the nurse assistant to do what they told him. As a Nigerian male, Ikem felt that he should not have to take directions from females, despite his lower professional ranking. Unless someone with this cultural disposition can be placed under the supervision of another man, it will be difficult to maintain a viable working relationship on the floor.

A Team Approach

Josepha DeLeon, a Filipino nurse, did not get along well with her coworkers. The nursing staff on her unit was composed of two Anglo Americans, two Nigerians, and Josepha. She felt her coworkers were taking advantage of her, because they would ask for assistance whenever they saw her. Josepha was angry over what she perceived as obvious discrimination. She cheered herself by reminding herself that she was a better nurse than the others; she could do her work without their help. In addition, she was not lazy like they were. She took care of her patients; the other nurses insisted that their patients take care of themselves.

One day, Rena, one of the Anglo nurses, was unusually friendly, so Josepha opened up to her. As they got to know each other better, Josepha shared her feelings of being taken advantage of. Rena explained that it was common procedure for the nurses to help each other with their work. Rena confided that the others thought Josepha was being snobbish and proud because she never asked for help. They saw what Josepha had interpreted as laziness on the part of the others as being team players. Rena also explained that American health care providers believe that independence is important and encourage self-care among their patients.

Josepha was stunned by Rena's revelations. Rena offered to help bridge the communication gap between Josepha and her coworkers. Rena explained to the others that Josepha was trying to save face by never asking for help; she didn't want them to think she couldn't do her job. Josepha began to teach her patients self-care and to ask her coworkers for assistance. Over time, the cross-cultural misunderstandings were resolved, and Josepha's coworkers became her best friends.

Leadership

157   Problems also arise from the traditionally passive female roles valued in most Asian cultures. Myung Soon Park, a Korean charge nurse in intensive coronary care, was an excellent worker. She was quiet, industrious, and knowledgeable. She gave the patients good care and was proficient in using the specialized equipment in the unit. In her role as charge nurse, however, Myung Soon was perceived as incompetent. She was unable to lead. She did not offer strong guidance to her staff. She did not counsel or reprimand them. She was indecisive and became apologetic when anyone made a mistake.

Although Myung Soon's personality was partly to blame, her submissiveness was consistent with the traditional role of Korean women. Korean culture is hierarchical, and the ideal woman is passive and subservient. She is taught to avoid conflict and maintain harmony. These values made it difficult for Myung Soon to perform the functions of a good charge nurse. Her coworkers liked her personally but were frustrated by her professional performance.

Myung Soon was aware of the problems she was having. Counseling helped her to realize she could not handle her job. She resigned as charge nurse but continued on as a staff nurse.

Passive Versus Assertive Behavior

A few examples have been given of the passive, submissive behavior of Filipino and other Asian nurses. Many other nurses, however, report the complete opposite. They say that Filipino nurses, for example, can be very assertive, to the point of aggressiveness. What accounts for this discrepancy?

As in any culture, people are born with personality traits that fall along a continuum. Different cultures, however, value and reinforce different aspects of the continuum. If a child is by nature passive and the culture reinforces passivity, socialization will be easy. If the child is by nature assertive, socialization will be difficult but possible. If when that child grows up, he or she moves to a country where assertiveness is valued, years of socialization to be passive may be suddenly undone, as the individual's true nature comes through. The assertiveness may even be exaggerated as a result of years of repression.

Thus, passive Filipino nurses are the ones who were by nature passive even before being socialized in that direction. It will be very difficult to train them to be assertive. The aggressive ones are most likely those who were socialized to be passive against their inherent nature and who now find in America cultural permission to be assertive.

Hierarchical Cultures and the Meaning of Criticism

Lourdes Balmonte was a sixty-year-old Filipino patient with pulmonary tuberculosis. Her physician had ordered strict home isolation, but she was not complying with the order, so the county health department issued an order that stated that if she did not remain in her home, she would be confined in a treatment facility or jail, according to the California Code of Regulations. Josephine, a middle-aged Filipino nurse with the county health department, was asked to act as translator when Rebecca, an Anglo American county health supervisor, served Mrs. Balmonte the medical order. Josephine agreed, both out of respect for her supervisor, and because she was still on probation at the job and wanted the chance to impress Rebecca with her interpreter skills. Unfortunately, it didn't work out that way. 158

Several times during the session, Rebecca stopped to criticize Josephine. First, she criticized her for smiling and talking in too friendly a manner to Mrs. Balmonte. "This is a legal matter and must be taken seriously," she informed Josephine. She also disapproved of the way Josephine was doing the interpreting. Josephine's translations were often much longer than Rebecca's statements. Each time this happened, Rebecca would pause and give Josephine a look of annoyance.

After the session, Rebecca pulled Josephine aside. She thanked her for helping out and said she had done a good job, but then pointed out some things that Josephine should remember next time. First, she explained, "Smiling and making friendly gestures will make the patient take the matter lightly." Then she said that she should translate only the exact words and not embellish on the speaker's statements. Josephine was devastated by Rebecca's criticism, and two months after the incident was still worried that it would affect her probationary status.

What went wrong? What Rebecca didn't realize was that the dynamics of the situation put Josephine in a very awkward position. Filipino culture is very hierarchical, and the elderly are accorded great respect. Even though Josephine was only translating for Rebecca, she felt extremely awkward having to scold Mrs. Balmonte for disregarding the doctor's orders. Smiling and making friendly gestures was Josephine's way of conveying respect. She felt she had to go beyond merely translating Rebecca's words, for there are many English words that lack an exact counterpart in Tagalog. Josephine felt that the only way she could translate Rebecca's meaning was by citing examples. In addition, she had to use both Tagalog and the Ilocano dialect from the region Mrs. Balmonte was from.

Did Josephine explain all this to Rebecca? No. Rather than defend her actions, Josephine merely listened quietly to Rebecca's criticisms. It would have been against Filipino cultural norms to "talk back" to her supervisor. Instead, Josephine has been afraid that the incident will result in her not getting the permanent position once her probationary period is over. She feels caught between her values and her job, and fears that honoring her values will cause her to lose her job. In all likelihood, Rebecca has forgotten the incident, or, if she remembers it, assigns little or no importance to it. Because of the hierarchical nature of Filipino culture, criticism from a supervisor carries much more impact than it does in our more egalitarian culture. Rebecca probably saw her comments as helpful; Josephine saw them as questioning her ability to do her job.

This situation underscores the need for cultural competence training. Rebecca needed to understand some of the difficulties in translating from one language to another, as well as the awkwardness of putting Josephine in a position where she had to "scold" an elder. Had an older or male Filipino been available to act as translator, it would have been a better choice. Josephine needed to understand that criticism has a different connotation in American culture and that it is acceptable to offer an explanation for one's actions without appearing to show a lack of respect. Practice in cross-cultural communication skills is essential.

Hierarchical Cultures and Offering Help

Another incident involving status differences concerned an Anglo nurse   159
who was in the habit of helping out nurses' aides when her own work was
done. All the aides but one accepted Sylvia's assistance gratefully. When
Sylvia offered to help Celina, a Filipino aide, with the difficult care of her
quadriplegic and stroke patients, she declined. Celina was insulted, because in the hierarchical culture in which she had been raised, a supervisor would offer to help only if she felt the worker could not do her job
properly. Sylvia responded, "Don't be silly! It's crazy to do this alone. You
could get a bad back." Celina took the words "silly" and "crazy" literally
to mean that Sylvia thought she was mentally ill, a condition that is highly
stigmatized in Filipino culture. No wonder she was insulted. Celina also
interpreted the original offer of help to mean that Sylvia thought she was
slow and incompetent. Her *amor propio* (self-esteem) had been wounded.

Sylvia learned of Celina's reaction from another Filipino aide. Celina
had not said anything directly to Sylvia because she wanted to avoid conflict and show respect for authority—important values in Filipino culture.
Although Sylvia had at first perceived this as "going behind her back," she
later learned that the use of a third party go-between is common in many
Asian cultures. The next time Sylvia saw Celina, she apologized, saying
that she had not understood how Celina felt. Celina explained that she
had been raised with certain ideas and was having trouble adjusting to
American ways. For example, Filipino nurses feel they have failed if they
do not complete all their work on an eight-hour shift. American nurses
will simply tell those on the next shift that they were very busy and could
not finish everything. By the end of their discussion, Celina and Sylvia
came to an understanding and never had any more problems. It is important to realize that words and actions can carry greater significance than
we might intend.

Medicine

The Role of the Doctor

A cross-cultural misunderstanding between a Middle Eastern male physician and an Anglo American female patient sheds interesting light both
on the roles of men and women in Middle Eastern culture and on the roles
of doctors and patients.

Roberta Hansen had been admitted for pneumonia. Abbas Mehraban   160
had been called in to consult when her own physician found some lab
results that he could not explain. Dr. Mehraban questioned her about her
symptoms, and then told her how he was going to treat her condition. He

neither explained his rationale nor included her in the decision-making process. When Ms. Hansen tried to question him about her treatment, he gave her only vague responses. She became increasingly angry and yelled at him, using profanity. Her behavior angered the physician so much that he resigned from the case.

Most Americans can probably understand why Ms. Hansen was angry, but what about Dr. Mehraban? In the Middle East, doctors are seen as authority figures and their decisions are not to be questioned. Ms. Hansen breached proper Middle Eastern etiquette regarding patient and physician roles. Dr. Mehraban needed some teaching on the relationship between American patients and their physicians, including the patient's "right to know."

Although by American standards Dr. Mehraban would not be considered a "good" doctor, there are other cultures in which he would. In many Native American and Asian cultures, a "good" doctor does not need to ask the patients a lot of questions. The doctor should be able to diagnose the patient by reading the proper signs. This is in direct conflict with the American approach, which values physicians who *ask* their patients a lot of questions and *listen* to the responses. "Good" American doctors may thus unwittingly lose the respect of some their patients. Perhaps they might judiciously choose to have the nurse ask questions of the patient before they begin their examination.

The American legal and medical systems recognize the patient's right to know all the details of his or her condition. The high incidence of medical malpractice suits also dictates that physicians share all possible complications of any surgical procedure or medication. Such openness and honesty can have a negative effect when dealing with patients from other ethnic groups.

In China and Japan, where doctors are seen as authority figures in a hierarchical and patriarchal society, patients are told little about their condition. Lawsuits are extremely rare. The physician is expected to know best and to use good judgment. If the patient has cancer, the family might be told, but the patient is rarely given the diagnosis. Asians have a tremendous fear of cancer, perceiving it as a death sentence, even though many forms can be successfully treated. Patients told they have cancer often mistakenly assume the situation is hopeless and give up. Loss of will to live can lead to premature death.

Imagine the situation of a Chinese or Japanese patient new to the United States who is told he or she has cancer. The physician may believe it is easily treatable through a combination of surgery, radiation, and chemotherapy. The patient, knowing that doctors never reveal a diagnosis of cancer to a patient, assumes the worst. He or she is going to die immediately. The psychological ramifications can be devastating. In such a case, it might be advisable to use a technical medical term other than cancer and begin by emphasizing the success of treatment.

Language and Communication Problems

Speaking in the Native Language in the Workplace

One of the problems that is mentioned most frequently in my workshops is that of nurses speaking their native languages in the hospital. This is a very interesting issue, with legitimate explanations on both sides.

The American nurses dislike it when coworkers speak in their native language for a number of reasons. Most important, when, for example, a Filipino nurse speaks to a coworker in Tagalog in front of a patient, the patient may think they are talking about him or her.

Harry Davisson, a Vietnam veteran, was in the recovery room following surgery. Two nurses in the room were speaking to each other in Tagalog about their weekend plans. Mr. Davisson was disoriented due to the anesthesia. He thought he was in a prison in a foreign country. When he later told his family about this, they were quite upset and went to speak to the charge nurse. They felt that the two nurses had added unnecessarily to their father's anxiety. A staff meeting resulted. Such incidents can be easily avoided by strictly following the rule of only English around patients.

It is less critical, but still hurtful, when nurses speak in their native tongues around other employees. American nurses frequently report feeling left out when they walk into a room and several Filipinos continue to converse in Tagalog. They see it as extremely rude.

When this issue comes up in groups, I usually ask the Filipinos to explain why they speak in Tagalog at work, even though they can speak English. Some of their answers are to be expected; others are surprising. Among the expected answers: away from their native land, it brings them a sense of home and belonging. As one Filipino stated, "Speaking our own language reassures Filipinos that even though we are here in the United States, we still have something that bonds us together, something that we have in common that gives us a sense of belonging." In an emergency situation, they feel they can communicate more quickly in their native tongue. Some things, like jokes, do not hold up in translation. They may be embarrassed by their thick accent in English.

I've heard two other explanations that were less predictable. One is that in Filipino culture it is important to show respect to your superiors in the hierarchy—for example, anyone who is older than you. Tagalog has different words that do this; English does not. It could therefore be seen as rude for a Filipino to talk to an elder in English. Another explanation has to do with the fact that, in the Philippines, speaking English is associated with higher social status. If you are Filipino and speak to another Filipino in English, you will be seen as conceited, as acting as though you are better than the other person.

In discussions of the topic at hospital workshops, Filipinos often seem surprised that the other nurses don't just ask to join in. Anglo Americans say they could never do that; it would be rude. They want to be invited. I was recently reading an interesting book by Sarah Lanier, *Foreign to Familiar*. She contrasts hot-climate "inclusion" cultures with cold-climate "privacy" cultures. In inclusion cultures, individuals know they are automatically included in conversations, meals, and any other activities of the group; it is rude to hold a private conversation. In privacy cultures, private conversations are acceptable and people are expected to ask permission to interrupt a conversation. It's clear that such a distinction may be in operation when an Anglo nurse enters a break room and finds a group of Filipinas in conversation. They may assume she knows she's included, while she may feel she cannot join in without an express invitation.

It is important for native English speakers to realize that Filipinos are not intending to be rude when they speak in Tagalog in the presence of others. But Filipinos must also realize that it can be very distressing to patients and can make non-Filipino coworkers feel excluded. Open discussion of all perspectives is usually quite effective. The most equitable solution is to allow hospital employees to speak in their native tongues when on break, as long as no one else is around. When nonspeakers enter the room, they should immediately switch to English. Under no circumstances, however, should they converse in anything other than English around patients (unless, of course, the patient is fluent in that language).

Open Communication

The next example underscores the importance of open communication. Making assumptions is dangerous, while asking questions can lead to greater harmony.

162   Natasha was an Eastern Orthodox Christian nurse from Russia. She was the only non-Filipino staff member on the unit. The Filipino nurses organized a potluck dinner one night, and kept inviting her to have some of the Filipino delicacies they had brought. The problem was that it was in the 40-day period before Easter, when Eastern Orthodox Christians do not eat meat. Many of the Filipino delicacies have meat in them. Rather than tell them the truth, she would simply refuse, saying, "Thanks, I'll have some later in my break." Finally, they just made up a plate for her with her name on it. This created conflict for her, since she felt it was disrespectful not to eat food that is given to you, but eating it would go against her religious beliefs. She finally decided the only thing to do was tell them

the truth. When she did, they burst out laughing. They had perceived her refusal as some sort of discrimination—as if she was "too white" to touch their food. They also thought it might be because she was anorexic; she was very thin. It never occurred to them that it could be a religious issue. This incident broke the ice and now their communication is much more open and filled with questions about each other's religion and culture.

Demeanor

Eva, a Chinese nurse, was caring for a young girl. Eva had been directed   163
by the intern to keep the girl under close observation because she was becoming diaphoretic and pale. After two hours, these conditions continued to worsen, and she was breathing abnormally. Eva was alarmed, but tried to stay calm and composed when she called the patient's doctor. The physician was unavailable, so she spoke to his associate. She said, "The patient is looking dusky. Can someone come to look at this patient?"

Three minutes passed, and the patient's condition had worsened, yet none of the doctors had arrived. Eva eventually had to call a "code" over the phone, which summoned every doctor at once.

Afterward, Eva was chided by her nurse manager for not indicating the seriousness of the patient's condition when she called the doctor. She should have used the word "now" emphatically, and conveyed a sense of emergency by her tone of voice.

Eva was offended at first, but then realized it was a cultural problem. As a Chinese woman, she had been raised to control her emotions and to remain calm in an emergency. Since that incident, she has learned to employ more "American" communication skills and call for help more assertively when necessary.

When "Yes, I Understand" Means "No, I Don't"

Marsha, an Anglo nurse, attempted to assess the knowledge and techni-   164
cal skills of the critical care nurses in her hospital. Most were from China, Laos, Korea, Vietnam, and the Philippines. The first phase of testing involved a written exam focusing on general principles. Confusion reigned, and the scores were low. Thinking the problem lay in the language of the test, Marsha rewrote the exam. In the new version, the nurses had only to answer yes or no to questions about their knowledge of a specific procedure (e.g., "I understand the principles of hemodynamic monitoring"). Over 90 percent of the questions received a "yes" response. Disturbed by the contradictory results of the two tests, Marsha interviewed several of the test takers, asking open-ended questions that required them to demonstrate their knowledge. Although their English was proficient, many were

unable to answer correctly. Why did they say they understood procedures and principles they clearly did not?

Recall the discussion in Chapter 2, "When 'Yes' May Mean 'No.'" The Asian nurses were probably too embarrassed to admit they did not know something. Education is highly valued, and a lack of knowledge indicates a lack of education. The result is a loss of self-esteem. The lesson here is the same as earlier—try to avoid asking yes or no questions. Ask that people *demonstrate* their knowledge instead.

165   Speaking of exams, Celine was involved in an incident with Malea, an older Filipino nurse who was taking a CEU class in order to renew her nursing license. As Celine passed the nursing station, she saw Malea asking two younger Filipino nurses the answers to some of the questions. They answered several questions for her before making excuses about having to get back to work. Celine noticed them rolling their eyes when Malea wasn't looking. When Malea later asked Celine for help, she refused. For Celine, it was a matter of integrity. She saw Malea as "cheating." She felt the younger Filipino nurses helped Malea out of respect for elders and avoidance of conflict. It's likely that for Melea, it was a matter not of cheating, but of the kind of sharing that is expected in a culture that values *inter*dependence.

"Please" and "Thank You"

166   Patty, an Anglo nurse, had been working with Maria, a Korean nurse, for two years. Their relationship had been rather hostile. Patty felt that Maria was a very bossy person, never saying "please" or "thank you." Maria was also perceived as rather cold and standoffish, as evidenced by the fact that she would rarely call her coworkers by their first names, especially the older ones, even after being asked to do so. Patty decided to interview Maria for a class assignment in order to understand her better.

When discussing her values, Maria explained the importance of respect in Korean culture. People will call each other by their last names, and use special terms when addressing people older than themselves. However the hierarchy works two ways. When asking something of someone younger than yourself, it is unnecessary to say things like, "please," and "thank you," since you are in the higher position and can act more informally. The respect is understood. Because Maria was older than many of the other nurses, she rarely said "please" or "thank you," assuming it was understood. It wasn't; the others merely thought she was rude.

After the interview, Patty realized that her impression of Maria had been totally wrong, and they soon became friends. Nurses must recognize that what is polite in one culture may be seen as rude in another. Open discussion of cultural differences, however, can help alleviate such problems, as it did in the case of Patty and Maria.

Leslie reported that her hospital had recently hired five new Korean *167* nurses. Unfortunately, they did not get along well with the rest of the nursing staff. They rarely said "please" or "thank you" and were generally perceived as rude. Leslie was reading an earlier edition of this book and suddenly realized that the Korean nurses were older than the other nurses on the unit and probably felt that "please" and "thank you" were understood. Leslie then showed the other staff nurses the section on "Please" and "Thank You." She reported that morale on the unit is much improved. Sometimes, all it takes is a little understanding.

"With Your Permission"

An American physician and professor, consulting in Japan, was about to *168* address a group of university physicians; it was fully understood by all that he would give his talk in English. He nevertheless prepared a brief introduction in Japanese, concluding with the statement, "My Japanese is limited so, with your permission, I will continue in English." When he asked his Japanese secretary if his statement was grammatically correct, she seemed uncomfortable, and upon further questioning she reluctantly admitted that, grammar aside, it was not appropriate for someone of his stature to ask the audience for permission, and that this would diminish the audience's ability to respect anything else he said. Instead, she suggested, he should merely announce that he would continue in English. In this context "asking permission" was entirely pro forma—in American culture, it would be seen as a polite gesture. In Japan, however, it was considered inappropriate from someone in a position of authority, and would likely result in a loss of respect for the person doing the asking. It is easy to see how a Japanese physician working in an American hospital, who believes that asking is inappropriate, would likely be perceived by subordinates as rude and could inadvertently cause major conflicts with other staff.

Religious Conflicts

Medical personnel also face conflicts between their duty to patients and their own religious beliefs.

Elisa, a nurse of the Jehovah's Witness faith, was temporarily transferred *169* to the intensive care unit, where she admitted a patient with gastrointestinal bleeding. He required several units of blood. Elisa refused to hang the blood. It was against her religious beliefs even to participate in a blood transfusion. Reluctantly, she did agree to watch it infuse after someone else started it.

Carmen, a Filipino nurse, was informed that she was to be the circu- *170* lating nurse on a therapeutic abortion. She immediately began to cry and told her supervisor that she would leave work unless her assignment was changed. Carmen was a devout Catholic and refused to participate in an abortion. Joyce, her supervisor, was upset. Other Catholic nurses had worked on abortions before. Besides, she was short of personnel and cases were already running over schedule. Joyce agreed to find someone else to circulate, but she asked Carmen to gather the equipment and supplies for the case. Even this was a problem. "If I set down the room, it's just the same as if I were doing the case," she explained. "I have assisted or aided in taking a life." Joyce finally changed her assignment, but not without some resentment.

A number of the medical students I taught said they would have problems performing abortions. In order to best serve the needs of their patients, they should be able to discuss, without prejudice, the various options available to the pregnant woman, and be prepared to refer their patients to someone who is not uncomfortable with the procedure.

171 David, an RN from the step-down unit, applied for and received a position as an ICU/CCU staff nurse. When he received his new schedule, he went to the unit director to ask to have his schedule changed. He was scheduled to work on Saturdays. As an Orthodox Jew, he needed Saturdays off in order to observe the Sabbath. The unit director refused his request, saying that it would cause them to be understaffed on Saturdays. Rather than compromise his religious practices, David decided to go back to the step-down unit. The unit director could have handled this situation better by asking if any of the other nurses would be willing to trade days off with David. When some of the other ICU/CCU nurses who had Saturdays off found out what happened, they said they would have traded with David. Unfortunately, the unit director didn't think to ask.

It is often very difficult for people to understand others' religious practices, especially when they cause inconvenience. But it is best, whenever possible, to avoid giving assignments that conflict with individuals' religious convictions. Jehovah's Witness nurses, for example, can be assigned to coronary care or well-baby units, where there is rarely a need to hang blood. Days off can be traded. Nurses assigned occasional duties that conflict with their religious beliefs can arrange to switch tasks with a coworker. If their beliefs get in the way of their job too often, however, they should be advised to look for a new job.

Summary

Given the vast cultural diversity of the health care staff in American hospitals, it is sometimes surprising that more conflicts do not occur. The major problems seem to stem from the different roles that doctors and nurses are assigned in different cultures. These are often accentuated by gender role differences. Thus, male physicians from male-dominated countries tend to be even more authoritarian than American male doctors, and female nurses from such countries tend to be more submissive than American nurses. Rules of polite behavior vary cross-culturally, and are often a source of misunderstanding.

Because rules of behavior are rarely made as explicit as rules of grammar or rules of the road, conflicts and misunderstanding abound. In most cases, such problems can be avoided or resolved through cultural education. Doctors and nurses from foreign countries could be required to participate in an in-service on the culture of the American hospital system. In addition, workshops in which staff are led to discuss the way things are done in their culture, in which participants can feel free to ask questions and share their feelings, are often successful in alleviating conflicts and misunderstandings.

Key Points

- One source of staff conflict is the fact that in many cultures, men have much higher status than women, as do physicians compared with nurses. This can create conflict between American-born nurses and foreign-born physicians.
- The scope of nursing in the United States is much broader than that in other countries in that it includes both patient advocacy and psychosocial care. It also requires critical thinking skills.
- Foreign-trained clinicians need to be trained in the "culture" of American medicine and nursing.
- American nursing is based on a team approach, while Asian nursing is based on a hierarchical one. This is the source of much conflict and misunderstanding between American- and Asian-trained nurses, particularly with regard to the meaning of offering help.
- American patients often expect to be a partner in the decision-making process. In other countries, physicians often take on a more paternal role.
- When foreign-born nurses speak in their native tongue at work, they do so for many reasons; they don't realize that nurses who speak only English feel excluded.
- Many problems between staff could be resolved through more open communication.
- Try to avoid asking yes or no questions; when checking competence skills, look for a demonstration of skills.
- Words like "please" and "thank you" are often thought to be understood, and thus unnecessary to say, in hierarchical cultures.
- Try to avoid giving assignments that conflict with individuals' religious convictions.

Chapter 9
Birth

Increasingly, people enter the world in a hospital. Birth is an emotional and generally painful occasion imbued with cultural ritual and thus, once again, we find the potential for misunderstanding and conflict, as well as opportunities for cultural sensitivity.

Ante Partum

Pregnancy Taboos

A classic anthropological theory, formulated by Bronislaw Malinowski, states that under conditions of chance or uncertainty, when things cannot be controlled by knowledge, people will turn to magic. Pregnancy certainly fits that condition, and thus it is not surprising that there are numerous beliefs regarding what one should and should not do during pregnancy. One of the most common taboos involves reaching your arms over your head. Doing so is thought to result in the cord being wrapped around the baby's neck. This belief is found among African Americans, Anglo Americans, Asians, and Hispanics.

172   An Anglo student once told me that when she was pregnant she was warned against raising her arms. As a nurse, she knew there was no medical connection between the activity and the presumed result, so she ignored the warnings. Her son was born with the cord wrapped around his neck. Fortunately, the hospital staff were able to save him. She said that the next time she became pregnant, she was careful not to lift her arms above her head, even though she knew there was no medical basis for it. Why take a chance?

This case illustrates the probable origin of many of the pregnancy taboos found around the world. Throughout human history, childbirth has been a dangerous enterprise. There is much that can go wrong during pregnancy, much that we have little or no control over. After carrying a child for nine months, learning that the child is dead at birth must be devastating for the mother. The first question that must come to her is "Why?" If she can figure out why the baby died, she can prevent it from happening again. Looking back over all the incidents that occurred during pregnancy, you find one that makes some sense to be connected to the baby's death. You then avoid that behavior the next time you are pregnant, and warn other women as well. If the next child is born healthy, that is seen as proof that the connection was valid. And thus, a taboo is born. Pregnancy taboos include such things as avoiding lunar eclipses to prevent the baby from being born with a deformity (Mexican), postponing a baby shower until after the birth to prevent the baby being stillborn (Sephardic Jewish), and avoiding tying knots or braids, which can result in a difficult labor (Navajo).

Miscarriage

Bella took care of Anna Boswell, a Romany (Gypsy) woman in her mid-twenties who had come in for a procedure following a miscarriage. Her physician had written orders for her to be discharged. Bella noticed that female relatives surrounded the patient. They asked Bella numerous questions about how much bleeding would occur, and argued against her being sent home. Bella explained that bleeding was normal, and that if any complications arose, Mrs. Boswell could call her physician. Yet she begged to be allowed to remain in the hospital, offering cash to stay.

173

Why were they all so concerned about normal bleeding, and so adamant about remaining in the hospital? It reflects the Rom concept of *marime*, or impurity. The Rom believe that a woman is "impure" for six weeks after giving birth. (Note that six weeks is the length of the traditional lying-in period, and the time biomedicine says it takes the woman's uterus to return to normal after childbirth.) As long as Mrs. Boswell was bleeding post-miscarriage, she was considered "polluted." It also explains why no males were in the room. Men are to avoid women while they are *marime* so they do not become contaminated. Culturally, it would be much easier for her if she were to stay in the hospital until the bleeding stopped and she was once again *wuzho* (pure).

Dietary Prescriptions and Food Cravings

As described in the chapter on diet, many Asian and Hispanic cultures practice a system of hot/cold body balance. Pregnancy is generally thought to be a hot condition, and thus foods which are considered "hot" are restricted so as not to exacerbate an already out-of-balance body. Unfortunately, many foods that are high in protein are considered to be hot foods. It is important for physicians to carefully assess the pregnant woman's diet to make sure she is getting enough protein. Many Hispanic women also avoid iron supplements and prenatal vitamins, which are considered hot. A culturally competent physician will recommend that she take them with a neutralizing "cold" beverage, such as fruit juice.

Food cravings are a common feature of pregnancy. I've been told that among many African American women it is believed that unsatisfied food cravings can cause birthmarks on the baby. One example a student gave me was a woman who craved fried chicken, but whose husband refused to go out and get it for her. Their baby was born with a birthmark in the shape of a drumstick.

Some women crave and eat nonfood items, a condition known as pica. Mexican American women often crave magnesium carbonate or the ice that forms in the freezer. Unsatisfied cravings (*antojos*) are thought to cause injuries or birth defects in the infant. Among African American women, the traditional pica was for clay dirt, which was later replaced by Argo laundry starch.

Physicians should be aware of the prevalence of pica, and question pregnant patients about it in a nonjudgmental manner.

Prenatal Care

A common complaint of labor and delivery nurses is that many women do not seek prenatal care. Although this can sometimes result in problems, the primary difficulty is a conflict in perception. Americans are raised to see pregnancy and birth as medical conditions; births usually occur in hospitals under the supervision of doctors. Medical culture also values education (thus, childbirth classes) and a future time orientation (preparation for the coming birth). Prenatal care is an essential part of this package.

One nurse reported that in the small California town in which she lives, Hispanic women often do not come in for a prenatal visit until they are well into their second trimester. This is the case even though the health care staff repeatedly try to "educate" the women, using translators. The nurse who shared this wondered if it was due to stubbornness on the women's part, or because translators did not adequately relay the information during their previous pregnancy. Neither is the most likely explanation. Pregnancy is generally seen as a "normal" condition rather than an illness and thus not necessarily requiring the assistance of a physician. Elder women provide the support and information needed. Time orientation is focused on the present rather than the future; hence a frequent lack of prenatal care. Although health care professionals should strive not to impose their values upon their patients, if a woman who has just given birth can be predicted to have high-risk pregnancies in the future, health care providers should take the time to explain why prenatal care will be important next time.

A Vietnamese nurse said that Vietnamese women believe that pregnancy is a natural process and, like many Hispanic women, therefore do not seek prenatal care. They also may avoid prenatal vitamins, thinking they are too "hot" (in the yin/yang sense) for the fetus. Instead, they will eat more "cold" (yin) foods during the last trimester. These foods include eggs, steamed rice, and pork.

Labor and Delivery

Labor Pains

Individuals respond differently to pain, although cultural norms often dictate how it is expressed. This holds true for the pains of labor.

Miguela Coronel, a Filipino woman, was delivering her baby. Her contractions were very strong and closely spaced. The baby was positioned a little too high, and there was some discussion of a possible caesarean section. Despite her difficulties, she cooperated with the doctor's instructions and labored in silence. The only signs of pain or discomfort were her look of concentration and her white knuckles.   174

Doris Davis, an African American woman, lay in the delivery room across the hall, moaning and groaning. Although the delivery was progressing normally, her cries increased in intensity. Finally, her bloodcurdling yells resounded through the halls. The hospital personnel compared the behavior of the two women and naturally rated Mrs. Davis's unfavorably. Why was she acting like such a baby? Why couldn't she control herself as Mrs. Coronel did?   175

Cultural differences account for the behavioral differences. Miguela Coronel's culture values stoicism; Doris Davis's culture does not. Filipinos believe that a woman must experience pain and discomfort as a part of childbirth. To express these feelings, however, brings shame upon her. This is true in most Asian cultures. One of my students from mainland China once explained to me that any woman, "even a queen," would be ashamed to cry out in childbirth. A nurse who works frequently with Hmong patients noted that it is imperative to monitor their facial expressions very closely to determine if they've entered Stage 2 (pushing) because they are very stoic, rarely uttering a word during the process. As Anne Fadiman describes of the mother in *The Spirit Catches You and You Fall Down* (1997), moaning or screaming is thought to thwart the birth.

The culture of African Americans does not place such restrictions upon its women. Varied emotional expression has always been a part of Black culture. Mrs. Davis was culturally appropriate in expressing her pain. Another Black woman might have suffered in silence and still have been culturally normal.

176   Maricela still remembers the time she assisted Galilahi Hayes, a Cherokee patient, while doing a rotation at a birthing center. Although it was her first baby and she was already four centimeters dilated when she came in, she was in complete control. Her grandmother, a Cherokee healer, was attending her, along with her mother and sister. Despite not using any pain medication, Mrs. Hayes barely made a sound during the ten-hour labor. When the time came to deliver the baby, her grandmother helped her into a squatting position while the midwife sat on a stool at the side of the bed. After twenty minutes of pushing, the baby was born into the grandmother's hands. Maricela said it was the most amazing birth she had ever witnessed.

In contrast, Mexican women are notorious for loud behavior during labor and delivery. It is often possible to identify a Mexican woman in labor simply from the "aye yie yies" emanating from her room. Although this chant can be annoying to nurses and patients alike, it is actually a form of "folk Lamaze." To repeat "aye yie yie" several times in succession requires long, slow, deep breaths. "Aye yie yie" is not just an expression of pain; it is a culturally appropriate method of relieving pain. However, it is important, as always, not to stereotype. As a third-year medical student doing her obstetrics rotation noted, although the two Hispanic women she observed giving birth to their first child were loudly yelling, another Hispanic woman having her fourth child was completely silent during labor and delivery. It is important to remember that there are always individual differences; some cultures simply allow free expression while others discourage it.

177   Women from some cultures may profit greatly from emphasizing their pain during childbirth. A labor and delivery nurse reported that the most difficult patient she ever attended was Robabeh Farag, an Iranian woman, who yelled and screamed for the entire duration of her labor. After she delivered their child, her husband presented her with a three-karat diamond ring. When her nurse commented on the expensive gift, she responded dramatically, "Of course. He made me suffer so much!" Iranian custom is to compensate a woman for her suffering during childbirth by giving her gifts. The greater the suffering, the more expensive the gifts she will receive, especially if she delivers a boy. Her cries indicate how much she is suffering. A young Iranian doctor recently told me that when his wife has a baby, he will present her with a diamond ring or a watch.

American nurses value cooperation; a cooperative patient is one who is stoic and follows directions. Uncooperative patients, like Robabeh Farag, are often avoided. How can hospital personnel deal with the variety of expressions of women's pain during labor and delivery? As one nurse put it, there are techniques for controlling pain that are more effective than yelling, but the delivery table is hardly the place to educate women in coping skills. If nurses understand why patients behave the way they do, however, they can be more supportive.

As for the patients themselves, it might be very disconcerting for an Asian woman accustomed to controlling her emotions to labor next to a highly expressive Mexican or Middle Eastern woman. Ideally, women might be placed in rooms with women from cultures similar to theirs. Unfortunately, this is not always possible. Sometimes, a brief explanation of cultural differences in the expression of pain might help, particularly for a first-time mother who is laboring next to a woman from a more expressive culture.

Labor Attendants

It is currently standard American practice for a woman's husband to assist her in labor and in the delivery of their child. Husbands are expected to be helpful and to attend to their wives' needs. Unfortunately, things do not always work out this way.

Naomi Freedman, an Orthodox Jewish woman, was in labor with her third child. She had severe pains, which were alleviated only by back rubs between contractions. Her husband asked Marge, a nurse, to remain in the room to rub his wife's back. Because she had two other patients to care for, Marge began to instruct him on how to massage his wife. To Marge's surprise, he immediately interrupted her, explaining that he could not touch his wife because she was unclean. Marge, assuming he meant she was sweaty from labor, suggested that he massage her through the sheets. In an annoyed tone, he again explained that he could not touch his wife because she was unclean. He then left the room. 178

Marge later learned from Mrs. Freedman that "unclean" referred to a spiritual, rather than a physical, condition. According to the Orthodox Jewish tradition, the blood of both menstruation and birth render a woman unclean and her husband is forbidden to touch her during those times.

Labor and delivery nurses must do everything for the Orthodox Jewish patient whose husband will not participate. This often generates resentment toward both the patient and her husband. Nurses sometimes try to avoid being assigned to Orthodox patients or assign another Jewish nurse to attend to them. As always, a good solution is education. If nurses understand why an Orthodox husband cannot get involved in his wife's labor, they may be more accepting.

An Arab husband can be similarly unhelpful during his wife's labor and delivery. After his wife Azar was admitted to the unit, Ahmed Ramzy told the nurse that he would wait outside. Realizing that her patient did not speak English, she asked him to stay and act as translator. At first, he refused, insisting that it was a woman's place to help in birthing, not a man's. 179

Since there were no Arab women available to translate, however, he reluctantly agreed to stay.

During her entire labor, Ahmed ignored Azar except to translate as requested. She was obviously having a difficult time, expressing her pain quite loudly, but he did nothing to comfort her. The staff grew angry with him. It was in fact inadvisable to insist that he stay with his wife during childbirth. Because it was inappropriate for him to be there, he felt extremely uncomfortable and did little to help her situation.

Some nurses have reported that Middle Eastern men often do accompany their wife or sister in the delivery room, but not to assist her. Rather, they are there to "protect" her virtue.

180   A similar case involved a young Mexican couple. Judging from her "aye yie yies," Juanita Guerrero was in a great deal of pain. When the nurse insisted that her husband, Carlos, attend to her, he very reluctantly entered the room. Rather than help soothe her by holding her hand, speaking gently to her, or wiping her brow, he stood in the corner. He looked up, down, everywhere but at her. The nurse became very angry. She felt that because he had gotten her into this position in the first place, he should be willing to comfort her.

181   In another instance, Julio Gomez, a fifty-one-year-old father-to-be for the sixth time, became so upset when the staff nurse insisted he join his mother-in-law and sister-in-law in attending his wife in the delivery room that security had to be called. Fortunately, the security guard was an older Mexican man who understood why Mr. Gomez preferred to be in the waiting room with his brothers, uncle, and sons. He explained to the staff nurse that the husband's responsibility was to be strong for his wife—*outside* the delivery room.

182   In Mexico, it is inappropriate for a husband to attend his wife during delivery. It is a woman's job—ideally the job of her mother. This may be related to the extreme modesty of Mexican women. American nurses who have difficulty believing that the modesty of traditional Mexican women can extend to her own husband should be told of the eighty-five-year-old Mexican woman with a tattoo of a small cross on her upper thigh. No one in her family—including her husband and daughters—had ever seen it. It is likely that during all the years of her marriage she had undressed in another room and made love in the dark. She told the nurse who was caring for her that she had done it in her wild and crazy youth.

Whatever the reason, a number of cultural traditions dictate that a husband not see his wife or child until the delivery is over and both have been cleaned and dressed. For those who find these cultural practices hard to understand, consider suddenly being forced to watch one's parents have sex. How would we feel? Would we stand there and coach them? Wipe their sweaty brows? Or would we stand in a corner, looking up, down, everywhere but at them? Sexual relations occur in the presence of children in some parts of the world but are taboo in American culture, just as it is taboo for a Mexican man to watch his wife give birth, though it is a common practice for American men. Younger, more Americanized Mexican couples may want to participate in the delivery process together, but it should not be assumed that the husband is the proper person to coach his wife in this situation.

In general, traditional Latina women often prefer that their mothers attend them in labor. This is also true of Asian women, although sometimes the mother-in-law is considered more appropriate. A Korean nurse shared this information in class one day, to the general shock and horror of the rest of the class. As she explained, traditionally, when a Korean woman marries, she goes to live with her husband's parents and spends much of her married life taking care of the needs of her in-laws. This is reversed during childbirth. Then, a mother-in-law must attend to the needs of her daughter-in-law, both during delivery and throughout the month-long lying-in period.

Caesarean Section

Chue Hong, a Hmong refugee woman, was pregnant with twins. Early in   183
labor, it was discovered that the second twin was lying across the uterus rather than head down. The attending physician recommended a caesarean section. The woman's husband and mother refused, stating their fear that she would die during surgery. Although the doctors and nurses continued to try to persuade the patient and her family that she should consent to the surgical delivery, they remained adamantly against it. As a result, the first twin was delivered without problem but the second twin died. The next morning, the husband returned and requested the placentas, explaining that they had to be separated in order to protect the live infant from death.

Why was the family so opposed to a caesarean section? Perhaps because, like many non-Christian rural Southeast Asians, they feared that souls are attached to different parts of the body. During surgery, they can leave the body, causing illness or death. In such a situation, there is little that the health care team can do except respect the wishes of the patient and family. This case resulted from a conflict in beliefs, and, in the United States, the patient has the right to refuse medical care.

Postpartum

Burying the Placenta

Farhana Setrak, a young Muslim Arab woman, was giving birth in a rural   184
hospital. Two older women accompanied her. She was very expressive in

her pain. During the long labor, several staff members heard the women talking about a burial. Although they didn't quite understand what she was referring to, the news quickly spread throughout the unit. There was much speculation on the part of the staff, especially since the women grew quiet right afterward. Were they fearful that they had been overheard? The women also wanted to know how soon after delivery the new mother and baby would be released. The staff grew concerned. Why was the family so secretive? Why were they so eager to leave the hospital?

Mrs. Setrak gave birth to a baby girl. Speculation continued, especially since some staff members knew that Arab culture often prefers sons to daughters. Was the family planning on killing the baby girl? Was that the "burial" they referred to?

Fortunately, no. It was the burial of the placenta that concerned the family, a fact known to the physician but one he had failed to communicate to the rest of the staff. Once the staff understood the situation, mother, baby, and placenta were quickly discharged so they could perform the ritual burial.

Many cultures have a tradition of burying the placenta. In her book *The Spirit Catches You and You Fall Down* (1997), Anne Fadiman describes how the Hmong word for placenta also translates to "jacket." It is this "jacket" that the soul must don at death in order to make the dangerous journey to the place where it will be reunited with its ancestors and await rebirth. Without the placental jacket, the soul is doomed to wander, alone and naked, for eternity. That is why the placenta must be safely buried. A traditional Arab belief holds that the future fertility of a woman is connected to the disposition of the placenta. Should something happen to it, the woman might be rendered sterile. This belief does not appear to be currently widespread among Arabs, and it is not known why Jasmine and her family wanted to bury the placenta, but health care personnel should not be surprised if a patient requests to take the placenta home. Holy Cross Hospital in Maryland has worked with the health department and its own infection control department to allow the placenta of African women to be stored in a container for them to take home for burial (see http://www.openhere.com/current/392093892.stm (2002)).

Umbilical Cord

In some cultures, parents may want to keep part of the umbilical cord. A Vietnamese student shared that in Vietnam the umbilical cord is dried and kept for good luck. Her mother still has her dried umbilical cord in a small box. Others put it in wine to drink. A Japanese student said there is a similar custom in Japan. Traditionally, the cord is dried and placed in a small box that the mother keeps for a lifetime; it is usually buried with her as proof that she gave birth to children and brought spirit to the future. The student said that when she herself gave birth in the United States, she would have liked to do the same, but was ashamed to ask. She thought it would be nice if nurses would remember to ask.

Breastfeeding

It is well known that the colostrum that fills a new mother's breasts before her milk comes in is rich in antibodies that fight infections to which newborns might be subject. Western doctors and nurses emphasize the importance of feeding infants colostrum. Many ethnic groups, however, refuse to do so.

Sofia Salgado, a Mexican American, gave birth to a son. The nurse   185
wheeled the baby into her room and handed him to her to be nursed. Instead, Mrs. Salgado pointed to her breasts and said, "No leche, no leche" (No milk, no milk). Pedro, her husband, explained to the nurse that she would bottlefeed now and breastfeed when she returned home.

According to the nurse who related this example, most Mexican women who gave birth in a hospital near the Mexican border followed the same pattern—early bottlefeeding, later breastfeeding. Because colostrum is so important, this practice worries health care professionals.

Many Mexican women believe they have no milk until their breasts enlarge and they can actually see it. Some perceive colostrum as "bad milk" or "spoiled" and thus not good for a baby. Many do not realize that nursing stimulates milk production. Still others are very modest and are embarrassed to expose their breasts while nursing in the hospital.

The best way to deal with this situation is through education. Explain the importance of colostrum to the baby's health. If the mother's concern is to provide "real" milk for the baby, tell her that nursing on the colostrum will help it to come more quickly. The new mother should also be given privacy while nursing her infant.

Similar advice could be given to the Vietnamese mother who refused to breastfeed in the hospital, explaining that she would do so when she returned home. The Vietnamese also believe that colostrum is dirty and often delay nursing until after their milk comes in.

Postpartum Lying In

Angela Wong, a Chinese American woman, had had a caesarean section   *186*
the day before. She was covered with eight blankets and sweating profusely; her patient gown was drenched. When Celia, the nurse's aide, tried to remove the blankets and offered her a sponge bath, she refused both. Lourdes, one of the other nurses on the unit, explained to Celia that Mrs.

Wong was practicing the traditional postpartum lying-in period. Lourdes then spoke to her about the importance of movement to recovery and in preventing pneumonia and deep vein thrombosis. In an example of cultural compromise, they came to the agreement that Mrs. Wong would take a short walk once a day, and that every couple of hours she would move in bed and practice deep breathing. Lourdes showed cultural sensitivity in respecting traditional practices, while at the same time promoting the kind of care she felt was necessary.

187   Maria Salazar was a thirty-two-year-old recent immigrant from Mexico with an infected caesarean section. She asked Tovya, her nurse, for some water. When Tovya grabbed the bedside pitcher to refill it, she discovered it was full. When Tovya pointed this out to her, she answered in Spanish, "Yes, but I have a fever and a cough, if I drink that cold water I will get even more sick." Tovya, who spoke some Spanish, was taking a course in cultural diversity at the time and was elated to see hot/cold beliefs in action. She then emptied the ice water and refilled it with warm water. Curious, Tovya asked her if there were any changes she would like to see in her treatment. Mrs. Salazar nodded her head. She said she didn't understand why the nurses kept insisting she do things that would make her ill—things like taking a shower. Didn't they understand she had a fever and had just delivered a baby? And why did they want her to spend so much time walking, when she knew she should stay in bed and rest as much as possible?

Angela Wong and Maria Salazar were both practicing versions of the traditional lying-in period observed throughout much of Asia and Latin America. For a period of time after a woman gives birth, her body is thought to be weak and especially susceptible to outside forces. The new mother is encouraged to avoid both exercise and bathing. These traditional practices come into direct conflict with Western health care, which promotes exercise and bathing for new mothers as soon as possible following childbirth.

The traditional practice in China is called "doing the month." It is important to keep the room warm, lest cold or wind enter the new mother's joints. Bathing is considered dangerous for similar reasons. No matter how hot the weather, a traditional Chinese woman will want the windows closed and the air conditioning off.

In Asia, health is believed to depend upon keeping the body in a state of balance. As stated earlier, pregnancy is generally thought to be a hot condition. Giving birth causes the sudden loss of yang, or heat, which must be restored. The most effective way to do this is to eat yang foods, such as chicken. Cold liquids should be avoided lest the system receive too great a shock.

Traditional Asian thought has it that the price for not "doing the month" is aches, pains, arthritis, and other ailments when one is old. Although practical circumstances may prevent a woman from observing the entire month, many want to practice at least a shortened version of it. This explains why the patients in the cases described above refused ice water in preference for warm and rejected bathing or exercise, insisting on keeping extremely warm.

As noted above, in Mexico the lying-in period lasts for six weeks, the time believed necessary for the womb to return to normal. The customs involved are essentially identical to those of the Asian practice: the woman is to rest, stay very warm, and avoid bathing and exercise. Special foods designed to restore warmth to the body are prescribed. Disregarding these practices is believed to lead to aches and pains in later life.

Another problem nurses encounter during the postpartum period involves Pakistani and East Indian women. It is traditional for them to have a female companion who does everything for the woman—feeding her, taking care of her hair, pouring beverages, and all infant care except breastfeeding. If no one is available to do these things for her, a Pakistani woman may expect the nurse to fill that role. This can lead to anger on the part of nurses, who tend to see such patients as demanding and lazy. Instead, they should realize that it is simply the way traditional Pakistani women have been raised to behave after childbirth. They may not know it is done differently in this country.

There are three additional points to be made about the postpartum lying-in period. First, it is designed to give a woman a period of rest between childbirth and returning to work. The women who practice this custom are usually Asian and Latin American. In these cultures women traditionally did not return to office work, but went back to physical labor in the fields. Because they usually had large families, it might be the only time they had to rest.

Second, avoidance of bathing may also have practical origins. In many countries the water is impure and filled with harmful bacteria. Bathing could introduce these organisms into the body and cause illness. Although conditions in the United States are different, the custom continues.

A third point involves the ways different generations adhere to customs. Sometimes, in order to avoid her mother's nagging, the daughter may comply with the cultural traditions when the mother is present. When the patient is alone, she may be more receptive when a nurse suggests bathing, exercise, and so forth.

Compromises can be made. Although it is important for a patient to drink fluids after childbirth, hot tea and hot water with lemon deliver the same amount of liquid as ice water without violating custom. Using boiled water (cooled down) may make a sponge bath more acceptable. (This was done in China to remove impurities.) The patient should be kept covered and given socks or slippers to walk in. It is important to explain the reason for bathing and exercise and not to assume that the patient will follow orders that violate the traditions and wisdom of her own culture.

Bonding

Maternal-infant bonding has become a major concern of Western health care professionals in recent decades. Poor bonding has been associated with failure to thrive, child abuse, and psychological problems. It is therefore not surprising that doctors and nurses become concerned when they observe cultural beliefs and practices that appear to reflect poor bonding. However, they often do not.

188   An example is the case of Ngo Lien, a Vietnamese woman who came to the hospital to deliver her fifth child. After giving birth to a son, she refused to cuddle him, although she willingly provided minimal care such as feeding and changing his diaper. The nursery nurse, feeling sorry for the "neglected" baby, picked him up, cuddled him, and stroked the top of his head. Mrs. Ngo and her husband became visibly upset. The baby, who had jaundice, had to remain in the hospital for several days after Mrs. Vo went home. She did not visit her baby even once during the time he remained in the hospital.

In the past, nurses who worked in areas with a large Vietnamese population often referred these mothers to social services. Eventually, however, they came to understand that the apparently neglectful behavior did not reflect poor bonding, but instead indicated cultural belief and traditions. Many people in the more rural areas of Vietnam believe in spirits. Because spirits are particularly attracted to infants and likely to "steal" them (by inducing death), it is important that parents do everything possible to avoid attracting attention to their newborn. For this reason, infants are not verbally fussed over. They are sometimes even dressed in old clothes to "fool" the spirits. The apparent lack of interest new parents demonstrate reflects an intense love and concern for the child, rather than the opposite.

A Vietnamese nurse also pointed out to me that Vietnamese women are socialized not to show emotion in public, and thus may not be displaying the emotional attachment they feel while health care providers are in the room. That doesn't mean they don't play with the infant when they are alone.

Mrs. Ngo and her husband were probably distressed over the nurse's attention to their baby for two reasons. First, they may have feared having attention drawn to their baby. Second, Southeast Asians view the head as private and personal. It is also seen as the seat of the soul and is not to be touched. Not only did the nurse risk attracting the attention of dangerous spirits, but she also stroked the child in a forbidden area.

Why did Mrs. Ngo not come to visit her son in the hospital after she was discharged? She was probably practicing lying-in and was at home resting while her internal organs resumed their normal position in her body.

Nurses can best deal with Vietnamese mothers by following their lead. If the parents do not fuss over the child, nurses should not either. In any event, they should avoid touching the infant's head. And as long as a mother can feed and hold her baby properly, they should not be concerned about an apparent lack of interest; it is merely an illusion.

Nurses were similarly disturbed when a woman from India refused to hold her babies except to feed them. Shankari Prabhu, a young Indian woman, gave birth prematurely to twin girls. Although the father was out of town on business, numerous other relatives were there, including the mother-in-law, aunts and uncles, nieces and nephews, and cousins.

Shortly after the delivery, Indira, the father's sister, came to speak to Edith, the nurse, explaining that Mrs. Prabhu was too tired to speak with her, but did plan to breastfeed the babies. Edith explained the importance of breastfeeding to the sister-in-law, and emphasized the importance of the mother spending time with the babies.

The next day Indira spoke to Edith again, giving her the names of the babies to put on the crib card. Although Edith knew enough about East Indian culture to realize that Mrs. Prabhu was practicing the lying-in period and had designated her sister-in-law to care for the infants, she reiterated the importance of having her spend time with the babies. She also explained that it was not enough for Indira to tell her the babies' names; that information had to come from the parents. Realizing the cultural importance of Indira's role as caregiver, she encouraged her to change the babies' linens and diapers, and hold the girls. But she was adamant in insisting that Mrs. Prabhu visit the babies because she was concerned about bonding.

Mrs. Prabhu finally came to visit her babies the next evening. She held them only briefly, and then passed them on to one of the many family members who were there with her. When Edith questioned her, she remained passive and allowed family members to respond for her. Fortunately, Edith had enough cultural competence to put aside her ethnocentric expectations that the mother should take full control in caring for her infants. This is not an expectation or common practice in Indian culture. The only care many Indian new mothers provide for their infants is to nurse them. A family member takes over its other care. In a variant of the lying-in period common in Asia and Latin America, the new mother is encouraged to rest in bed and eat a special diet including large amounts of milk, cooked butter, ghee (clarified butter), and high-protein foods.

189

Edith was able to adjust her expectations, thus creating a more pleasant situation for the patient and her family, as well as a less stressful situation for herself.

Baby Naming

190   When the subject of baby naming came up in class, Leila, a Hindu nurse from India, shared her own experience. She said that when she and her husband had their first son, they wanted to name him in the traditional Hindu manner, which meant waiting until he was seven days old. Before choosing a name, they would have to consult an astrologer who would give them a list of auspicious letters, based on the baby's time and date of birth. These letters would be given to her husband's sisters, who would then choose a name beginning with one of the letters on the list.

What they had not counted on was the response of the hospital. Despite the fact that Leila is a nurse, she did not realize the importance placed on filling out the birth forms. When they refused to fill in the baby's name, the nurse reported her to the head nurse. This resulted in visits from the hospital administrative nurse, the chaplain, and the social worker. They all seemed concerned about Leila's plans for the baby once they got home. When she asked the social worker why everyone seemed so disturbed, the social worker admitted that they were worried that she wasn't bonding properly with the baby—why else would she not have named him?

Leila and her husband were both shocked and embarrassed that anyone would think they did not want their child. She quickly explained the Hindu tradition to the social worker, who noted the information for the nursing staff. Leila also recommended that, in the future, a patient who refuses to fill out the child's name should be asked *why* before any misunderstandings result.

Leila was told to call the hospital as soon as they named the baby, but apparently the hospital could not wait. On the morning of the seventh day, Leila received a call from the social worker, wanting to know the child's name so the forms could be completed.

When Leila asked her mother and grandmother why they were to wait until the seventh day to name the child, they told her that it is the day the stump of the umbilical cord falls off, and is thus the baby's first day of life. It is also the first time that the baby really opens his eyes and looks around. Although they did not mention it, it is probably related to high infant mortality rates.

This custom of delaying the naming of the baby is found in many Asian cultures. Traditional Chinese will often give the baby an unattractive nickname at birth, such as "Little Doggie," or "Ugly Pig," to make the child seem less attractive to any spirits who might want to steal the infant.

Suk Luu, a Chinese man from Vietnam, shared that his mother attributes the fact that his daughter grew up to be healthy, talented, and intelligent to her "ugly" name; her "real" name was for use only on her birth certificate. As the girl's grandmother explained, her ugly name ensured that no devils paid attention to her; who would be jealous of an "ugly name girl"? In contrast, Luu's older brother was given a name that meant "intelligent" or "bright and clear." His mother pointed out that the devils were clearly jealous; his brother suffered serious illnesses for many years and died at the age of only thirty, as a military prisoner in South Vietnam.

Rejection

Occasionally parents will reject a newborn. Such was the case with a Middle Eastern couple after the wife, Salomi, gave birth to a baby girl. At the moment of delivery, while the doctor and nurses were oohing and aahing over the infant, her father turned and abruptly left the delivery room. The mother herself would not hold or even look at her child. When a nurse approached the lobby where many of the woman's relatives had earlier been anxiously awaiting the birth, she found that they had all left. Later, she held her child, but she refused to lavish any loving attention upon her.

191

The nurse who reported this incident could not understand why parents would respond so negatively to such a joyous event. A Middle Eastern acquaintance later told her the reason. The couple had two daughters but no sons. Males are extremely important in Middle Eastern culture because they carry on the family name and all wealth is passed on through them. Many groups trace descent through the male line only, unlike our own system, which recognizes both the mother's and father's sides of the family. Even in groups that have adopted more Western patterns of inheritance, the traditional importance of the male may remain. A third daughter was a great disappointment.

There is little that the staff can do in such a situation, other than refer the parents to social services—and that may not be entirely welcome. Parents will rarely change ideas that have years of cultural tradition behind them. The important thing for nurses to do is to watch for signs of neglect.

Infant Care

In yet another case, a nurse attempted to explain baby care techniques to Middle Eastern parents. Because the new mother was not feeling well, the nurse began to explain everything to her husband. To the nurse's surprise, he refused to listen, stating that in his country men did not get involved in child care; it was a woman's job. Although economic and other

192

factors may intervene, there is generally a very strict delineation of sex roles in the Middle East. Childrearing is a woman's responsibility. A man deals with his children later on in their lives. In such situations, it may be best to wait until a new mother is well enough to listen to instructions rather than try to explain things to her husband.

Belly Buttons

American medical professionals fear germs. For this reason, they are almost obsessively concerned with cleanliness. A custom practiced by Mexicans and other groups to create an attractive belly button is thus likely to disturb them. A coin is applied to an infant's navel and the area is wrapped tightly with a cloth to keep the coin in place. Sometimes the job of keeping the navel flat is left entirely to the bellyband. In any case, a protruding belly button is considered unsightly. Loving mothers will do what they can to ensure that their babies are attractive.

Health care professionals are concerned about the possibility of infection from a dirty cloth or coin. To respect their tradition and address health concerns, mothers who practice this custom should be taught the importance of using clean cloths and wiping the coin with alcohol before putting it on the baby's body. Most mothers are willing to make the minor adjustments necessary to ensure the health of their children.

Birth Control

A chapter on birth must also acknowledge efforts to prevent the event. Limiting the number of children is an extremely complicated issue in many cultures. Often, women and men take different positions on the issue, particularly in cultures where women have the primary responsibility for raising the children and men's major access to status and prestige is through the number of children they sire. Although a woman's status in such cultures may also derive from her role as a mother, women generally take the more practical stance.

193   Carmen Rosales, a twenty-four-year-old Mexican woman, was ready to deliver her sixth child in six years. She begged her obstetrician to perform a tubal ligation after the delivery. Hospital policy at that time, however, required her husband to sign a consent form for the procedure, and he would not allow it. Mrs. Rosales was concerned that they would not be able to feed another child; she was not even sure they could feed this one. But her husband wanted as many children as she could give him. She begged the physician to tie her tubes and not tell her husband.

He refused. Women who had been sterilized at their own request had sued the hospital. The husband would learn later that his wife had had a tubal ligation. Rather than admit it had been done at her insistence and risk losing her husband, she would claim that she had not known what she was signing or had been coerced. For this reason, many hospitals refuse to sterilize women without their husband's consent. (Interestingly, few, if any, hospitals require the wife's consent for a vasectomy.)

A forty-five-year-old Mexican woman named Luna Ortiz was advised by her obstetrician that another pregnancy might prove fatal. Her eighth pregnancy (and third caesarean) had caused a thinning of her uterine wall. Rather than have her tubes tied while she was in the hospital, Mrs. Ortiz said she would have to discuss the matter with her husband. "He will decide what to do." Unlike Mrs. Rosales, Mrs. Ortiz accepted the authority of the male to make all major decisions, including whether to have more children, regardless of how it affected her health. 194

Summary

Different cultures have different traditions regarding the process of birth. Some cultures dictate that a woman suffer the pains of labor in silence; others encourage her to express or even exaggerate her pain. The husband, mother, or mother-in-law may attend the birth. Some cultures have postpartum rituals that a new mother must observe that contradict the recommendations of Western medical science. Some bathe and exercise as soon as possible, while others are taught to lie in bed and avoid showering and physical activity. Some have customs that may appear to reflect a lack of bonding but, in fact, do not. Although doctors now encourage immediate breastfeeding, women in some cultures believe it is necessary to wait several days lest the "dirty" antibody-rich colostrum harm their child. Finally, many cultures do not share our advocacy of birth control, in part because children are a major source of self-esteem for those who would otherwise have no access to status.

Some of these differences affect the health of the mother or child but others do not. Health care professionals must learn to recognize the difference. Detailed explanations and compromise are necessary when good health is the issue; cultural relativism must be exercised when it is not.

Key Points

- Most pregnancy taboos originated in the desire to control the outcome of pregnancy.
- Pregnancy is considered a "hot" condition in cultures that practice a system of hot/cold body balance (many Asian and Hispanic cultures). Because foods that are high in protein may be perceived as "hot" and thus avoided, physicians should carefully assess the pregnant woman's

diet to make sure she is getting enough protein. The same is true for prenatal vitamins. If they are too "hot," they can often be neutralized by taking them with a "cold" beverage.

- Prenatal care may be avoided because many women see pregnancy as a "normal" condition and thus not requiring the assistance of a physician.
- Some cultures dictate stoicism during labor; others allow free expression of pain.
- In many cultures, female relatives are the preferred labor partner. If the husband seems unwilling to be in the room with his wife, do not force him to be.
- In some Southeast Asian cultures, surgery may be avoided due to the beliefs of the patient.
- In some cultures, patients may want to keep the placenta or the umbilical cord.
- Some women may want to postpone breastfeeding, believing that colostrum is bad for the baby. Patient teaching may be necessary.
- Many Asian, South Asian, and Hispanic women may practice a postpartum lying-in period in which they are to rest, stay warm, and avoid bathing and exercise. Compromise when possible.
- Do not be concerned if Southeast Asian women do not appear to be bonding with their infant, as long as they hold and feed the baby properly. If they are not fussing over the infant, follow their lead.
- In many traditional Asian and South Asian cultures, baby naming may be delayed for up to a month.
- Be prepared to compromise. For example, rather than tell a mother not to use a bellyband on her child, make sure it is clean and not too tight.

Chapter 10
End of Life

In the past most people died at home, cared for by their families. Today, however, people are dying more frequently in hospitals, cared for by professionals. Thanks to improved medical technology, people are also taking longer to die. The end of life is often fraught with difficulties for most patients and their families. In addition, there are complications that can occur because cultural traditions vary significantly in terms of a variety of issues, including whether or not to reveal the diagnosis to the patient, attitudes toward removing life support, expression of grief at the time of death, attitudes toward organ donations and autopsies, and beliefs and customs surrounding the moment of death.

Dying

Revealing/Withholding a Negative Diagnosis

One of the first cultural issues that arise with regard to the end of life is whether or not to reveal a terminal diagnosis to the patient. From the perspective of American culture, which values individualism and autonomy, this is not even a question. Of course the patient is told if she or he has a terminal condition; it is one of the basic patient rights to know. However, the situation becomes complicated when the patient is from a culture that values the family over the individual. Studies have found that 52 percent of Mexican Americans feel that dying patients should not be told their prognosis, and 65 percent of Korean Americans believe such information should be withheld (see Kagawa-Singer and Blackhall 2001). In many Asian countries, including China and Japan, it is customary for the physician to reveal a cancer diagnosis only to the patient's family, and leave it up to the family whether or not to tell the patient.

In some cultures, it may be seen as insensitive to tell a patient he or she is dying. It may be thought to create a sense of hopelessness and hasten the dying process. A Mexican American woman explained that the stress of knowing your condition would only cause you to get worse. The very devout may believe that only God knows when someone will die. Among the Hmong, to tell someone they are dying is thought to curse them. How could you know they will die unless you plan to kill them yourself?

For the health care staff, however, honoring the patient's culture may mean ignoring the American values of autonomy and individualism as well as creating potential legal complications. One solution is for the physician to discuss with the patient—ideally, before the need arises—to whom the patient wants information about his or her condition to be given. Does the patient want the physician to speak directly to a family member, or to him or her? How much does the patient want to know about his or her condition? Whom does the patient want the physician to speak to for decisions regarding treatment? It is important that any conversations regarding how much the patient wants to know be held in private, in order to ascertain the patient's true feelings.

The state of Washington passed a law that allows patients to waive personal consent authority for making their own medical treatment or nontreatment choices. They may sign a document that says they waive their consent authority freely and voluntarily, and do not wish to be informed of the nature and character of the proposed treatment/procedure; the anticipated results of the proposed treatment/procedure; the recognized alternative forms of treatment/procedure; or the recognized serious possible risks and complications of the treatment/procedure and of the recognized alternative forms of treatment/procedure, including nontreatment. They may also assign authority for decision making to a third party. Recognizing the patient's "right *not* to know" is an important step in cultural sensitivity.

195   Suken Hashimoto, a seventy-eight-year-old Japanese woman, was scheduled to receive chemotherapy for cancer. Normally, her nurse would explain to a patient why she was receiving chemotherapy, but Mrs. Hashimoto did not know she had cancer. Her physician had carefully discussed Mrs. Hashimoto's plan of care with her son; he had told the physician and the nursing staff not to let his mother know her diagnosis. The staff had a hard time understanding this wish, and felt they needed to call in the ethics committee. Before this, however, they asked Mrs. Hashimoto if she wanted to know her diagnosis and why she was receiving chemotherapy medication. To their surprise, her answer was no. She said, "Tell my son. He will make all of the decisions." The situation was resolved by having her sign a durable power of attorney for her son to make all her health care decisions. This is something hospitals can routinely do at the beginning of a hospital stay. Some patients will choose to be informed; others may prefer to defer that right.

196   Kioko, a Japanese student of mine, said that in the mid-1990s she went to Japan to care for her father when he was diagnosed with end-stage

stomach cancer. The physician told the family of her father's poor prognosis and advised them not to tell her father the truth, because it would cause him to lose hope and hasten the dying process. After working in an American hospital for ten years, Kioko found it difficult to withhold the information, and felt guilty about it. However, she said that because she was raised to respect her family's opinion over her own, she abided by their decision.

A sixty-four-year-old Latino male with a poor prognosis had family *197* members at his bedside around the clock, despite strict visiting rules. Whenever the nurses asked them to leave, they would argue and insist on staying. When one of the nurses finally asked about their concerns, the patient's daughter explained they were afraid that one of the staff might tell their father that he was dying. The family felt that being told death was imminent would cause him to lose the will to live, a will that would provide him strength to fight the disease.

The problem was solved by documenting their request in the nursing process notes and verbally passing on the information during shift change. They also informed the physician and nurse practitioner about the family's wishes. The patient was told that his condition was critical, but that they were taking it one day at a time and hoping for the best. When the patient died, the family expressed their gratitude to the staff and physicians for going along with their concerns and wishes. The staff did well by respecting the family's wishes, but it would have been better to ascertain the desires of the patient by finding out from him how much he wanted to know.

It is also important to remember that not all members of the same culture will make the same choices. I had two Filipino students in my class who had recently lost a grandparent. In one case, the family followed the more traditional pattern of withholding that information from the patient. Afterward, they were pleased with their choice, feeling that their loved one was able to live out her days without the added burden of knowing she was dying. In the other case, the family decided to tell the patient. They, too, were content with their choice, knowing that the patient was able to make her final arrangements and say goodbye to everyone. Two Filipino families, two different choices, both leaving the family feeling satisfied. This underscores the importance of both not imposing American values on others, and not stereotyping. The culturally competent health care provider will neither assume that the patient does *not* want to know, nor impose American ways and tell the patient everything. Instead, she or he will come to the situation knowing the cultural possibilities and ascertain what the individual patient wants.

Acting in such a culturally competent manner can help physicians avoid two potential problems, as described in the following cases.

198   I presented a workshop to physicians at a hospital, and one of the topics I spoke on was the issue of family members wanting information to be withheld from the patient. An older physician came up to me afterward and shared that when he was a young physician, he had such a case. He didn't know how to handle it, so he simply avoided the patient. More than thirty years later, he still feels guilty.

199   A nursing student told me about a physician who strongly feels it is his moral and legal responsibility to tell patients their diagnosis. This attitude has created problems with several families who did not want their family member to know. Some of these patients frequently missed appointments; others never returned. It is likely the family members refused to bring them in to this physician in order to "protect" them from hearing their diagnosis.

Hospice

A growing trend in care of the dying is hospice. Unlike Western medicine, which is dedicated to preserving life as long as possible, hospice care emphasizes death with dignity. To that end, one of the major goals is pain relief. Another is to help the person deal with the psychological issues they may be facing. Hospice care can take place either in a dedicated facility or in the home. Although by allowing patients to die in their own home, surrounded by loved ones, hospice more closely approximates the conditions of dying in more traditional cultures, it is primarily utilized by Anglo Americans. Part of the problem is that many mistakenly believe that hospice care is provided only at special facilities and they prefer to take care of their loved ones at home, rather than "abandon" them to such a facility. In fact, the reality is quite the contrary. Most hospice care is given at home, where family members can continue to care for their loved one with the aid of a visiting hospice nurse who can provide palliative pain medication. There are additional cultural variables that may also play a role.

Because hospice is for "terminal" patients, some might feel it would show a lack of faith in God. This is an attitude held by many Muslims. If you have no faith in Allah, why would Allah save you? Others, as in the following case study, may want to "protect" the patient from a terminal prognosis.

200   Mrs. Hidalgo, an elderly Mexican woman, was dying of cancer. Her doctor spoke with her family about receiving hospice care. They liked the idea of having the hospice personnel provide her with medication to reduce her pain; however, there was a problem. In talking with the hospice organization, the family learned that before the hospice would accept Mrs. Hidalgo as a patient, she had to sign informed consent, acknowledging that she had a terminal condition and would die within six months.

Because the family would not allow Mrs. Hidalgo to see the form (and prognosis), hospice care could not be given.

Current Medicare Conditions of Participation require that an informed consent be obtained from the patient. The reasoning is that when patients elect hospice, they are relinquishing their Part A (hospitalization) benefit. One person cannot do this for someone else. Although some programs have ignored this requirement and conspired with the family to avoid informing the patient, it can create numerous problems. Besides conflicting with one of the most important values of the American health care professions—honesty—when the patient does find out, they lose trust in the hospice staff. Ethical programs, she explained, do not lie to the patients by either omission or commission. She suggested that hospice personnel explain to the family that this informed consent can be gently obtained and the person needs to know only that they are giving up their hospitalization benefit in favor of symptom management and comfort. Most hospice election statements refer to the fact that the patient has a "life-limiting illness" or something along those lines, rather than stating they are dying. She added, however, that most people know that they are seriously ill and not getting better and are relieved when the truth is in the open.

Another reason why non-Anglo ethnic groups may underutilize hospice is that hospice emphasizes the use of pain-killing drugs; this may be a problem for those who especially fear addiction, such as Filipinos and East Indians. Recall the Filipino nurse (case study #63) who halved the doctor's prescribed dosage when administering pain medication to her dying mother. It is essential that health care personnel explain to the family the true nature of addiction and why this will not occur in the case of their loved one.

Many traditional cultures feel it is the duty of the family to take care of its own members. This duty is particularly important in many Asian cultures, where filial piety is highly valued. Calling in hospice may be perceived as not fulfilling one's responsibility. In such cases, involving family members as much as possible in the patient's care will be important. It should be emphasized that hospice is meant to assist rather than replace the family, and that the family should appear to be in control of the patient's care.

An additional, though less significant, impediment may be that because hospice emphasizes the psychosocial needs of the dying patient, individuals from cultures that emphasize keeping personal issues within the family (e.g., Mexicans) may not feel comfortable discussing them with outsiders.

Perhaps because hospice allows patients greater control over their own death, it is a better fit with the worldview of the dominant American culture, which views nature as something that can be controlled. For many other ethnic groups, including those in the Middle East and Latin America, life and death are up to the will of God. *Qué será será.*

Palliative Care

201   Matilda Salazar, an extremely ill Hispanic patient, was dying as a result of sepsis, acute respiratory distress syndrome (ARDS), and multiple organ failure. Her family asked that a *curandera*, a traditional healer, be allowed to come pray with her and massage her with oil. Dr. Edgar, a culturally sensitive physician, not only agreed to this but requested he be called to the bedside when the healer arrived. Using an interpreter, Dr. Edgar spoke with the *curandera* about the rituals that would take place. He stayed to watch from the corner of the room as the *curandera* chanted, prayed, and massaged oils into Mrs. Salazar's body. Although the ceremony did nothing to affect the patient's prognosis, the family and patient seemed more at peace afterward, and the experience improved the family's rapport with the physician. When the time came for Dr. Edgar to tell the family there was nothing else they could do for Mrs. Salazar, they accepted it calmly and began saying their goodbyes. After she died, the family remained grateful to the doctors and staff for respecting their traditions. This case is important because it shows how respect for a patient's cultural traditions can have a positive effect on the relationship between the staff and the patient (and family). It also underscores the fact that the point of medicine doesn't always have to be to cure, but to *care* for the patient.

Advance Directives and Removing Life Support

A culture's worldview will also have a strong influence on the willingness of an individual or family to learn about or consent to "do not resuscitate" (DNR) orders, or to advance directives.

Advance directives are the written directions that a patient gives to family members and health professionals to guide decision making about end of life care, including the use, or not, of extraordinary measures to prolong life. A relatively new phenomenon, advance directives are legally binding in some states. Nurses, in their role of patient advocate, as well as physicians have the responsibility to ascertain the wishes of the patient regarding the use of and adherence to advance directives. Depending on cultural beliefs about health care practices and treatments, as well as the meaning of life and death, patients may accept or reject the option of advance directives.

Although it is difficult for anyone to actively allow a loved one to die, cultural and religious influences play an important role in determining whether or not a family member is willing to remove life support. Jill Klessig

(1992) studied the effect of values and culture on life-support decisions and found that members of several cultural and religious groups were reluctant to withdraw life support, for a variety of reasons. These groups included Muslim Iranians, Orthodox Jews, Korean Americans, African Americans, Mexican Americans, and Filipino Americans.

Muslim Iranians were generally opposed to removing life support, not only because is it seen as an obligation to seek medical attention, but also because only Allah can decide when someone will die. Note that starting life support is using the "gift" of technology that has been given to man— it is not seen as interfering with God's will the way *removing* life support is. Even if a patient is suffering, this is not a reason to remove life support because suffering is an opportunity to show courage and faith in Allah.

An example can be seen in the case of Noor Gatrad, an elderly Iranian woman. Mrs. Gatrad was slowly dying. The staff felt that nothing could be done to improve her condition, and that her son's refusal to sign a DNR order and his insistence on doing everything possible to prolong her life was causing the patient to endure needless suffering. Her son steadfastly held to his decision, despite the assistance and recommendations of the ethics committee. Her nurse shared this case with me during a course I was teaching on cultural competence. She said that at the time, she felt only frustration and could not understand Mrs. Gatrad's son's behavior. After learning about Iranian attitudes toward the removal of life support, she suddenly understood. Such knowledge might have enabled the staff to feel less stress while caring for Mrs. Gatrad.

Orthodox Jews also generally want to prolong life support. Because there is no belief in an afterlife, and life itself is considered sacred, it should be preserved whenever possible. However, because suffering is not thought to bring redemption, it is acceptable to remove life support if the patient will die within seventy-two hours.

Klessig found that Korean Americans were generally opposed to removing life support because stopping it (although not starting it) is seen as interfering with God's will. In addition, stopping life support, even if that is the wish of a parent, may be thought to dishonor family members in the eyes of relatives or community, due to the importance of filial piety.

She found that African American families were more likely than Anglo Americans to want life support continued. Some distrusted the largely white medical community, and feared that life support would be withdrawn early for racist reasons. Others were very religious and believed that God could provide a miracle cure, as in the following case.

A fifty-two-year-old African American man named William Jefferson was admitted to the critical care unit with a diagnosis of pneumonia. Upon admission, he was offered an Advance Directive, which he refused, saying that God would help him with his illness. His lung cancer had gone

202

203

into remission after radiation treatment; he believed that God had helped him through that illness, and would help him through the current one. He thought that signing a Do Not Resuscitate form or Advance Directive would be a sign of giving up or losing faith in God. Unfortunately, he died ten days later, after enduring a great deal of suffering.

Klessing also found that Filipino Americans and Mexican Americans were often opposed to withdrawing life support. Catholicism strongly influenced their attitudes. It is seen as morally wrong to encourage death with any action or omission ("suicide"), and if the illness is punishment by God, one should not interfere with the opportunity to redeem one's sins through suffering. It is important to note that traditional respect and courtesy toward physicians may lead patient or family to agree with a doctor who suggests removing life support, even when they are opposed to it.

204   The following case sheds some additional light on Filipino attitudes toward DNR. Agusto Joaquin, a sixty-five-year-old Filipino man, had been diagnosed with metastasized lung cancer. He and his wife had arranged a final trip to the Philippines, but he went into respiratory distress a few days before the scheduled flight. According to the doctors, he had but days to live. For the past two days, he was alert and oriented, but unable to be weaned off the ventilator. The doctors recommended that his code status be changed toDNR and that he be extubated and moved to a hospice facility. The family became quite angry at the suggestion, and refused. The physicians requested a social worker and interpreter for a family meeting. Because Emilita, a nurse at the hospital, was the only person on duty that day who spoke Mr. Joaquin's dialect, she was asked to interpret. She met with the doctors and social worker prior to meeting with the family. The oncologist raised the question of how to proceed asking the patient about DNR status and hospice care. Emilita was taking a class in cultural diversity at the time and was able to offer some pertinent suggestions.

She explained that major decisions are often decided by the family, rather than the individual. In addition, Filipinos might be reluctant to put family members on DNR status because this could be seen as disloyal to the patient. Sending a family member to a hospice facility could be seen as *walang utang na loob*—lack of sense of indebtedness. It is generally expected that Filipinos take care of their own family. Emilita suggested that they give the family time to discuss the issue of code status among themselves, and to let the team know when they had made a decision. She also recommended that the patient be discharged and hospice care be provided in the home.

Four days after the meeting, the family came to a decision to follow Emilita's recommendations. Mr. Joaquin's code status was changed to DNR, he was extubated, and his family took him home. A discharge planner arranged for home hospice care. A difficult situation had been resolved to everyone's satisfaction through the application of cultural competence skills.

Klessig found a dual attitude among Chinese Americans: it is acceptable both to stop life support and to do everything possible to extend a patient's life. Because the family is valued over the individual, if life support is an economic or emotional burden on the family, the patient who forgoes it is seen as performing an act of compassion, which is highly valued. In contrast, among Buddhist Chinese, there is a precept that prohibits killing and a concern that stopping life support will interfere with a person's karma. Issues of filial piety may also be involved.

Other, more unusual, circumstances can contribute to a refusal to remove life support, as the following case illustrates. Ngoc Ly, a twenty-five-year-old Vietnamese man, was hit by a car while riding his bicycle to work. Paramedics were able to resuscitate him, but the physician at the local trauma center determined that Mr. Ly was clinically brain dead. He placed him on life support until the family could be notified.

205

An interpreter explained Mr. Ly's condition to his wife and parents. They nodded in understanding and quietly left the hospital. Normally, the staff neurosurgeon would then have pronounced Mr. Ly dead and removed him from the ventilator, but he was suddenly called to surgery.

Later that afternoon, Mr. Ly's family met with Dr. Isaacs, the physician they had spoken to earlier. Dr. Isaacs intended to tell them of the plan to pronounce Mr. Ly dead and discontinue the ventilator, but the Lys had other plans. They informed him that they had consulted a specialist who said this was not the right time for him to die. Dr. Isaacs was confused. What kind of specialist would make such a recommendation? An astrologer who had read Ngoc Ly's lunar chart advised that his death be postponed until a more auspicious date.

The physician had never encountered a situation like the one now facing him. Fearing legal repercussions if he did not abide by the family's request, he agreed to keep Mr. Ly on life support until further notice. A little less than a week later, the Lys called to tell him that Ngoc could now die.

Most members of the staff were stunned by this incident. Mr. Ly's body was starting to decompose and smell. People looked up books on astrology and questioned Vietnamese coworkers. They learned that many Asians take astrology seriously. When an important decision is to be made, they will often consult a *bomoh* or *dukun* to interpret the astrological charts.

Although most people cannot predict or control the date of their death, simply knowing when someone has died can be helpful in terms of knowing what fate has in store for the deceased's descendants. If a person dies at the "proper" time, his or her children will be rewarded with good health and goodwill. If the time is inauspicious, the children will suffer financial losses, unhappy marriages, or similar negative fates. A *bomoh* can tell people what the future holds for them so they can be prepared.

The Ly family had an opportunity denied to most people. By delaying removal of Ngoc Ly's life support, they could influence the fate of his descendants for generations. How could they not do everything possible to bring good luck to his children?

Death

The Moment of Death

The moment an individual makes the transition between life and death is significant in many cultures. Many Americans feel it is important to be with their loved one at that instant, so that they do not feel alone.

206   The opposite is the case in the Sephardic (Spanish Jews) tradition. When Leon Taranto, a thirty-seven-year-old Sephardic man, lay dying, his family made a point of leaving his room for five minutes every hour. Like many Sephardics, they believed it is too hard for the dying to let go of life in the presence of loved ones. By leaving the room regularly, the dying patient is given the opportunity to pass on, unencumbered by the emotional ties created by family members. Mr. Taranto made the transition when his family was out of the room.

Other customs are followed by the Roma (Gypsies), as illustrated in the following cases.

207   Philip Maturo, a Romany (Gypsy) king in his late seventies, was brought to the hospital and diagnosed with pneumonia. The severity of his illness necessitated an oxygen tent. Clan members caused pandemonium; they crowded into Mr. Maturo's room, blocked the doorways, and filled the cafeteria with their coffee cups and cigarette smoke. This behavior, however, was merely a nuisance. The greatest problem was that they insisted on keeping a candle on the shelf at the head of Mr. Maturo's bed. The nurses lived in fear that it would be lit while the oxygen was turned on and cause an explosion. Many animated discussions were held on this point, but the Roma were adamant. If their king died, the candle would be lit at the moment of death to guide his spirit to heaven. Fortunately, Mr. Maturo recovered and the hospital survived.

208   Another hospital witnessed a different Rom custom regarding death. When the end was imminent, the clan received the hospital's permission to move the king outside, bed and all. They felt this would help free the soul of their dying leader, now unencumbered by walls and ceilings.

Concern for the ability of the spirit to soar to freedom is common in many cultures. One nurse who worked at a hospital close to the Hoopa Indian reservation in northern California told of how, when someone died, the nurses would open the windows to allow spirits to leave. The importance of this custom to the Native Americans made it difficult for her when she moved to a hospital where none of the windows opened.

In an example of how cultural sensitivity can be advantageous for both the patient and the clinician, Christina said that the most memorable death she ever participated in as a nurse was that of Mr. Shi, a practicing Buddhist. When the time came to remove the ventilator, she helped the family dress him in a suit that had had its buttons removed, to enable the soul to slip out easily. She was given a bag of coins to place in his left hand, and a bag of food to place in his right hand, sustenance for the journey. Finally, she was told to place a coin in his mouth. After Mr. Shi was extubated, his entire family came and took many photos of him after his final breath. Christina was asked to return the bag of money, but the deceased kept the food, coin, and suit.

Reyna also had a positive experience helping the family of an elderly male Vietnamese patient who died from a chronic illness. It was Thanksgiving, and when she saw that he was about to die, she called her husband at home and had him read to her about Vietnamese culture with regard to death from her course text. She was amazed to see that the words in the text so accurately described the scene that was unfolding before her. The eldest son made all the decisions and arrangements. He requested that Reyna bathe and dress his father in his own clothes. Reyna said the other nurse looked at her as if she were crazy for doing this. Steeped in the importance of culture from the class she was taking, she said she was keenly aware of why she was doing it, and how important it was to the family. She watched as his son placed a small gold medallion in his mouth. His family asked her to place several items in his pockets, including a handful of play money and simulated food items.

Later, several of her coworkers told her that if they had been in her shoes, they would have told her to tell the family to do it themselves. Although she said her first instinct was to chastise her coworkers for their callousness, instead she used it as an opportunity to explain the cultural significance of her actions. Acting in such a compassionate—and culturally competent—manner not only helped the patient's family, but made Reyna feel like she had contributed something important to this family.

Expression of Grief

Individuals express grief over the death of a loved one in a number of different ways. Furthermore, culture may influence whether it is more appropriate to cry and wail without restraint or to present a stoic face to the world. Anglo American culture tends to value emotional stoicism. Jacqueline Kennedy was praised for the way she maintained her composure in public after her husband, President John F. Kennedy, was assassinated. Hospital culture reflects the dominant culture and tends to find stoicism more admirable as well as easier to cope with, which can present problems when people from more expressive cultures die.

211   Mustafa Mourad, a Muslim Arab, was admitted to the oncology floor. A few weeks earlier he had been diagnosed with extensive colon cancer. His family kept him at home until he went into a coma. Upon admittance, it was determined that he was a "no code," but little else had been discussed. There had been no time to develop rapport. Six to ten family members were at his bedside throughout the night.

At 2 A.M., the daughter ran to get the nurse—he had stopped breathing. When the nurse confirmed that he had no pulse, several family members began to cry and wail loudly. The nurses tried to comfort them, but Mr. Mourad's son pulled them away. Soon the entire family joined in the wailing. The son asked the staff not to interfere, stating that the loud display was part of the grieving process. He added that it was necessary in order for his father's soul to be released.

The problem was that it was 2 A.M., and the wailing and crying were disturbing all the other, noncomatose patients, who were pushing their call buttons. They were angry, concerned, and frightened, and wanted to know what was going on. When the nurse asked the patient's son to have them please soften the noise, he became angry and accused her of being disrespectful.

The nurse had called Mr. Mourad's physician earlier to report the death. He instructed her to call the emergency room physician to pronounce the man dead. They were still waiting for him. Meanwhile, the nurse called the nursing supervisor. She also, unsuccessfully, tried to speak with the family about lowering the noise.

The doctor from the emergency room arrived nearly an hour later. When he requested they stop their wailing, they complied. He arranged to have the body moved to the chapel where they could continue their mourning without disturbing the other patients. The physician also instructed the nursing staff not to call the mortuary until told to do so by the family, which they did at 10 A.M. the next morning.

There are a number of cultural elements displayed in the Moustafa case. No plans had been made with the mortuary regarding the impending death because to do so would interfere with the will of Allah. The most disturbing element of the case for the staff was the loud crying. Wailing is an important cultural ritual. The nursing staff, unaware of this, was totally unprepared.

Another cultural aspect was the fact that the family ignored the requests of the nurses but complied with those of the physician. Arabs have a great deal of respect for authority—of physicians, not nurses. This is accentuated by the greater respect the culture has for men.

In this situation, the physician demonstrated an important understanding of cultural diversity and suggested a solution (moving to the chapel) that allowed the family to continue their ritual without compromising other patients. It is important to work within the culture, rather than impose solutions from outside it.

Postmortem Organ Donations and Autopsies

Most religions have rules regarding what can be done to the body after death. Although there will be variations according to how devout the family is, there are some practices that health care professionals can anticipate. Orthodox Jewish and Muslim patients may be opposed to organ donations and autopsies (unless required by law). According to Jewish belief, the body must be whole for resurrection if the messiah comes. For that reason, Jewish families may request that the deceased be buried with amputated limbs and bloody clothing, for example, if they died in an accident (see case study #71). Furthermore, many Jews believe that the body belongs to God, and we do not have the right to disfigure it without a good reason. There are mixed feelings regarding organ donation among Muslims. Those who are opposed say the body can still feel pain, and that life is a "trust," so you cannot donate part of your body to anyone else. It should be returned to Allah in the same shape in which it was given, and that was not with body parts missing. Those Muslims in favor of it say that because it can save a life, it falls under the Islamic doctrine that "necessity allows the prohibited." Hmong families are also likely to refuse autopsies and organ donations because they believe that whatever is cut will be missing when they are reincarnated.

Burial and Funeral Practices

Humans have disposed of the dead for at least the last 90,000 years. The earliest records we have of burials are associated with the Neanderthals of western Europe, whose skeletons have been found with the remains of wild flowers, animal bones (food for the journey to the afterlife?), and stone tools. Disposal of the corpse is important both as a public health measure and as a mirror of religious and cultural beliefs. The means of disposal, like most cultural traditions, often reflect both practical circumstances and ideology. The two most popular means of disposing of a dead body in the United States are burial and cremation. Generally, Muslims and Jews will be opposed to cremation, while Buddhists and Hindus may prefer it. The views of the Catholic Church have shifted on this issue.

Cremation used to be forbidden in the belief that the body must be whole for resurrection. However, in recent years, probably due to the practical influence of overcrowding and lack of burial space, it has been thought that as long as there is even a chunk of bone left, resurrection can occur. This is an excellent example of how cultures adapt to changing circumstances.

We can see how traditions regarding disposal of the body relate to both environmental conditions and beliefs regarding the afterlife. For example, among Orthodox Jews, cremation is forbidden. This reflects the Jewish belief that when the messiah comes, we will be resurrected, and need our bodies to be whole. It also reflects the ecological circumstance of the Middle East. There is not a lot of wood for burning bodies in the desert, but there is plenty of room for burial. This helps explain why there are so many similarities in Jewish and Muslim funeral traditions. Orthodox Jews are buried in a plain white shroud. The belief is that we are all equal in the eyes of God, and should thus appear that way. Judaism itself is a very egalitarian religion, compared, for example, with Roman Catholicism, which is very hierarchical. All members of the Jewish community are to assist in the actual burial by shoveling dirt onto the coffin. This reflects the strong value of community and the fact that Jews have always been outsiders and have had to rely on their own people.

Cremation is part of both Buddhist and Hindu traditions. From an adaptive perspective this makes sense. Japan, a traditional Buddhist culture, is a small but highly populated island. There is little room for burial, but there are plenty of trees to provide wood for burning bodies. Although India is a large country, there is tremendous overcrowding in the major cities. Cremation makes sense as both a public health measure and a way of disposing of corpses easily. I have one vivid memory of my seventh grade science class. The teacher had been to India that summer. On the first day of class, he described how in the mornings, the street sweepers would sweep up the bodies of the dead, along with the garbage. I've never forgotten that image, and for me it underscores the practicality of cremation. At the same time, both Buddhism and Hinduism believe in reincarnation. Given the ideological belief that we are born into new bodies in our next life, there is no need to maintain the integrity of our current bodies. Again, the practical and ideological merge to create a tradition.

Numbers and Death

Most Americans would be uncomfortable if they were assigned to room 13, because the number 13 is considered by many to be "unlucky." Many buildings do not have a 13th floor, at least, not one labeled as such. In Japan, while most high-rises do have a 13th floor, they lack a 4th floor, due to the association of the number four with death.

A young Japanese woman named Kieko Ozawa was being wheeled into operating room 4 when she noticed the number over the door. She began to cry softly. The nurse became concerned and asked what was wrong. Kieko was embarrassed but explained that the Japanese character for the number 4 is pronounced the same as the character for the word "death." Already concerned about her health, Kieko was disturbed to be wheeled into a room labeled "death."

Although she said it was just a silly superstition, Kieko was unable to let go of her fear. The surgery went well despite the room number, but the patient suffered needless anxiety. Had the hospital personnel mentioned to Kieko that she was being scheduled for room 4, her feelings might have become known in time to reschedule her into a different operating room. Room number 3, for example, would have been appropriate because 3 in Japanese characters also means "life."

The same is true for the Chinese and for Koreans. In fact, one hospital situated in a largely Chinese neighborhood realized that they needed an in-service workshop on cultural diversity when a Chinese man on their board of directors became quite upset during his hospitalization. He had been put in room 444.

Whenever possible, avoid putting Chinese, Japanese, and Korean patients in rooms with the number 4. As a side note, 4 is not the only number with special significance for the Chinese. They regard numbers 8 and 9 as lucky. The character for 8 signifies wealth and the character for 9 means long life. (For the Japanese, however, 9 may represent "suffering.") In Hong Kong, most of the expensive luxury cars owned by the Chinese include the number 8 on the license plate. The Chinese pay extra money and wait in long lines to get a plate with that number. An expensive car without an 8 is generally owned by a foreigner.

The number 4 is not a universally negative number. Although it has negative connotations for the Chinese and Japanese, the opposite is the case for the Navajo, who see much of the world in terms of four. Phrases are repeated four times in their ritual chants, pollen is thrown to the four directions in many of their ceremonies, and they revere four sacred mountains. A Navajo might find it easier to remember to take medicine four times a day than three or five times.

Summary

Although this chapter has only touched upon some of the issues that face caregivers when working with dying patients, it demonstrates the importance of culture in shaping people's attitudes and behavior in the face of death. At the same time, remember that culture does not explain everything; peoples' responses at this momentous life transition are often purely personal.

Key Points

- Because it is common in some cultures to withhold a negative diagnosis/ prognosis from the patient, it is important to discuss with the patient— in private, and ideally, before the need arises—to whom the patient wants information about his or her condition to be given. Does the patient want the physician to speak directly to a family member, or to him or her? How much does the patient want to know about his or her condition? Whom does the patient want the physician to speak to for decisions regarding treatment?
- When raising the subject of hospice care with families, make sure they understand that care can be provided in the patient's home. This will allow family members to continue to care for their loved one.
- Cultural and religious influences play an important role in determining whether or not a family member is willing to remove life support. These influences can include the belief that only God can make that decision, the belief that suffering is an opportunity to show courage and faith in God, the need to show filial piety, and distrust of the white medical establishment.
- Many cultures have beliefs regarding the moment of death, including whether or not someone should remain at the bedside and what needs to be done to free the individual's soul.
- Many cultures have specific practices regarding how the body should be prepared after death. Health care providers can play an important role in assisting families at this time.
- There are cultural variations in the expression of grief, as well as attitudes toward organ donations and autopsies (see Appendix 2).
- Traditions regarding disposal of the body relate to both environmental conditions and beliefs regarding the afterlife.
- Numbers can have significance for people; 13 may be seen as unlucky by many Americans; 4 by many Asians is associated with death.

Chapter 11
Mental Health

The mental health profession is paying increasing attention to the effect of culture on individual psychology. Many graduate programs in clinical psychology now offer courses on treating clients from culturally diverse backgrounds. Knowledge of the range of what is considered "normal" is essential to effectively treating both private practice clients and hospital patients. Unfortunately, psychiatric diagnoses of foreign patients are often inaccurate, due to health care workers' ignorance of cultural patterns. This chapter will address some issues that relate to the mental health of patients.

Mental Illness

Defining Mental Illness: Deviation from the Norm

One definition of mental illness is behavior that deviates significantly from the norm. Because each culture values different behavior in its members, what is considered normal in one culture may be perceived as deviant in another. In a culture that values emotional control, expressiveness can be seen as a sign of instability. In a culture that values independence, the desire to live with one's family after adolescence may be seen as something that needs to be worked on in therapy. When diagnosing patients it is essential to distinguish mental illness from culturally supported behaviors and personality traits.

The following case took place in 1974. Current laws and cultural change make it unlikely that it could happen today, but the role of culture makes it an extremely relevant case example.

Chio Yamamoto, a forty-six-year-old Japanese immigrant woman, was committed to a state mental institution by her husband on the basis of what he termed a major personality change and uncharacteristic behavior. The problems began after her three children went to college. Mrs. Yamamoto decided she wanted to attend college as well, something that was rare among Japanese women at the time. When her husband learned of her intentions, he had her committed. Her primary diagnosis was "chronic undifferentiated schizophrenia" with an acute psychotic episode and a secondary diagnosis of "hypochondria with multiple somatic complaints." Clearly, she did not belong in an institution simply because she wanted to attend college. Then why was she diagnosed with psychiatric problems once in the mental hospital? Probably it was due to her behavior, which, though consistent with Japanese culture, was misinterpreted as psychotic.

The staff at the institution documented her "noncompliant" behavior. She was "sullen," quiet, and would not participate in group therapy. Furthermore, she would not make eye contact with anyone. She also had multiple somatic complaints with no medical basis. These included vague abdominal pains, extremely poor appetite, and general weakness.

What were the cultural bases for these "symptoms"? At that time in Japan, women were raised to show respect for authority and to be submissive. It would have been culturally inappropriate for Chio to have questioned the therapists who were treating her. Eye contact is to be avoided in order to show respect. It is not surprising that she was extremely withdrawn in therapy; to call attention to yourself and talk about your feelings is completely antithetical to the Japanese notions of inconspicuousness (consider the Japanese saying, "the nail that sticks out gets hammered down") and emotional control. In addition, mental illness carries a tremendous stigma in Asian cultures. Chio must have certainly been burdened with the shame of her diagnosis, causing her to withdraw even further.

Rather than express her feelings, Chio somaticized them. Psychosomatic complaints are common among the Japanese, who are allowed few acceptable outlets for their anger. Stomach pains are commonly associated with emotional distress. It is difficult to eat when your stomach hurts, and if you don't eat, you become weak. Thus, the chain of her "symptoms."

Chio was falsely institutionalized for eight months. Though it is now much more difficult to commit someone against his or her will, the error was compounded by a lack of understanding of Japanese culture on the part of the psychiatric hospital staff.

215   Culture can add a layer of complexity to psychiatric diagnoses. Miya Fukui, a Japanese woman who had been living in the United States for more than thirty years, was admitted to an inpatient psychiatric hospital. She had been referred by the emergency department for attempting to commit suicide "for no reason" by overdosing on Tylenol. The physicians at the psychiatric hospital assumed her attempted suicide was due to depression.

Sonya, her nurse, had a long discussion with Mrs. Fukui. She said that she had been unhappy in her marriage but stayed with her husband for the sake of her three children, who were now grown. Just recently one of her daughters was arrested for drug trafficking. The shame Mrs. Fukui felt over the arrest was so intense that she chose to kill herself rather than live with it.

Sonya explored with her patient the concepts of honor and shame in Japanese culture. Although Mrs. Fukui still felt suicidal, and her shame was increased by her failure to die on her first attempt, she developed a strong enough bond with Sonya to connect with her for safety. Why did she trust Sonya to that degree? Because Sonya was the only clinician to try to understand her perspective. Mrs. Fukui thanked Sonya for "understanding" her.

Sonya then spoke to the psychiatrist and treatment team and shared Mrs. Fukui's perspective. Together, they were able to address all Mrs. Fukui's issues with her family and help them understand her situation as well. Sonya's cultural competence in asking the right questions may have saved Mrs. Fukui's life.

Consider another case, this time involving a Hispanic woman. Rosa Valdez was a forty-seven-year-old woman who, though born in the United States, considered herself Puerto Rican, because that is where her family was from. Spanish was her primary language. She was a long-term patient in a state psychiatric hospital, diagnosed with "schizoaffective disorder-depressed type" along with borderline, histrionic, and dependent personality traits. Although she clearly suffered from mental problems, hers is a case in which a lack of understanding of cultural traits may have affected her personality disorder diagnosis.

Puerto Ricans often tend to be vocal, expressive, and dramatic. When seen through the perspective of a culture that values rational, controlled behavior with a minimum of emotional expressiveness, such behavior could be interpreted as dramatic and attention seeking; in other words, histrionic traits. Puerto Rican females were traditionally taught to be modest, submissive to males, and demonstrate a strong sense of closeness to the family; such traits could well be interpreted as dependent in a culture that values independence and individuality.

One of her psychiatric "symptoms" was that she would not make eye contact when speaking with the psychiatric nurse. In fact, Puerto Rican women of her generation were taught to lower their eyes and avoid eye contact. It should not be misinterpreted as a lack of ability to relate to others.

Ms. Valdez often complained of physical symptoms; she claimed she felt "feverish or that her eyes "felt funny," or that she suffered from a stomachache or headache. It is common in Puerto Rican culture to convert emotional feelings to physical symptoms. As Rosa explained, in her culture you are not expected to talk about feelings. She referred to her psychiatric illness and depression by saying, "My heart is hurting me."

When she spoke of her family, it was of the large, Latino, extended family, which includes aunts, uncles, grandparents, and cousins. Although she would have liked to return to them, her prognosis made it unlikely. Each time she progressed to a point where she could be discharged to a personal care boarding home, she regressed quickly and was returned to the hospital. It is likely that the hospital had taken on the role of her family—the traditional, hierarchical family structure in which her needs are all taken care of, but where her illness frees her from any obligations or expectations.

Again, it is not that the patient had been misdiagnosed as mentally ill on the basis of culturally normal behavior. Rather, some of the traits she displayed are not necessarily symptomatic of psychiatric illness but part of her cultural upbringing. Her culture confused her diagnosis.

217   In the next case, behavior that is seen as normal in one culture is perceived as abnormal in another. Esperlita, a Filipino nurse, began acting strangely. Her aunt and uncle had died in a fatal car crash on their way to Reno. A week after the funeral, Esperlita began to see visions of them. She would hear someone calling her name, smell the scent of her uncle's hair dressing, and feel a cold breeze on her face. The experience disturbed her so much that she began having trouble sleeping and was losing her appetite.

Esperlita shared her experience with Jackie, an Anglo American nurse, who strongly advised her to get psychiatric help. Jackie believed that the stress of her relatives' death was leading Esperlita to a nervous breakdown.

Esperlita related the same story to Araceli, a Filipino coworker. Araceli had a completely different interpretation. She thought that Esperlita's dead relatives, having died in a foreign country and lacking the proper burial ritual, were having trouble making their journey into the next world. Or perhaps they simply wanted to say goodbye. Whatever the explanation, Araceli saw the experience as normal, not as a sign of impending psychosis.

Convinced of Araceli's interpretation, Esperlita and her family offered masses for her departed aunt and uncle over the next two weeks. They also lit candles on their graves each night. At the end of two weeks, the voices, visions, and scents disappeared, Esperlita could sleep undisturbed, and her appetite returned.

What is interesting about this case is the difference in the interpretation of the same behavior by an Anglo American and by a Filipino. The former's culture does not allow for the existence of spirits; the latter's does. Seeing spirits is not interpreted as a sign of mental illness in cultures where people believe spirits exist.

Diagnosing and Treating Mental Illness

218   As mentioned in the first two case studies above, diagnosing mental illness can be complicated by the fact that in many cultures, including Puerto

Rican and Asian groups, emotional stresses are converted to physical symptoms. Consider the following case. Canh Cao was a thirty-four-year-old Vietnamese woman who was treated by a medical student at a public health clinic. She had made several visits for various physical complaints—abdominal pain, backache, headaches. She was diagnosed with somatoform pain disorder—preoccupation with pain in absence of physical findings.

Several months later, Cao attempted suicide. She was sent for evaluation to a psychiatrist, who at that point diagnosed her with depression. She had been depressed all along, but the medical student was both inexperienced and unaware of cultural issues, so he missed it.

It is often difficult to diagnose depression in Vietnamese American patients because they will tend to focus on physical complaints rather than underlying emotional problems. As I've mentioned, mental illness carries a great stigma in Asian cultures, and thus individuals will tend to somaticize their problems and report only the physical symptoms. Health care workers need to be aware of this.

Also remember that when dealing with refugees from any country, you must consider numerous other conditions that can affect their mental health, including homesickness, concern for the future, loss of family members, adjustment to a new culture, language problems, and job dissatisfaction. These factors can all lead to depression and suicide attempts.

The Stigma of Mental Illness

Maria Kim was a twenty-four-year-old Korean woman, admitted after overdosing on Valium and Xanax. She was also diagnosed with decreased blood pressure. Celia, the admitting nurse, was Filipino; Roberta, the charge nurse, was Anglo American. Celia called Roberta to request a room assignment. Roberta reminded Celia that Ms. Kim would have to be admitted to the intensive care unit for constant observation, as per procedure with all overdoses, because such patients are considered a threat to themselves. Celia explained that the patient's physician, a Korean named Dr. Chee, had insisted that the overdose was accidental. Roberta would have questioned Dr. Chee's pronouncement, but Celia's Filipino background would not allow her to insult his authority in that way. Roberta compromised by assigning Maria Kim a room in front of the nurses' station, where she could be observed.

The patient was extremely withdrawn and would not speak. She crawled under the bed covers, while her brother stood watch all day. At 5:00 P.M., Dr. Chee arrived, noted that her blood pressure was now stabilized, and discharged her. When Roberta suggested to him that Kim have a psychiatric evaluation, he simply replied that it was an accident and that the family wanted to take her home.

219

Although Maria Kim's behavior seems to indicate that she was extremely depressed and probably suicidal, the fact that her physician was also Korean influenced the way the case was handled. Because of the stigma associated with mental illness in Asian cultures, people with such problems are generally taken care of by the family. Dr. Chee recognized this, and did not stigmatize her with the label "depressed" or "suicidal." Her problem was handled by her family, who watched over her and took her home with them.

Roberta, the Anglo nurse, was uncomfortable with merely letting Ms. Kim go without evaluation. Lacking the automatic and absolute respect for the authority of the physician that her coworker held, Roberta sent a social service referral on the patient for follow-up. The results are unknown.

Why is mental illness so highly stigmatized in Asia? As a Korean student explained to me, mental illness is thought to be inherited. If it were known that someone in the family was mentally ill, no one would want to marry into that family. When I've mentioned this in class, students from other Asian countries have nodded in agreement. This is consistent with the fact that in Asian cultures the group is the primary unit. It is not just individuals who marry, but families.

When I was teaching a class of nurses from mainland China in the 1980s, they were quite astounded to learn that many Americans sought psychotherapy for minor problems. They believed that you were either sane or hopelessly mentally ill. There was no middle ground, no category of "neurotic," only that of "psychotic." I once met a Chinese psychiatrist in Los Angeles. When I mentioned that it was surprising to me to hear the combination of "Chinese" and "psychiatrist," he nodded understandingly and said that his parents were ashamed that he was a psychiatrist due to his association with the mentally ill. To hide their shame, they told their friends only that he was a "doctor."

Stress and Mental Health

Discussing Emotional Problems

Although mental illness carries a stigma for most Americans, a distinction is made between psychosis and the stresses of everyday life. Seeking counseling to deal with such stresses does not carry the same burden of shame for most of us. However, talking about personal problems to strangers is not something that is comfortable for everyone. Few African Americans will turn to therapists, because most therapists tend to be white, and they may distrust white institutions in general. Furthermore, it is difficult for a white person to fully understand the stresses of being Black in America. Often, African Americans will turn to the church instead. As mentioned earlier, many Puerto Ricans and Asians will somaticize their feelings and seek treatment for physical symptoms instead.

One might think that having a counselor of the same ethnic background as the patient/client would make it easier to talk, because the counselor would have a better understanding of the cultural stresses. This is not the case. Ethnic communities tend to be very tightly knit, and the (unfounded) fear that the therapist will talk within the community might keep the client from opening up in therapy.

Many Italians and Hispanics will turn to their families, rather than dis-   220
cuss their personal problems with strangers. A fifty-five-year-old Mexican American woman named Maria Ibañez was admitted to the coronary care unit with chest pain. She appeared withdrawn and was crying. When asked what was wrong, she shook her head and replied, "Nothing." She gave brief answers to Dr. Mandel, the physician who took her family history, but offered no additional information. Her crying continued even after her chest pain ceased, so Dr. Mandel asked why she was depressed. Still she did not answer.

Eventually Mrs. Ibañez's thirty-five-year-old daughter Cecilia arrived and explained that her mother had been in a state of emotional upset since her father had left home two weeks before. At this Mrs. Ibañez cried out, "No, no! You must not say anything. It's private." Her daughter quietly replied that she could not stand to see her mother suffer so and that she was frightened by her chest pains. Dr. Mandel then suggested that Mrs. Ibañez might want to talk with the staff psychiatrist. In response she exclaimed, "No! No other people should know about this!" Dr. Mandel drew Mrs. Ibañez closer to him, held her hand, and gently said, "Okay. But we need to talk about this." Cecilia, who was visibly disturbed, pleaded with her mother, "Please, Mama."

Why was Mrs. Ibañez so reluctant to discuss the problem that was most likely causing her chest pains? A Mexican nurse on staff later explained that Mexicans feel personal matters should be handled only within the family. They should not be discussed with strangers. Furthermore, a traditional Mexican woman's status is in large part derived from her role as a wife. If her husband leaves, she is nothing. Mrs. Ibañez's pride and embarrassment probably prevented her from talking about the situation. Her daughter, a second-generation Mexican American, was more Westernized and thus more open with outsiders about personal matters.

As it turned out, Mrs. Ibañez did not have a heart attack and was transferred to the post-coronary-care unit the next day. The nurse attending her case stopped by her room several times before she left. Although she still did not want to discuss her husband, she had stopped crying and was feeling somewhat better emotionally. What she needed most from the staff was nonintrusive warmth and support. In this case, the underlying emotional nature of the problem was discovered, due to the intervention of the more Westernized daughter and the sensitivity of the physician. However, had they not been involved, it is easy to see how the somaticization of Mrs. Ibañez's emotional condition could have easily masked the real problem.

It is important for health care providers to remember the strong connection between the mind and the body. People often somaticize their emotional stress. The potential for this is further increased when culture dictates a withholding of feelings. It may take a great deal of sensitivity and luck to get patients to discuss their feelings with health care providers. Whenever possible, try to involve culturally appropriate individuals, such as clergy members, traditional healers, or more acculturated family members.

Psychotherapy is not common in most cultures. In traditional, non-Western societies, mind and body are not seen as separate. The same healer—be it shaman or *curandero*—will treat the problem, without distinguishing between emotional and physical ailments.

Acculturation and Mental Health

Depression and anxiety are very common in immigrant populations. Individuals are often alone, without their extended family. They are frequently busy trying to make a living, with little time to talk to one another. Although there are medications to treat depression and anxiety, patients often don't want to take them because of the stigma associated with any kind of mental illness. This is particularly true in Asian populations. A Korean physician has found that when she tells Korean patients that it sounds as if they're suffering from depression, they often break down and cry. Although counseling would generally be appropriate in such a situation, she said she rarely refers them, because they won't go, due to the stigma of "mental illness." She finds she has more success if she herself does supportive counseling. Patients will often spend some time talking with her. She typically assures them that anxiety and depression are very common; they won't be on medications forever, but the medications will help them get through the difficult time. She says it may take a few visits to convince patients to take medication, but eventually, they usually do. She also encourages them to look for support in their church or community. Traditional healers can be helpful as well.

221   While Myra was doing a psych rotation, she cared for Zulema Herrera, a Mexican patient who had been diagnosed with major depression. Mrs. Herrera was also experiencing delusions and her husband had her hospitalized because he was afraid she might harm their daughter. Mrs. Herrera

had moved to the United States two years earlier. She was not responding to medication, and the psychiatrists were considering electroconvulsive therapy. Mr. Hererra disagreed with their diagnosis and plan; he believed his wife was suffering from *susto* and needed treatment from a *curandero*.

A team of psychiatrists, nurses, and social workers met to discuss her situation. The nurses and social workers felt that Mrs. Herrera's illness was related to the stress of being in a new country and far from her family in Mexico. They thought she would benefit from seeing a *curandero*. They physicians reluctantly agreed but insisted they meet first with her husband and the *curandero* to discuss what would take place. They decided to allow the *curandero* to treat Mrs. Herrera with prayer, massage, and herbal teas.

After the *curandero* performed his healing ritual, Mrs. Herrera was noticeably less depressed and was more responsive to the therapy prescribed by the psychiatrists.

With the increasing numbers of immigrants in this country comes the growing problem of children who are raised at home with one set of cultural values and are exposed to another set at school and with friends. This can create stress for first-generation Americans.

Tammy Tang was born in China, but her family moved to the United States when she was in elementary school. Her parents were very traditional. When she was in college, she still lived at home. In fact, she attended the specific college she did because her parents would not let her enroll in any university that was too far from home for her to commute. She was not allowed to date and had a very early curfew. If she were living in China, these restrictions would not have been a problem; however, she was living in the United States. Most of her friends could date and stay out as late as they wanted. Many lived in the dorms or had their own apartments. Tammy felt a tremendous inner conflict. She respected and wanted to obey her parents; at the same time, she wanted the freedom enjoyed by most American college students.

She felt further trapped by her inability to discuss her feelings with anyone. It had been deeply ingrained in her that you should never talk to outsiders about your problems; you discuss them only with your family. But her family *was* her problem. How could she talk to them? It would be completely disrespectful.

I know of Tammy's situation because she was a student in one of my classes. As part of a class requirement, she had to keep a journal. There were several entries in which she discussed her dilemma and the fact that she had often considered suicide as a solution. When I read these entries, I immediately asked Tammy to come see me. I told her that I understood her situation, and strongly advised her to seek help at the student counseling center. Therapists who have worked with clients caught between cultures say that the most effective approach in dealing with such problems is a direct one: discuss the conflicts as resulting from cultural differences. It is not about being a "good" or "bad" person, but what is valued in different cultures.

The wise health care provider will recognize the potential for such problems with their adolescent patients. The stress created by intergenerational, intercultural conflicts may be a complicating factor in presenting health problems. Social workers who are trained in cultural diversity may be needed. However, because people from many immigrant cultures have strong feelings against any kind of psychotherapy, either because "mental illness" is highly stigmatized or because personal problems should not be discussed with outsiders, any counseling sessions will have to be scheduled when the family are not around.

The Supernatural

Healer or Psychotic?

223   Juan Gutierrez, a fifteen-year-old Mexican American, was referred to the inpatient psychiatric unit of the hospital by his school psychologist. She noted that he had a history of seizures and was currently experiencing visual and auditory hallucinations as well as evidencing delusional thinking. Although they were very loving parents, the Gutierrezes were not in favor of the decision to hospitalize Juan and did not want him treated with medication. They did not share the hospital staff's view that he was mentally ill, despite the fact that he heard voices in his head, alternatively complimenting and criticizing him, and was constantly being distracted by things he alone could see. The staff also noted that Juan was experiencing delusions of grandeur, with his belief that he was born destined to be a *curandero*. In fact, his family reinforced this belief and interpreted what the staff saw as his "psychotic" symptoms as signs of his "calling."

Fortunately, the hospital staff in this situation acted in a culturally appropriate manner. Although they did not share Juan's interpretation of his symptoms, and proceeded to put him on antipsychotic medication, they did follow the recommendation of a Mexican American therapist who suggested that a *curandero* meet with Juan and his family.

The meeting had a very positive effect on the mood and attitude of the entire Gutierrez family. Juan's symptoms showed gradual improvement, and he began to participate in the hospital's program of structured activities with his peers. Not long afterward he was able to be discharged home, on continued medication and with an appointment at his community mental health facility. In all likelihood, Juan also continued to see the *curandero*.

Supernatural Healing

Clara Sandoval, a seventy-one-year-old Mexican woman, was referred to   224
a geriatric assessment program by a local psychiatrist. He had been treating her for severe depression using antipsychotic and antidepressant medications. They had not helped. In the past year she had lost forty pounds.
She often lay awake at night, crying and screaming. Her doctor recommended inpatient hospitalization with electroshock therapy, and sent her
for assessment. Though uncomfortable with the doctor's recommendation, Mrs. Sandoval's family agreed to abide by the geriatric assessment
program's recommendations.

When the geriatric assessment team arrived at Mrs. Sandoval's home,
they found her in a darkened room filled with religious icons. She was
wearing a six-inch crucifix around her neck. During her two-hour interview, Mrs. Sandoval wrapped her rosary around her hand and began to
beat her chest. She frequently referred to the "evil ones" who were steal-
ing her soul and the "voices" that haunted her in the night. Her affect
during the interview ranged from flat and unresponsive to near hysteria.
Mrs. Sandoval's family added that although she had been a devout Catholic, she refused to go to mass during the past year and would not accept
any visits from the local clergy.

When they spoke with the parish priest, he told the assessment team
that it was not uncommon for elderly Hispanic women to fear possession
and punishment for past sins. He supplied them with the name of an
exorcist who had successfully treated some of these cases. The exorcist
visited Mrs. Sandoval on three occasions. Although it is not known what
he did during those visits, when the geriatric assessment team visited
Mrs. Sandoval a month later, they found her remarkably improved. Her
antidepressant medication appeared to be working, and she had gained
ten pounds.

Exactly what happened in this case is unclear. What is known is that an
obviously religious woman had been suffering from depression, was hearing voices, and feared that her soul was being taken by "evil ones." Medication was ineffective in treating her condition. After three visits from
an exorcist, she was on the road to recovery. The important point is that
treatment within the framework of Mrs. Sandoval's belief system was effective in a way that traditional psychiatric treatment was not.

A similar situation occurred with Carlos Gonzales, a twenty-two-year-   225
old Mexican American inmate of the county jail. He was referred to medical services with symptoms of a heart attack. When the doctor examined
him, he discovered no cardiac abnormalities. Gonzales was then sent to
the mental health section, where he appeared to be in a state of acute
fear. He clutched his left side, and his garbled Spanish was incoherent.

From his appearance and vital signs, alcohol withdrawal was suspected. He was sent back to the medical service.

Shortly thereafter, he was returned to the mental health service. He lay on the floor, conscious but shaking violently, a look of terror covering his face. He claimed to be dying and begged Regina, the nurse, to inform his mother. Asking Carlos if he believed in God and getting an affirmative answer, Regina reached for a Bible. She quickly tore out a picture of Jesus and held it over his heart. Slowly he calmed down. When asked if he wanted a cigarette, Carlos surprised everyone by getting up and following Regina to her office.

Still clutching Jesus' picture to his chest, Carlos explained that he had been cursed by a former lover in Mexico. When he ended the relationship, she consulted a *bruja* (witch) who put a spell on him that would cause him to die of a heart attack. Regina called Carlos's home and spoke with his sister, who confirmed the story.

As the night wore on, Carlos gradually stopped shaking but remained fearful. Regina finally convinced him that his belief in God, coupled with the prayers of his family, would counteract the curse. By morning, he was fairly calm, perhaps because he was still alive.

Interpreting the incident from an etic perspective, one might suggest that Carlos experienced heartburn that evening. Mindful of the curse, he thought his symptoms signaled a heart attack. His Catholicism may have also contributed to his guilt, punishing his "love" affair with a "heart" attack. From an emic perspective, the *bruja* worked a powerful spell.

Anthropological Perspectives on the Supernatural

From an anthropological perspective, it is somewhat difficult to discuss cases involving the supernatural. If one acknowledges the reality of the supernatural, one is not being scientific; if one does not, one is being ethnocentric. If in fact such things as spirits and witchcraft exist, the responses of Carlos Gonzales and Mrs. Ibañez are perfectly normal, and do not belong in a chapter on "mental health," except in terms of how their behavior is interpreted by the dominant American culture.

The symptoms Juan experienced are certainly consistent with that of receiving a spiritual "calling." In fact, it is common for shamans to experience psychotic episodes before they begin shamanizing. It is through these episodes that they learn to control their entrance into and out of altered states of consciousness that psychiatrists refer to as "psychotic." Often the problem with psychotics is that their perceptions do not "match" those of the rest of us; they therefore cannot function in our society. It has been argued that by acknowledging "hallucinations" and "delusions" as real—as evidence of communication with the spirit world—non-Western societies provide a place for psychotics to function. That view, however, is rather ethnocentric. If we are to be culturally relativistic, we should not dismiss entirely the possibility that there is a spirit world and that some people have the ability to connect with it.

Because we do not recognize shamanic healers, witchcraft, or "evil ones" in our own culture, we have no framework for understanding the experiences of Clara Sandoval, Carlos Gonzales, or Juan Gutierrez beyond that of psychosis. It is unknown what the visiting *curandero* said or did with the Gutierrez family. At the very least, however, it is clear that the fact that the acknowledgment by hospital staff of the family's belief system made them much more cooperative and comfortable. From the medical perspective, it was the medications that helped Juan, but his attitude after seeing the *curandero* certainly may have contributed to a faster and smoother recovery, as well as to his willingness to participate in the medical treatment plan.

The lesson to be learned from all these cases is that whatever one's personal worldview, it is far more effective to treat patients in the context of their belief system rather than just one's own.

Summary

The crux of the mental health issue rests with what is considered normal. Because this varies across cultures, behaviors that are perceived as normal in one culture are deemed abnormal in another. This becomes a problem in the United States because of the vast numbers of people from diverse cultures living here. Although there are some individuals who would be considered mentally ill in *any* culture, there are many who are labeled mentally ill because their beliefs or behavior are inconsistent with cultural norms, or who are misdiagnosed because what is perceived as culturally appropriate varies so greatly. For example, a person who has visions of the dead may be perceived as abnormal, normal, or even special, depending on the beliefs of the culture. Health care providers who understand the worldview of their patients will generally have much more success in treating them.

Health care workers also need to be sensitive to the fact that mental illness is highly stigmatized in many cultures; patients with emotional problems may be reluctant to discuss them with strangers. This can be a particular problem for the children of immigrants, who may feel unable to discuss the stress they experience resulting from the conflict between American culture and that of their parents. In all cases, what is called for is greater awareness and sensitivity on the part of the health care provider.

Key Points

- Because each culture values different behavior in its members, what is considered normal in one culture may be perceived as deviant in another.
- In many cultures, emotional stresses are converted to physical symptoms.
- Mental illness is highly stigmatized in Asian cultures.
- Remember to get the patient's point of view on his or her condition.
- In many cultures, people turn to family members or church for emotional support, rather than professionals, and may resist talking to health care providers about their personal problems.
- Acculturation can be a source of stress, as can intergenerational conflict.
- Many cultures believe in the supernatural.

Chapter 12
Traditional Medicine: Practices and Perspectives

People have been healing the sick long before the advent of biomedicine. Neanderthal burials from 65,000 years ago show evidence of healed wounds and the presence of plant pollen from species known to have healing properties. Even chimpanzees—our closest living relatives—have been observed chewing a particular species of leaf that appears to expel some sort of tapeworm.

Many people grow medicinal plants in their own gardens or obtain them from a neighborhood or professional healer. These plants may be used as first aid, to treat wounds and burns, aches and pains, upper respiratory infections, earaches, and chronic conditions. Most people will try home remedies, passed on from grandparents and parents, before coming in to the doctor. In many cases, home remedies are effective and save a trip to the physician. However, in other cases, they don't do the job, and the patient shows up in the emergency department or the physician's office. Because these remedies sometimes leave unfamiliar markings on the body, they can lead the clinician to a misdiagnosis. In other cases, they can have negative interactions with biomedicine. In rare cases, they may actually harm the patient.

It is the intent of this chapter to familiarize health care providers with some of the more common traditional remedies, along with a brief look at several traditional health care systems, including Ayurvedic medicine, Chinese medicine, Mexican folk medicine, and African American folk medicine. Also examined will be the kinds of errors that result from the fact that traditional remedies are often used differently from biomedical remedies. The examples of cultural competence in this chapter lie largely in the integration of traditional and biomedical approaches to healing.

Traditional or "Folk" Remedies

Coining

A Korean man named Sung Kim was brought into the emergency room, unconscious. His chest was covered with red welts. The family did not speak

English, and there was no interpreter available. The staff assumed that Mr. Kim's lack of consciousness was related to the red welts, that both were symptoms of the same condition. They were not. Unfortunately, by the time they discovered what Mr. Kim was suffering from, it was too late to save him. Had they known to ignore the welts, they might have saved his life.

227   A Vietnamese girl named Kathy Dinh was in her first year at an American elementary school. She was not feeling very well one morning, so her mother rubbed the back of her neck with a coin. She then felt well enough to attend school. Later in the day, however, she began to feel worse and went to see the school nurse. When the nurse discovered the welts on Kathy's neck, she immediately assumed she was seeing a case of child abuse and conscientiously reported the Dinhs to the authorities. The situation was finally straightened out, but it created a great deal of needless embarrassment for Kathy's family.

The patients in these two cases had experienced a traditional Asian form of healing known as coin rubbing. There are several variations, including heating or oiling the coin or other metal object, such as a spoon, but they all involve vigorously rubbing the body with a coin. This produces red welts on the affected area, which can distract health professionals from the real problem or be mistaken for abuse.

It is not that Asians never abuse their children, but rubbing them with coins is not the way they do it, any more than Americans abuse their children by having thin pieces of metal wrapped around their teeth and tightened until their teeth move out of place. Braces are often applied for primarily aesthetic reasons. Coin rubbing, at least, is an attempt to heal. Apparently, it often works; only the failures show up in the medical system.

Underlying this practice is the belief that the illness in the body needs to be drawn out. Rubbing the body with a coin produces a raised red area, giving the appearance that the illness has been brought to the surface of the skin. It is believed that red marks will appear only on people who are ill, which is seen as further support for the effectiveness of the technique. Many Asian Americans claim that they still practice coin rubbing because it brings relief from colds and other ailments.

While conducting a continuing medical education (CME) class for physicians, I showed a film on patient diversity, which had a segment involving coining. A Vietnamese physician in the audience shared with me that he had experienced coining the week before. The physician was born in Vietnam but came to America at a young age; he had no accent. He looked to be in his late twenties or early thirties. After my lecture, I asked him more about it. He said he had been experiencing migraine headaches, body aches, and general flu symptoms. First, he tried aspirin, but that didn't help. Next, he tried naprosin. When that didn't work, he went to the strongest pain reliever he knew, Fiorinal. When that didn't help, he had his mother use coining on his chest. The coin was dipped in eucalyptus oil and then rubbed until welts formed. He explained that if he weren't sick, no redness would appear. He claimed that the coining was effective whereas the other remedies were not; his symptoms were gone by the next day. He said that when he's ill, he'll try Western medicine first. If that doesn't work, he'll turn to traditional medicine.

It is important that health care professionals become familiar with the practice, lest they become distracted from the real problem or mistakenly make accusations of child abuse. When such welts are observed, if the patient and family do not speak English, it would be a good idea to pull out a coin and mime rubbing the body with it. That, along with a questioning look, would probably convey the message. If the patient or family nods in agreement, the marks should be ignored. If it is necessary to write a report on the marks, a note should be made indicating that they may be the result of a traditional healing practice.

Cupping

Another healing method that produces similarly misleading results is cupping. John Bagdasarian, a forty-six-year-old Armenian, was brought into the critical care unit with a diagnosis of acute myocardial infarction (heart attack). While doing a physical assessment, the nurse found round red marks all over his upper back that looked like burns. The staff speculated about the source of the marks. Theories ranged from birthmarks to some form of torture or sadism. An Armenian physician finally cleared up the mystery. The marks were a result of cupping.   228

The patient's family had tried to cure him of his chest pains by heating a glass and placing it on his body. The vacuum created under the glass caused the skin to rise and left the red marks. When cupping did not stop the chest pains, his family brought him to the hospital.

The traditional form of cupping is that which the Bagdasarians practiced. A more modern version uses a suction pump to create a vacuum under the cups. In both cases, the skin is drawn up into the cup, increasing circulation and leaving a large, circular bruise. It is commonly used to treat sore muscles and respiratory problems.

Marianne Bernstein, a middle-aged Anglo American woman, was sick with flu, bronchitis, and pneumonia. She could not stop coughing. She went to her physician for treatment, and took three rounds of antibiotics. Despite that, she continued to cough. She finally went to an acupuncturist who performed cupping on her. Her coughing relented that day and continued to improve. Although it may have been due to the antibiotics finally kicking in, or to the disease finally running its course, or perhaps   229 to the Chinese herbs she took for the next week, Marianne was convinced that the cupping was primarily responsible.

I include this example for two reasons. One is to point out that traditional remedies may be used by patients from other cultures. Traditional Chinese medicine has experienced great popularity among upper-middle-class Anglo Americans. Two, to point out the possible efficacy of traditional "folk" remedies.

Cupping is said to be particularly successful for treating sore muscles and is frequently practiced for that purpose in many parts of the world, including Asia, Latin America, Russia, and parts of Europe, and it is taught in acupuncture colleges in the United States. As with coining, however, health care professionals who are not aware of the practice can easily misinterpret the marks it leaves.

Fevers

Current medical wisdom has it that the most effective way to reduce fever is to cool the body. This is done by removing regular blankets and placing an "ice blanket" under the patient. In contrast, many cultures believe that the best way to treat a high temperature is to sweat it out. These conflicting theories are the source of another common cultural conflict in the hospital.

230   Hiroshi Tomita, a Japanese business executive on a trip to the United States, was admitted to the hospital with a 102-degree fever of unknown origin. According to standard procedure, his nurse, Jean, removed the blankets from the bed, leaving only a sheet to cover him. She explained that it was to keep his temperature from going up. She gave him a glass of cold apple juice, but he only took two sips. At 9 P.M., the doctor examined Mr. Tomita and prescribed a mild analgesic every four hours for temperatures greater than 101 degrees and a cooling blanket for temperatures greater than 102 degrees. When his temperature rose to 103 degrees at 10 P.M., Jean ordered a cooling blanket, per the doctor's instructions. At this point, Mr. Tomita asked for his blankets, but Jean refused, once more explaining why. She put the ice blanket under him and left the room. In a few minutes, Mr. Tomita complained that the ice blanket was too cold and asked for his regular blankets. For the third time, Jean patiently explained the treatment. He did not say anything; he simply curled up under his sheet. When Jean returned a half hour later to check on him, he was sitting up in the chair with all the blankets wrapped around him, covered with goose bumps and shivering. By midnight, his temperature was up to 105 degrees. Jean gave him his second dosage of acetaminophen. Mr. Tomita continued to ask for his blankets and to get out of bed. Jean was at the point of putting restraints on him to keep him in bed.

She asked him why he did not want to stay in bed. He explained that in Japan, people with fevers were covered with warm blankets and given plenty of hot drinks. Cold juice was particularly inappropriate. This approach, found throughout Asia, is probably based on the Chinese notion of hot and cold balance, or yin and yang. Mr. Tomita was experiencing chills, which logically should be treated with heat, not cold. Furthermore, it is believed that fevers must be sweated out, again necessitating measures that produce greater warmth.

Reflecting on his comment, Jean asked herself what she did when suffering from a temperature and chills. She realized that she did exactly what her patient wanted—she piled lots of blankets on herself, turned the electric blanket to the maximum temperature, and drank hot liquids!

She then called a team conference. Most of her colleagues admitted to similar behavior, but no one wanted to take responsibility for going against medical orders. Realizing that she could no longer treat Mr. Tomita against his beliefs and wishes, Jean decided to call the admitting doctor. It was now 1 A.M. The physician was angry at being awakened. He impatiently listened to her story, was silent for a moment, and then agreed to a change in orders: discontinue the cooling blanket, administer analgesic tablets every three hours if the patient's temperature rose above 101 degrees, and keep the patient as comfortable as possible.

Mr. Tomita was extremely happy and grateful for the change in orders. His temperature came down after about three hours and eventually he removed the blankets on his own.

A similar case involved Rosa Torres, a twenty-nine-year-old Hispanic woman with a surgical infection. Her temperature was 104 degrees. She had piled six blankets on top of herself, curled up into a ball, and lay there moaning loudly. When Rebecca, her nurse, discovered the mound of blankets, she attempted to remove them. Ms. Torres vehemently refused. "No, I will get cold." Rebecca explained that the blankets were keeping her body temperature too high; she needed to remove them to reduce the fever. The explanation did nothing to change her mind, but Rebecca was determined and gently pulled off all but one blanket.

Shortly thereafter, Rebecca tried to take Ms. Torres's temperature rectally, per the doctor's orders. Again, she refused. She did not want her underwear removed and certainly did not want anyone to insert a rectal thermometer. Each of Rebecca's attempts to do so was met with screams. Rebecca tried to explain the importance of the greater accuracy of the rectal temperature, but Rosa did not care. Rebecca finally gave up, respecting Rosa's right to refuse. Another nurse on the unit, however, was not about to give in to the patient's desires and insisted that she remove her underwear. She managed to insert the thermometer despite Rosa Torres's cries and tears.

231

Although Rebecca did not understand the reason for Rosa's behavior at the time, she later learned from several Hispanic friends that it is believed that one of the greatest dangers during a fever is letting in cold air. Removing all the covers thus put the patient at risk. Second, the illness is seen as a kind of poison. Keeping the blankets on causes the body to sweat out the poison; thus, the fever goes down and the illness disappears. Ms. Torres's refusal to remove her underwear and have her temperature taken rectally was probably due to the modesty typically found among Hispanic women, along with the discomfort and sense of indignity involved.

Unlike the previous example, in which the nurse finally did respect the patient's wishes, in this case Western medicine won out. Rosa Torres was labeled a difficult patient because of her desire to adhere to her traditional beliefs regarding treatment of disease. Rebecca later suggested that the doctor could have been called to change the order from a rectal to an oral temperature. She still felt it was necessary to remove the blankets but thought that if she had understood Ms. Torres's reasons, she might have been more empathetic.

232   In another case, a Mexican American mother refused to use cooling measures in caring for her febrile infant, despite medical instructions to do so. Mrs. Lopez had called the hospital because her infant's temperature was very high. She was told to give the baby a mild analgesic and a cool bath and then to bring her in. Mrs. Lopez ignored both cooling instructions and, to the consternation of the medical staff, brought the child wrapped in several layers of blankets, outer garments, undershirt, and several pairs of socks. When asked why she did not follow the instructions given her, she replied, "He must sweat the fever out. Besides, he could get pneumonia from the night air and die."

Nurses who work in hospitals serving a large Hispanic population say that they see this behavior quite frequently. In fact, the sight of a family walking up to the registration window with a bundle of blankets in their arms usually prompts the nurses to prediagnose the child as having a fever and admit it right away. Immediate action is necessary to make sure the baby does not have a seizure while the family is registering.

Parents are generally willing to listen to the nurses' explanations on how to treat fevers in infants. The problem is often with their own parents. One young woman explained that she knew she should not wrap her baby so heavily, but her mother-in-law "made her do it." She had attended some parenting classes and knew the proper procedure, but felt it was too difficult to fight the whole family. Health education is the only way to deal with such situations, but it will not be easy to overcome years of tradition.

233   Another example occurred with an African American woman and her tiny grandson. The child was brought into the hospital by his mother, Mary Wilson, and grandmother, Adele Wilson. The nurse explained that she

would put the naked infant in a cool mist tent and bathe him in cold water to reduce his temperature. His mother was quiet, calm, and cooperative. She indicated her concern by asking several questions about her son's condition.

Adele Wilson, however, did not appear to be listening. She got up from her chair, looked into the tent, and said, "You forgot to give him a blanket. That thing is real cold inside." The nurse again explained that she was keeping him cool because of his high temperature. Mary Wilson tried to calm her mother-in-law, seeing that she was becoming hostile. "Mama, it's okay." Mrs. Wilson responded, "What you talkin' 'bout? They got you believing in this foolishness too. I'm gonna put his blanket on him 'cause he is cold. I raised all my nine children and I never put one in no icebox. You know you need to wrap him so he can sweat the fever out. Hot chamomile tea would bring that fever down."

Most of the nurses dealt with the grandmother by avoiding her. They could not talk to her without arguing. How might they have handled the situation? They might have begun by asking her how she would have treated the child. They could have acknowledged her approach, which comes from years of use of natural remedies within the African American culture. They might also have incorporated her recommendation of chamomile tea. Mrs. Wilson's hostility may have been a reaction to what she perceived as racism on the part of the white nurses. A bit more respect on the part of the nurses might have helped.

Medications

Applying the Medication Directly to the Site

A common source of cross-cultural misunderstandings involves the use of Western medications, which often differs from the application of traditional remedies. It is essential that complete explanations be given to patients regarding how to use medication. Florence, a Black nurse, was doing home care for a thirty-year-old Mexican woman named Lena Menendez, who had recently had a caesarean section. Mrs. Menendez spoke little English. Her mother, Gloria Flores, was staying with her to help with the baby. During her first visit, she wanted to make an assessment evaluation and change the dressing on the incision site.

234

When Mrs. Menendez removed her underpants, the first thing Florence noticed was the absence of a pad or gauze covering the gauze inside the wound. When she looked more closely, she discovered a bloody white cheesy substance on the gauze and in the corners and edges of the wound. Florence had no idea what it was. In her mind, she considered the possibilities: semen? intestines? When she removed the old dressing, she was relieved to find that it was not her intestines. She could find no evidence of infection, and after cleaning the wound, decided it was just a dirty wound.

When Florence returned the next day, she noted more of the white, bloody, cheesy substance. This time, she asked Mrs. Menendez what it was. Her mother answered for her, replying, "Her medication—the one with the powder in it. The nurse said it was for infections." Florence was astounded. She explained that the medication was to be taken by mouth. Mrs. Flores said, "No, in my culture, we mix the powder and put it where the infection is. In order for the wound to heal, the powder goes in there." Florence then spent several minutes explaining to Mrs. Flores and her daughter the difference between American medicine and traditional Mexican medicine. It was unfortunate that the nurse who had given medication to her had neglected to explain how it is used. Moreover, Florence should have asked about it on the first visit.

Do not assume that a patient will understand how to take the medication prescribed. Medicines are used in different ways in different countries, and confusion can result. Alternately, people simply may be unfamiliar with the administration of medicinal products, as evidenced in the next two cases.

235   One nurse related the case of an angry Mexican woman who became pregnant even though she faithfully took her birth control pill every day. Questioning revealed that the woman had inserted the pills into her vagina. Her action may have seemed logical to her; unfortunately, it was not effective.

236   Another Mexican woman became pregnant while using contraceptive foam. Although the failure rate with foam is much higher than with birth control pills, that was not the cause of her pregnancy. No one had explained to her how to use the foam. Since the directions on the can were in English, which she did not understand, she and her husband did what made sense to them—they applied the foam to his penis before he inserted it into her vagina. Again, when giving information on the use of any kind of medication, it is extremely important to give clear and complete instructions on its use.

Filling a Prescription

237   Health care practitioners are often frustrated when patients do not follow through on their prescriptions. Sometimes this apparent lack of adherence can result from cultural factors. Recall the case (100) described earlier involving Mrs. Nguyen, the sixty-five-year-old Vietnamese refugee. In addition to her lung problems, she was also dehydrated and malnourished. She ate little and did not comply with the dietitian's recommended liquid supplement.

While interviewing the patient regarding her condition and health care practices, the nurse learned that she was drinking rice water as a remedy for her gastrointestinal tract. Although her physician had given her a prescription for medication, Mrs. Ngyuen was not familiar with the procedure of having a prescription filled, and had put the prescription with the rest of the indecipherable papers she had received at discharge.

There is an important lesson in this case. Realize that recent immigrants may not be familiar with the system of having prescriptions filled, since they may have always been given medications directly by the doctor. Be sure to explain the procedure.

In another example of "noncompliance," an Anglo American nurse named John was caring for an older African American patient named Robert Williams. Mr. Williams had been admitted for congestive heart failure. Apparently, he had not been taking several of the medications his doctor had prescribed. When John asked why, he explained that he only took his "breathing pill" (digoxin) when he became short of breath. He did not see why he had to take it every day, even when he had no symptoms. It is important that health care providers explain the reason for taking each medication, particularly those that have a preventive function.

Dangerous Substances

There is a long tradition of using folk medicine in many different cultures. Many current drugs, including digitalis, have been developed from native plants. Artemisinin, the most effective current antimalarial drug, was developed from a compound found in the wormwood plant and used to treat fever in China for 2,000 years. *Pasionara* (Passion flower), a traditional Hispanic remedy for anxiety, is an effective sedative, and, if the right species is used, very safe. The same is true of *zábila* (aloe vera) when used externally to treat burns. The traditional Hispanic chili pepper is the source of the well-known pharmaceutical capsaicin, a topical cream used to treat arthritis pain, oral pain, and atypical facial pain. However, many traditional remedies can also cause problems, as the following case indicates.

Mrs. Jimenez brought her twenty-month-old infant to see the doctor because the baby was suffering from diarrhea. During the history, she mentioned that she had given her son a yellow powder that she got from a neighbor. She wasn't sure what it was, but said that it came from Guatemala and is used for stomach ailments. The powder was probably *azarcón* or *greta*, a compound that contains lead and can cause neurological disturbances including seizures, coma, and death.

While many traditional remedies are helpful, and many of those with no proven scientific benefit are at least not harmful, some can be considered dangerous. Sometimes this is due to inadvertent side effects caused by the potency of the main ingredient. For example, PC-SPES, a patent formula that contains eight different herbs and is used to treat prostate cancer, has been shown to stimulate estrogenic activity, which has resulted in some patients having a pulmonary embolism. In other cases, the problem is that the medicine has become contaminated with heavy metals, pesticides, and pharmaceuticals, such as steroids and benzodiazepines.

In 1998, the California health department analyzed over 250 Chinese patent medicines containing premixed herbs compressed into pills or capsules (Chinese Herbs 2000). Nearly a third of the products were found to contain toxic ingredients, including high levels of lead, mercury, and arsenic. A little over 6 percent were spiked with pharmaceutical drugs. One of the problems is that some of the herbs grown in China become contaminated during the farming process, particularly when the herb fields are located next to factories and absorb the pollution. Some of the specific medications found to have problems are Ansenpunaw tablets, which are advertised as "a brain tonic and sedative medicine," and "Double Dragon Pills." The Chinese *ma huang* herb, which contains ephedrine and helps breathing problems, caused heart attacks and strokes among some Americans using it as a diet aid. *Kava kava*, a Pacific Island anxiety-relieving tea, has poisoned the livers of those drinking a concentrated form.

The use of herbal remedies has gained much popularity in recent years among many populations in the United States, including middle-class Anglo Americans. A recent study (Holden et al. 2005) found that 10 percent of 238 rheumatology patients from three outpatient centers were at increased risk of hemorrhagic complications because they were using NSAIDs or corticosteroids in combination with supplements thought to have anticoagulant or antiplatelet effects. These included the popular remedies ginkgo biloba, garlic, and devil's claw.

All this should serve to underscore the importance of discussing with *all* your patients the drugs, herbs, and other remedies they may be taking. It is incumbent upon health care practitioners to ask their patients about this. But what if you don't believe in any of these alternative treatments? Realistically, you will probably not change your patients' attitude, especially if it's something they've grown up with. If you convey your negativity, all you will probably do is alienate your patient. What you want to do instead is make sure they don't do anything harmful, and allow them to continue anything that may be helpful or at least neutral. Many treatments, even if they have no proven pharmacological value, may have psychological value, and allowing your patients to continue to use them will help you gain their trust. Let them know that your primary concern is their health and well-being, and that you will not look down on them or criticize them for anything else they do, as long as they tell you about it.

You might try saying something along the lines of, "Many of my patients also see traditional healers who prescribe herbal remedies, or use home remedies that have been passed down for generations. Often they can be effective, but sometimes they can cause problems, especially when mixed with other treatments. That's why it's important that I know everything that you are taking to treat this or any other problem." An attitude of respect, rather than derision, is crucial.

"Folk" Diseases

Folk diseases are those diseases that are specific to a culture. A number of common Hispanic folk diseases will be discussed later in the chapter. However, at this point, I want to discuss one that is found in numerous parts of the world: evil eye.

Evil Eye

Belief in the evil eye is widespread throughout Central America, the Mediterranean, the Middle East, much of Africa, and parts of Asia. Although the beliefs and associated practices vary, the concept generally includes an evil that one person puts on another that causes the victim to fall ill. The motive is usually envy.

Jen, a second-year medical student, was on a pediatrics visit learning how to perform a newborn exam. As she followed the attending into the patient's room, she noticed that the baby's mother was sitting on the side of the crib talking in Spanish to her husband. The attending started to explain to Jen what is important to notice about a baby and what to look for on the physical exam, and proceeded to ask her questions about the causes of pneumonia and meningitis in the newborn period. As they were talking, the infant's mother came over to the crib. In an attempt to welcome her into our conversation, Jen said "hello," and proceeded to compliment her on her beautiful child. As soon as she finished the sentence, the mother said "thank you," but frowned, and her demeanor changed slightly—she stopped smiling, and looked nervous.

Jen wondered what she had done wrong, and suddenly realized that the family was Mexican, and her complementary words, intended as a tool to gain the mother's trust, resulted in causing her distress. Remembering what she had learned about Mexican culture and "mal de ojo" (evil eye), she touched the baby's hand, and looked back at the mother. The change was drastic—the mother smiled back at her, and nodded her head. She did not say anything, but her smile and nod tacitly communicated her gratitude for preventing "mal de ojo." Jen later commented to me that during the challenging period in medical school, while the medical student

240

is learning to become a doctor, it is often easy to focus on studying diseases, and to approach a patient with the perspective of having to figure out what is wrong and how to fix it. What medical students and doctors often forget is that patients' belief structure may be a very important part of their life, and unless this aspect is respected, they will not form a coalition with the doctor to help solve the mystery of their own sickness. She emphasized that knowledge of culture is an essential tool that should be understood and remembered alongside anatomy, pathology, and other important traditional medical school subjects.

Anthropologists have explained the evil eye curse in terms of the "theory of limited good," which is based on the idea that there are a limited amount of good things in the world, whether beauty, intelligence, wealth, luck, or health. If one person gets more, there is less of it in the world for others. Envy may dictate giving someone the evil eye. The victim's ensuing illness somehow helps even things out.

Belief in the evil eye can create distress and confusion between Mexican and American mothers. In Mexican culture, babies are considered weak and extremely susceptible to the power of an envious glance. It is not even necessary to wish a child harm; a simple compliment, unaccompanied by a touch, can bring on the evil eye. Touching the person while complimenting him or her, however, neutralizes the power of the evil eye.

Americans are raised to believe that germs cause disease. Mothers are uncomfortable when people get too close to their infants. Mexican mothers, in contrast, may worry when strangers admire their babies without touching them. The very act that is believed to protect a child from illness in one culture is thought to cause illness in another.

Each culture that believes compliments can cause the evil eye also has ways to neutralize them or protect against it. Putting a bit of saliva on one's finger and making the sign of the cross on a child's forehead when giving a compliment can prevent the evil eye in some (but not all) parts of the Philippines. In Ethiopia, spitting on a child while remarking on its good looks will prevent an inadvertent casting of the evil eye. Babies may wear special amulets to protect them against the evil eye. In Mexico, a "deer's eye"—a large seed pod with a bit of red yarn—may be used, in Greece and Turkey, a blue glass "eye" charm, in Italy, an animal's horn, and in the Middle East, a hand. Not all members of these cultures adhere to the belief, however, so it is important to pay close attention to nonverbal cues from the mother. Does she appear uncomfortable when you compliment her child? If so, she may believe in the evil eye (see case study #250).

241   When Ronnie learned about the evil eye, her attention was drawn to a baby brought in to the clinic where she worked. The infant had a blue "eye" amulet with small blue beads attached to his clothing with a diaper pin. When she asked the mother about it, she was told that it was to protect her baby from the evil eye. Ronnie told me that in the past she would have been reluctant to ask about the amulets for fear of offending. She now realized that she was less likely to offend if she simply asks. This is an important lesson for those who are learning to be more culturally competent. Most people are proud to share information about their culture with those who are truly interested. The trick is in how you ask.

Traditional Healers

Most cultures have traditional healers. Although their actions are based on a model of health and illness different from biomedicine, they can often be effective. The question many health care practitioners may have is, *why* are they effective? They operate outside the realm of Western biomedicine. Can it be that there is some validity to other healing models? For those who have difficulty accepting this possibility, consider the fact that the mind has a powerful influence over the body. The placebo effect has long illustrated that belief in the power of a "sugar" pill to heal, or faith in the abilities of a physician, can result in actual healing. Such power may be at work in the case of traditional healers. Culturally competent practitioners realize that collaboration between traditional healers and biomedical doctors can often result in better care for their patients, as the next two cases illustrate.

An eighty-three-year-old Cherokee woman named Mary Cloud was brought into the hospital emergency room by her grandson, Joe, after she had passed out at home. Lab tests and x-rays indicated that she had a bowel obstruction. After consulting with Joe, the attending physician called in a surgeon to remove it. Joe was willing to sign consent for the surgery, but it would not be legal; the patient had to sign for herself. Mrs. Cloud, however, refused; she wanted to see the medicine man on the reservation. Unfortunately, the drive took an hour and a half each way, and she was too ill to be moved. Finally, the social worker suggested that the medicine man be brought to the hospital.

Joe left and drove to the reservation. About three hours later he returned, accompanied by a man in full traditional dress complete with feather headdress, rattles, and bells. He entered Mrs. Cloud's room and for forty-five minutes conducted a healing ceremony. Outside the closed door, the stunned and amused staff could hear bells, rattles, chanting, and singing.

At the conclusion of the ceremony, the medicine man informed the doctor that Mrs. Cloud would now sign the consent form. She did and was immediately taken to surgery. Her recovery was uneventful and without complications.

What was responsible for her recovery? The hospital staff were sure it

242

was the skill of the surgeon; Mrs. Cloud was convinced it was a result of the power of the medicine man. In any case, without the medicine man, she would not have agreed to the surgery or, if she had, her attitude might have been so poor as to interfere with recovery. This is a perfect example of how traditional healers and physicians can successfully work together in the care of patients.

243   Another case with involving a successful collaboration between traditional medicine and Western medicine occurred in a prison health facility, thanks to the cultural competence of the nurse. Amy was assigned to care for Edgar Manuelito, a thirty-eight-year-old Native American. Although very ill, he was refusing food and medication, and did not allow the nurses to bathe him. His physician and most of the nursing staff expected him to die shortly. When Amy learned that he was Native American, she asked him if he would like a medicine man to come pray for him. His face lit up at her question. He asked if it would in any way be possible for her to arrange it. It took Amy ten phone calls, but she finally located a medicine man who was associated with the prison. She contacted him, and he said he would be happy to pray for Mr. Manuelito. The medicine man also told her about the seldom-used sweat lodge the prison had for its Native American inmates. A sweat lodge is used in a traditional Native American ritual. It is like an outdoor sauna, often made with tree branches. Stones are heated and water poured on them. There are usually several rounds of prayers used in this purification ritual. With some difficultly, Amy and the medicine man were able to convince the prison guards that it was important for Mr. Manuelito to visit the sweat lodge. The medicine man performed a traditional ritual involving burning incense and chanting. Mr. Manuelito then spent half a day in the sweat lodge. Although the other nurses thought Amy was "crazy" for arranging all this, Mr. Manuelito suddenly began to eat and take his medication. His health started to improve and he eventually recovered. Amy's culturally competent approach to his care probably saved his life.

One nurse, Leila, after taking a course in cultural competence, said that when she has a Mexican patient, she always asks whether the patient is following the advice of a *curandero* or *yerbera* (herbalist). If the patient replies affirmatively, she'll ask if she or he is following any special recommendations or taking any herbal remedies. Most of the Mexican patients she has treated thus far have been fairly acculturated, and none have replied "yes" to her questions. It is likely, however, that one day someone will. Such questions should be a standard part of the intake interview. The fact that none have said "yes" should also be a reminder not to stereotype individuals. Leila begins with the generalization that Mexicans may consult a traditional healer before seeing a physician, and then asks the individual to verify if the generalization can be appropriately applied in each specific instance.

Traditional Medical Systems

It is common for most individuals to seek out multiple health care practitioners for the same problem without sharing this information with their
medical practitioners because they fear offending them, or being ridiculed
by them, or because they don't think the information is important. This
can lead to problems, especially if they are taking herbs or treatments
that interact with medical treatment. An East Indian patient may be receiving treatment from an Ayurvedic practitioner while being treated by a
medical doctor. A Chinese patient may be taking herbs prescribed by a
traditional Chinese physician and medication prescribed by a family practice physician. A Mexican patient may be visiting a *curandera* or taking
traditional home remedies for a problem also being treated by her doctor. It is important that health care providers have some knowledge of
traditional medical systems and inquire about them. Again, however, it is
imperative that such queries be made nonjudgmentally. If patients feel
that they will be ridiculed, they will simply withhold information, information that may be crucial for the physician to know. It is important, also,
to have a basic understanding of some of these systems.

Ayurvedic Medicine

Ayurvedic medicine is a traditional Hindu system. *Ayurveda* (a Sanskrit
word meaning "Laws of Health") is the title of one of the four sacred
Hindu texts known as the Vedas. The notion of the whole person is emphasized, including the physical, psychological, and spiritual aspects—in other
words, body, mind, and spirit.

To summarize an incredibly complex system, according to Ayurvedic
theory the universe is composed of five elements—earth, water, fire, air,
and ether. The human body also has three humors, or *dosha*, which relate
to different aspects of bodily function: (1) respiratory system—air; (2)
digestive system (which produces heat)—fire; and (3) moisture in the
body—water. These must be maintained in a state of balance. If this balance is lost, then treatment might include foods, minerals, and herbs of
the proper forces to restore balance.

For example, if someone had asthma, the Ayurvedic physician would
observe that the element of air was excessively dominant. He would therefore prescribe a diet that excludes "air" foods such as rice and spices, and
would use a remedy that stimulated the other two forces. When diagnosing and prescribing, the physician also takes into account the patient's
character, age, nationality, and life and family circumstances.

Good health is maintained by paying attention to the five natural elements, and the life force, known as *prana*, which can be channeled to help

or heal. *Prana* can be thought of as "energy." It is similar to the Chinese notion of *chi*. The Ayurvedic worldview can be best understood through yoga, through which *prana* is received, transmuted, and transmitted to various parts of the body via the seven chakras, or "wheels of energy." They can be opened through yoga, meditation, and chanting or rhythmic breathing.

A student from India shared that medical treatment for children is largely based on Ayurvedic home remedies, passed on by family elders. Such traditional remedies are often given precedence over Western bio-medicine. However, when traditional remedies do not work, they will turn to biomedicine.

Traditional Chinese Medicine (TCM)

Chinese medicine has received a great deal of attention and interest in the United States over the past few decades. It has had a major influence on nearly all medical systems throughout Asia. The worldview that humans are a part of nature is reflected in the Chinese health care system. Rather than try to control nature by destroying germs as the Western health care system does, it seeks to restore a person's natural place within the natural system. It is based upon the principle of harmony and balance.

According to TCM, the two opposing principles in the universe are *yin* and *yang*. *Yin* is the female principle; it represents cold, darkness, and other qualities. *Yang* is the male principle; it represents heat, light, and so forth. When *yin* and *yang* (or cold and hot) are in balance, the individual is healthy. When they become out of balance, illness results. The goal of treatment is to restore balance, which can be achieved through acupuncture (a cold, or *yin* treatment, used for *yang* ailments) or moxibustion (a hot or *yang* treatment, used for *yin* ailments), and/or herbs.

244 Dak-Ho Yi, an elderly Korean man, was admitted for depression. The staff became concerned because he refused to take any of his medications. His family finally explained the problem. The nurses had been giving him juice or water to take his pills. That violated the hot/cold balance. Once they gave him hot tea instead, he took his medication without incident. It was a simple adjustment for the staff to make, once they understood the problem.

A diagnosis is made through an examination of the tongue and the pulses. Chinese medicine recognizes twelve pulses (readings are taken at three depths on each of the two pulses in each wrist), each associated with a different organ or system. Ted Kaptchuk's book, *The Web That Has No Weaver* (1983), is one of the better texts explaining Chinese medicine for the layperson. The title comes from the fact that Chinese medicine is less concerned with the *cause* of disease than with the pattern of disharmony.

Kaptchuk describes how the Chinese, if they were to see a web, would ask different questions from those an American would ask. Westerners are concerned with origins and issues of control. The Judeo-Christian Bible, for example, begins by answering the question "who created the universe?" Science addresses the same question, albeit with a different answer. Traditional Chinese religions do not have a god in the sense of a creator of the universe. In their view, it doesn't matter who created the universe; what is important to understand is the patterns that exist and constantly repeat themselves. If they saw a web, they would be more interested in the pattern of the web; most Americans who would want to know who created the web. For the Chinese, the universe is a web that has no weaver.

Kaptchuk gives the example of six patients with stomach pain. The Western physician would order upper-GI x-rays or endoscopy using a fiber-optic scope, and might diagnose all six patients as having peptic ulcers. Because they all have the same disease, they would all be given the same treatment.

The traditional Chinese physician might examine the first patient and find that pain increases at touch (by palpations) but diminishes with the application of cold compresses. He has a robust constitution, reddish complexion, and a full, deep voice. He seems assertive and aggressive. He is constipated and has dark yellow urine. His tongue has a greasy yellow coating. His pulse is "full" and "wiry." The diagnosis: Damp Heat affecting the Spleen. He might observe the second patient to be thin, with an ashen complexion and ruddy cheeks. She reports that she is constantly thirsty, and has sweaty palms. She has a tendency toward constipation, insomnia, and night sweats. She appears to be nervous and fidgety. Her tongue is dry and slightly red. This patient may be diagnosed with Deficient Yin affecting the Stomach. The third patient, with different signs and symptoms, might be diagnosed with Exhausted Fire of the Middle Burner, sometimes called Deficient Cold affecting the Spleen. All six patients would be given different treatments, according to their pattern of disharmony.

The bottom line is that Western medicine is concerned with the disease agents, which it tries to change, control, or destroy. Traditional Chinese medicine looks for patterns of disharmony that it tries to return to a state of balance. It's as though the Chinese are looking at the entire tree, while Western medicine is focusing on an insect on one of the leaves of the tree. Both approaches have value; they are different and reflect alternate worldviews.

Hispanic Folk Medicine

One important aspect of Hispanic folk medicine is based upon the theory of hot/cold body balance, as discussed in earlier chapters. Food, illnesses, and emotions are all thought to have the quality of being hot, cold, or neutral. What is considered hot and what is cold can vary from culture to culture, however. Often, diseases associated with vasoconstriction and low metabolic rates are considered "cold," while those associated with vasodilation and a high metabolic rate are considered "hot." Hot conditions include pregnancy, hypertension, diabetes, and acid indigestion. Cold conditions include menstrual cramps, pneumonia, and colic. To prevent illness, one should avoid extremes in diet and emotion. To treat illness, food or medicines with opposite qualities is used.

TRADITIONAL REMEDIES

245   Although it's not clear whether the following example is based upon hot and cold theory, it reflects the importance of food in the treatment process. It also serves as a good example of cultural competence. Peter, an RN, said that the majority of his Hispanic patients utilize herbal treatments. The one he hears about most frequently is *nopales* (cactus). He shared the example of Mrs. Gutierrez, a diabetic patient. She told Peter that eating *nopales* would lower her blood sugar, and pointed to the evidence in her lowered blood sugar measurements. Peter, curious to learn more, interviewed Mrs. Gutierrez. He learned that when she eats *nopales* with eggs at breakfast, she eats fewer tortillas. *Nopales* is a non-starchy vegetable that is also high in fiber. This causes her to get full more quickly, and thus eat fewer tortillas. Substituting fiber for starch is good for her diabetic condition, so Peter congratulated her on increasing the fiber in her diet and for eating more vegetables. Rather than challenge her interpretation, he encouraged her to eat *nopales* and other non-starchy vegetables. In this way, he was able to incorporate traditional diet into a culturally appropriate dietary plan for diabetes. Interestingly, a scientific study (Bacard-Gascon 2007) found that adding *nopales* to the traditional Mexican breakfast results in a reduction of glucose concentration in diabetics.

246   Luz Castillo, a thirty-five-year-old recent immigrant from Mexico, was in the hospital recovering from a repeat caesarean section. One of her concerns was that the staff would not allow her to give her newborn *manzanilla* (chamomile tea) to treat his colic. She was afraid that without it, her infant would suffer. According to a pediatrician I consulted, the only danger would be if parents used too much in place of higher-calorie breast milk or formula so that the baby didn't get enough calories. Allowing Mrs. Castillo to give the baby the tea, while cautioning her not to give too much, would have been a much more culturally competent approach.

247   *Manzanilla* tea is commonly used to treat other ailments, including indigestion, cramps, and stomach problems. Arturo Romero, a Mexican patient in his fifties, was hospitalized with a stomach problem. He wanted to take *manzanilla* tea to help it. When his nurse saw what he was drinking,

however, she immediately took it away from him and told him not to take *anything* the doctor had not ordered. Although I'm sure the nurse was trying to protect Mr. Romero's health, given the large number of Mexicans in the United States and the prevalence of the use of herbal teas, it would be helpful for health care providers to learn something about the more commonly used herbs. There is an excellent chart at http://www3 .baylor.edu:80/%7ECharles_Kemp/hispanic_health.htm.

And now, a warning.

A pediatrician working at a large urban county hospital shared the case 248 of a twelve-year-old Latino girl who presented to the emergency department with strep throat. She was in florid shock and died two days later. The doctors learned that an unlicensed physician had been injecting her twice a day with outdated tetracycline and outdated camphor. Although this in itself didn't kill her, it did contribute to her delay in getting health care from the hospital.

FOLK DISEASES

A number of folk diseases are recognized within the Hispanic culture. Folk diseases, also known as culture-bound syndromes, are a constellation of symptoms recognized as a disease in one culture but not in others. Some Hispanic folk diseases are of natural origin, others are of supernatural origin. Some of the more common "natural" folk diseases include *caída de mollera* (fallen fontanelle) and *empacho* (blocked intestine). *Caída de mollera* would generally be diagnosed as dehydration. It is commonly thought to be caused by the child falling or being dropped or bounced, or by pulling the nipple out of the child's mouth too vigorously. Symptoms include colic, listlessness, inability to suck, loss of appetite, vomiting, diarrhea, and fever. Traditional treatments include pushing the palate back in place by pushing on the upper palate; holding the child upside down over a pan of water; and applying a poultice, usually of fresh soap shavings, to the depression.

Alicia, a Mexican American student, shared that when she was a sixteen- 249 year-old mother, her infant would not stop crying one night. His soft spot was sunken, and he would not eat. She went to see her sister Graciela, who was ten years older, had three children, and had grown up in Mexico. Graciela took Alicia's baby and massaged his upper palate, abdomen, and back. Alicia was a bit disconcerted to see Graciela then swing her baby upside down. She wanted to tell her to stop, but she didn't want to hurt Graciela. She was surprised to see that her infant soon began to nurse and then fall asleep for the entire night.

Symptoms of *empacho* include indigestion/upset stomach, constipation, diarrhea, dizziness, nightmares, and migraine headaches. The treatment involves rubbing the stomach or pinching the back to dislodge the bolus of food. A purgative or tea may also be given. Physicians should note that *azarcón* or *greta* might be given to children suffering from *empacho*. These can be dangerous, because they contain lead and mercury oxides. Physicians should be sure to ask about them in a nonjudgmental manner, and calmly explain the dangers if being taken.

Common "supernatural illnesses" include *mal de ojo* (evil eye) and *susto* (fright/shock). *Mal de ojo,* as discussed earlier in this chapter, is caused by admiration or jealousy of a person with "strong eyes." It most commonly affects infants. Touching a child while complimenting him prevents giving the evil eye. Symptoms include a sudden reversal in the physical or emotional well-being of an infant, vomiting, fever, crying, restlessness, or nervousness. Treatment consists of a *limpia,* or cleansing, by sweeping the body with a raw egg to extract the "heat."

250   Sue Ramis, a home health nurse, received an angry call from Juanita Garcia, a Mexican American woman whose house she had visited the day before. As Sue was leaving, she innocently remarked that Mrs. Garcia's child was adorable. The next morning, the infant was crying and feverish. When Mrs. Garcia recalled Sue's compliment and the fact that she had not touched the child, she concluded that Sue had given him the evil eye. Being Anglo, Sue had no knowledge of the evil eye. She was innocent, except in the mind of Mrs. Garcia.

Susto is also known as "soul loss." It is caused by a traumatic experience, which can be major (e.g., witnessing a death) or minor (e.g., being startled). Symptoms include malaise, fever, insomnia, irritability, nightmares, depression, and anxiety, and can occur anytime from immediately after the fright or up to months later. The treatment, done by a *curandero,* involves a *limpia,* or "cleansing," and prayers.

251   Rowena first encountered *susto* several years ago. She was treating Concepción Montes, a Hispanic patient who had been diagnosed with Bell's palsy. A few days before the paralysis occurred, Mrs. Montes had suffered a great emotional shock and she was convinced that that was what had brought on her symptoms. Rowena spent a great deal of time trying to convince Mrs. Montes that the symptoms were *not* caused by *susto,* but were more likely a viral infection or immune disorder. Now, after taking a course in cultural diversity, Rowena realized that her approach might not have been the best one. She said that if this were to happen now, she would probably concede that the shock the patient had suffered (the *susto*) had weakened her immunity and made her more susceptible to the illness. This is a much more culturally sensitive solution, and is likely to increase the patient's faith in the caregiver.

Trust is a key factor in health care, because a lack of trust can lead to lack of adherence and poorer outcomes. Cultural sensitivity generally results in greater trust, which is why I've emphasized the importance of respecting the patients' beliefs, even if they conflict with your own and that of biomedicine. For an example of why this is so important, see the next case study.

Silvia Evangelista came to the United States from Mexico when she was 252 twelve years old. Now in her fifties, she was going over her past medical history with her new physician, Dr. Miles. She mentioned that she had had an emergency caesarean section years earlier. When Dr. Miles asked why she needed it, she explained that she had experienced *susto*, and her family had rushed her to the hospital. When she arrived there, she was so sick from the *susto* that she was immediately taken into surgery. Dr. Miles told Mrs. Evangelista that the scenario she had just described did not make any sense, and that it was medically impossible to believe her. Furthermore, he said, there was no such thing as *susto*. Mrs. Evangelista said she felt "dumb and belittled" by him, and refused to answer any more questions. It was the last time she saw Dr. Miles.

TRADITIONAL HEALERS

There are a number of traditional Hispanic healers. They include *curan-dero/as*, *parteras*, *sobadoras*, and *yerbero/as*. A *curandero/a* uses diet, herbs, massage, and rituals to treat illnesses. A *partera* is a midwife. A *sobador/a* is a folk "chiropractor" who treats the patient by manipulating bones and muscles. A *yerbero/a* is an herbalist who treats both natural and supernatural ailments.

Taryn was working in the emergency department when Mr. and Mrs. De 253 Canul, a young couple recently from Mexico, brought in their one-year-old son. Mrs. De Canul had accidentally slammed the door on the baby's right index finger. The father was concerned over whether Antonio would suffer from *susto*. Fortunately, Taryn was taking a class on cultural diversity and knew that *susto* was commonly treated by a *curandero*. She told the parents that they should not worry about it, but if it would make them feel better, they could take Antonio to see a *curandero*. They thanked Taryn profusely and told her that in the past, other nurses had told them they were crazy for taking their children to a *curandero*. By acting in a culturally competent manner, Taryn was able to build rapport with this family. If they had been in a more long-term setting, such trust would likely have led to increased adherence and better patient outcomes.

It is important, however, to remember not to stereotype patients. Just because someone is Hispanic does not mean they will utilize traditional healers. As one nurse shared, she often asks the family if they would like to have a *curandero* come visit the patient. Often they tell her, "That was only in the old country." Others inform her that they already consulted one before coming to the hospital. Use such information to generalize, not to stereotype. Keep in mind the possibilities for any particular ethnic group, and then see whether they apply to the individual in question. In the above case, the fact that the family was concerned about *susto* and had recently immigrated from Mexico made it more likely that they utilized traditional healers, but it can never be assumed to be the case.

A word of warning. Health care providers should be aware that in Mexico it is common for pharmacists to prescribe drugs, and thus many patients are used to buying drugs from storefront botanicas. Unfortunately, there are a lot of unscrupulous fake doctors and pharmacists out there, selling drugs to patients that may not be up to Federal Drug Administration (FDA) standards. Dosages may vary considerably, and there may be a problem with counterfeit drugs. However, these drugs are often cheaper than buying reputable pharmaceuticals, which contributes to their appeal. It's therefore extremely important that you make your patients feel comfortable enough to share the information with you.

Traditional African American Health Beliefs and Practices

Loudell Snow (1983) writes about traditional health beliefs and practices among lower socioeconomic class African Americans in the South. She found that illnesses were classified as either "natural" (based on how God intends the world to be) or "unnatural" (the work of the Devil). Physicians can cure only natural illnesses. Illness is generally seen as an attack by outside forces, which can be cured by the proper remedy, right physician, or more powerful healers. God can cure anything, if the patient's faith is strong enough.

254   As you may recall from case study #2, Emma Chapman was a sixty-two-year-old Black woman admitted to the coronary care unit because she had continued episodes of acute chest pain after two heart attacks. Her physician recommended an angiogram with a possible cardiac bypass or angioplasty to follow. Mrs. Chapman refused, saying, "If my faith is strong enough and if it is meant to be, God will cure me."

When Judy, her nurse, asked her what she thought had caused the problem, she said she had sinned and her illness was a punishment. According to her beliefs, illnesses from "natural causes" can be treated through nature (e.g., herbal remedies), but diseases caused by "sin" can be cured only through God's intervention. Remember, treatment must be appropriate to the cause. In addition, Mrs. Chapman may have felt that to accept medical treatment would be perceived by God as a lack of faith.

Mrs. Chapman finally agreed to the surgery after speaking with her minister, whom Judy called to the hospital. Another approach would have been to talk with Mrs. Chapman about her faith, emphasizing that God works through doctors and nurses as well as the patient directly. Utilizing the patient's belief system generally leads to better communication. In this case, medicine could not offer Mrs. Chapman a certain cure; it offered only the possibility of symptom relief and life extension. Someone could have suggested that if she prayed and had enough faith, God would see to it that the operations were successful. She might also have been told the following story:

A huge flood came and destroyed a tiny village. Almost everyone managed to escape in time except for one very religious man who believed that God would save him. He climbed onto his roof to wait. Soon a rescue boat came to help him, but he turned it away, saying, "God will save me." The next day, a second boat came, but again he refused to leave. He said, "My faith in God is strong; He will save me." On the third day, a helicopter flew by to rescue him, and again he turned it away. "God will save me." On the fourth day, the waters rose above his roof and he drowned. When he reached heaven, he demanded to see God. "Why didn't you save me?" he asked. "You've never had a more faithful or loyal servant than I." God responded, "What do you mean? I did try to save you. I sent two boats and a helicopter."

Although most cases of voodoo, an "unnatural" cause of illness, are limited to the American South, they can raise some interesting issues for health care providers. Chandra was a nineteen-year-old African American woman in a New Orleans intensive care unit with a stab wound to her pulmonary aorta. After several days, Carol, her nurse, sadly told the family that Chandra probably would not make it. The family asked if they could bring in a priest, a request to which Carol quickly acquiesced. What Carol didn't realize was that they were referring to a voodoo priest.

That evening, the voodoo priestess arrived in an elaborate costume. When she mentioned to Carol that she planned to kill a chicken as part of the healing ritual, the nurse quickly realized that this would be a problem with infection control. Live chickens were not allowed in the ICU, let alone freshly slaughtered ones! This presented a dilemma for Carol and the hospital. How could they provide for the spiritual needs of the patient and her family, while at the same time adhering to the necessary rules of the hospital?

Carol came up with a clever solution. She directed the voodoo priestess to an area outside the hospital where she could safely kill the chicken without compromising the standards of infection control and provided her with a jar in which to put the fresh blood of the chicken. The priestess did so, brought the blood back to Chandra's room in the jar, and sprinkled it around her body during the ritual she then performed.

The ritual made the family feel much better, knowing they had done everything that could be done for their daughter. Furthermore, the patient did not die, as had been expected. She spent the next thirty days in intensive care, but then was able to return home. The hospital staff attributed Chandra's recovery entirely to their ministrations and saw the voodoo

255

ritual as serving solely to benefit the psychological state of the family. Whatever the source of Chandra's recovery, the fact that Carol provided a cre-
ative compromise to the needs of the hospital on the one hand, and the
patient and her family on the other, certainly contributed to the well-being
of the patient.

In her research, Snow found that diet and emotional shock were believed to cause two conditions in the blood: high blood and low blood.
High blood would indicate too much blood; low blood is not enough.
Eating too many rich foods was associated with "high blood," and not
enough red meat with "low blood." Treatment generally involved diet and
home remedies; clear and white foods, such as lemon juice, pickle juice,
and garlic, were thought to lower "high blood," while red and rich foods
were thought to raise "low blood." Unfortunately, there was sometimes
confusion between doctor and patient when talking about high blood and
high blood pressure. A patient with these blood beliefs might hear the
physician's diagnosis of high blood pressure as a diagnosis of high blood,
and begin treating it with clear and white foods rather than medication.
A choice of pickle juice, high in sodium, would be a disastrous choice.
She describes a stroke patient who threw out her hypertensive medication
and treated her high blood condition by sleeping upright (so the blood
could drain back down), drinking a solution of honey and water (to "thin"
the blood), and having a minister pray for a cure. Snow also relates the
case of a hypertensive patient who stopped taking her medication when
the physician told her she had a low blood count. She thought that the
medication she was on had given her low blood, a condition that she
treated by stopping the pills that were meant to lower her blood pressure.

Although Snow wrote about such beliefs and practices in the early 1980s
and they may no longer be of great significance, they underline the importance of communication and show how easily miscommunication can
occur.

Summary

Most medical personnel believe that Western scientific medicine is superior to all other medical systems. In many cases, this may be true. It is
important to remember, however, that medical practitioners in other cultures have been treating patients with some success for centuries. Several
modern drugs, including quinine, were discovered in native "medicine
kits." Furthermore, scientific medicine has been notably unsuccessful in
curing many ailments, including the common cold.

Even in cases where Western scientific medicine is superior, if the patient
believes it is insufficient for treating the problem, it probably will be. The
mind has a powerful effect on the body and can influence both illness and

health. To treat patients successfully, it is extremely important to consider their beliefs, whether they are about the causes of disease, how it should be treated, what behavior is appropriate, or how the body is to be viewed.

Ideally, medical professionals everywhere will recognize the value of what other systems have to offer. They can then take the best of each and reach the ultimate goal of providing effective health care for all.

Key Points

- If you seen unfamiliar markings on a patient's body, ask about them rather than assuming they are a sign of abuse or a symptom.
- Be sure to give clear instructions on the use of medications; nonadherence may simply reflect a lack of understanding.
- Many traditional remedies are helpful, and many of those with no proven scientific benefit are at least not harmful. Allowing your patient to continue to use them will help you gain their trust and increase the chances they will listen to you when you tell them something *is* harmful.
- It is common for most individuals to seek out multiple health care practitioners for the same problem without sharing this information with their medical practitioners because they fear offending them, or being ridiculed by them, or because they don't think the information is important. It is important to ask respectfully.
- You can say something along the lines of: *Many of my patients also see traditional healers who prescribe herbal remedies, or use home remedies that have been passed down for generations. Often they can be effective, but sometimes they can cause problems, especially when mixed with other treatments. That's why it's important that I know everything that you're taking to treat this or any other problem.* An attitude of respect, rather than derision, is crucial.
- Collaboration between physicians and traditional healers is often in the best interests of the patient.
- Not everyone will adhere to traditional health care practices.
- Respect your patients' beliefs, even if they conflict with your own and that of biomedicine.

For more on medications, see Chapter 3.

Chapter 13
Making a Difference

In addition to looking at the ways in which cultural differences can lead to conflict and misunderstanding, this book has emphasized the things clinicians can do to provide more culturally sensitive care for their patients. Individual doctors and nurses can make a big difference, but for cultural competence to become an integral part of health care, hospitals and clinics must make changes as well. I'm delighted to report that many already are. In this chapter, I want to focus on some of the things that various hospitals and clinics are doing to provide more culturally sensitive care, as well as things they could be doing. It is my hope that health care facilities around the country will be inspired to adopt some of these changes and come up with more of their own. Making such changes may cost money in the short term, but in the long run, it should save money by reducing errors, increasing adherence and improving patient health, and building good will (which, incidentally, can result in fewer lawsuits). Hospitals that earn a reputation for providing more culturally appropriate care will also attract a larger client base. Hospitals have the opportunity to do well by doing good.

Language

As discussed in Chapter 2, CLAS standards instituted in 2001 require language access services in all federally funded health care facilities. Thus, patients are to be provided access to live or remote interpreter services 24 hours a day, seven days a week. Ideally, trained professional interpreters will be available at all times, but that is not always feasible. Having bilingual staff can help as well, although it is important that such staff receive training to be competent interpreters. They should also be remunerated for doing double duty because it can stress a work load that is already often filled to capacity. A list of staff who can provide interpretation services should be posted on every unit.

Some hospitals are using staff interpreters to provide interpreting in person, via phone and via video. It can be more efficient to use in-house interpreters via video or telephone, although there are times when in-person interpreting is preferable, such as when a relationship needs to be built, when giving bad news, when the patient is hard of hearing, when mental health services are being provided, when communicating with children, or when visual information is central to the communication. Video interpreting is considered by some to be the next best thing to an on-site interpreter for certain settings, although it can be very expensive. Telephonic services may be especially advantageous in sexual and repro-ductive health settings, when it may not be appropriate to have additional people in the room. For telephonic interpreting, dual receiver (or dual handset) telephones should be used. Another option is a cordless tele-phone with two handsets, each with headsets. Remember to sterilize them before and/or after each use. Ideally, every patient room should have such a phone hookup, but failing that, having several on rolling carts is often sufficient.

All hospitals should have signs and forms in multiple languages re-flecting the populations served. Facilities that want to show they truly value the populations they serve can also provide television channels in multi-ple languages. For example, one hospital in a predominantly Chinese neighborhood has a twenty-four-hour Chinese language news channel in patient rooms. Another hospital, which serves a Russian community, pro-vides magazines and literature in Russian. Most of the Russian-language magazines are donated. Even if they are slightly out of date, patients and family members appreciate them. Hospitals can post signs in family wait-ing rooms, requesting donations of magazines in various languages.

Diet

Hospital food is infamous for being bad, but it doesn't have to be that way. Some hospitals have begun buying food from local farmers, which means fresher, healthier food, often at lower cost. Others shop at Asian and His-panic markets to get food for their Asian and Hispanic patients. Many hospitals have added ethnic foods to their menu. For example, a hospi-tal in an area with a large Chinese population now serves *jook*, an easily digested rice porridge. Another hospital, also in a Chinese neighborhood, serves Asian-style porridges and stews, buying ingredients from a nearby Hong Kong market. Chopsticks are included with meals. A hospital with a predominantly Mexican immigrant population has menus printed in Spanish and English and offers pork chile verde, enchiladas, and burritos. Another hospital has menu selections for Russian, Jewish, Italian, and His-panic cultures, since they serve those populations. Dietitians download culturally specific recipes and incorporate them into the menu.

As discussed in the chapter on birth, many cultures have dietary prescriptions and prohibitions following delivery. Dietitians at some hospitals are making sure that warm teas are available for new mothers as an alternative to ice water. Other hospitals offer traditional foods such as *miyeok-guk*, a Korean seaweed soup rich in iron and protein and traditionally served to women after giving birth. Many hospitals are being more flexible about allowing family members to bring in food for their patients. Ideally, patient rooms would have a small refrigerator and microwave to accommodate that, along with culturally appropriate utensils, such as chopsticks.

Respecting Cultural Beliefs and Practices

An excellent way to demonstrate a commitment to serving culturally diverse populations in a sensitive manner is to provide amenities that respect cultural and religious beliefs and practices.

For example, as discussed in earlier chapters, two things of importance for many Muslims are female modesty and prayer. The typical hospital gown can create a great deal of discomfort for Muslim women (as well as many others) because they are so revealing. One hospital found that many of their female Muslim patients were either canceling or not showing up for their appointments as a result. In response, they designed a new two-piece gown that covers the legs, back, and arms. They button up the side, rather than tie in the back, for greater modesty. They're available to patients upon request. To accommodate prayer, Muslim prayer rugs are provided in the chapel/meditation room of a hospital serving a large Muslim population. It is important that hospital personnel make such amenities known to patients, otherwise, they will go underused. Signs placed on the walls of patient rooms, informing them of the amenities available, would be helpful. It is important, however, not to mention specific ethnic or religious groups on the signs, lest other groups feel slighted. For example, a sign could announce "Modest patient gowns and prayer rugs available upon request."

As discussed in the chapter on religion, any religious icons (such as crosses) that are hung on patient walls should be able to be easily removed. Space should be made for patients' own religious symbols.

One hospital took an unusual step to demonstrate their sensitivity to the beliefs of their Chinese population; they changed their main telephone number. Their old number, which they had had for several decades, contained the number 4 several times. As discussed in an earlier chapter, the word for the number 4 is pronounced the same as the word for death, and thus has the same negative connotation. The new telephone number has the number 8 three times; eight represents good luck and wealth.

Many Filipinos believe that heat loss can lead to illness and that by covering their head they can prevent illnesses that are caused by cold temperatures and exposure to outside air. While doing a class assignment, one of my students discovered this was a concern for many of his patients. He then took the initiative to contact the volunteer services manager. The solution they came up with was to offer knit stocking caps to the patients. Because the hospital was unwilling to take on the expense, the manager contacted several hospital volunteers who knit as a hobby. They were delighted to help out, and volunteered to keep the hospital supplied in brightly colored knit stocking caps at all times. My student then printed up a flyer to inform the staff of their availability. The caps are now offered to the patients when they are admitted. Not only has it brightened up the unit, but patient and family satisfaction has improved. This is an excellent example of how one person can make a significant difference in a hospital. It also serves as a reminder that money needn't necessarily be a deterrent to offering culturally sensitive care. Volunteers can be used to creatively help cut expenses.

In a clever nod to traditional games, a hospital serving a large Chinese population has mah-jongg, a Chinese game using small tiles, in the exercise room. Doctors use the game to work on patients' motor skills.

As discussed in the chapter on birth, women from a number of cultures may want to take home the placenta after they give birth; unfortunately, this conflicts with most hospitals' infection control policies. A hospital serving a large African population worked with the health department and hospital infection control to find a way to make this possible. They are now able to store the placenta in the hospital for the mother until she goes home and can take it with her.

One of the simplest and most effective things hospitals can do to accommodate patients from diverse cultures is to extend visiting hours. They can also provide reclining chairs for visitors to spend the night. Although many nurses may resist having family members underfoot, as described in Chapter 6, there are effective ways to involve family members that will help lighten their load. Of course, without private rooms, this will be problematic, but most newer hospitals are building private rooms, and enterprising nurses can create private rooms when they are available.

Flexible Scheduling

As discussed in the chapter on communication and time orientation, many people from developing countries have a present time orientation. That, along with other socioeconomic factors, often results in patients who are late for their appointments. The consequence is generally anger and frustration on everyone's part. Practitioners often feel insulted and taken advantage of when patients arrive late for their appointment and yet still expect to be seen. Patients resent being scolded for tardiness and don't understand the source of the practitioner's hostility. When one of the nursing students in my class learned about time orientation, she had an epiphany . . . and suggested and implemented a successful plan at the clinic where she worked.

Rather than have a specific appointment time, patients are given an appointment for either the morning or afternoon of a specific day. Within that time frame, they are be seen in the order in which they sign in. The morning session is from 8 A.M. to 11 A.M. Patients arriving at 11:00 are seen by 12:30. Those arriving after 11:00 are seen in the afternoon session, from 2 to 4 P.M. Since this new policy was instituted, clinic patient satisfaction has increased and practitioner frustration has decreased.

Showing Commitment to Cultural Competence

It is one thing to espouse an interest in cultural competence. It is another to truly support it. Facilities that are serious about providing culturally competent health care to their patients can demonstrate their commitment in several ways.

Educate Staff

The first is to provide education and training in language and culture for the staff. Continuing education courses can be offered on-site. Grand rounds can include topics on cultural issues. Monthly lunchtime discussion of culturally relevant topics can be organized. A bulletin board in the break room can include information about different cultures and health beliefs. If clinical staff members get involved in posting the information, it will increase the learning potential.

Motivate Staff

Clinical staff may need to be motivated to provide culturally competent care. One way to do this is to require that culture-specific nursing interventions be part of nursing care plans. Physician bonus pay can be made contingent upon participating in cultural competence training. Clinicians who provide culturally competent care and are specifically mentioned in the cultural competence category of patient satisfaction surveys should be publicly recognized and perhaps given a small award, such as movie theater tickets. Cultural assessments should be part of the patient intake form. This information should be included on the charge sheet to ensure that the information gets passed on from one shift to the next. (Remember that sensitivity in asking such questions is essential, lest people fear you are going to stereotype them.) If cultural competence is made part of the job description and thus part of the yearly evaluation, staff will be much more likely to pay attention to such issues.

At the same time, it's best to motivate clinicians by helping them see the importance of culturally sensitive care. They should be encouraged to share cultural aspects of their cases with their colleagues during rounds or shift report. A "Cultural Questions Box" at the nursing station can be a place to post questions to discuss at staff meetings. Because many of the staff at most hospitals are ethnically diverse, they should be encouraged to share information about their own cultures. A monthly potluck lunch in which staff members bring ethnic foods (remember, Anglo counts as an ethnicity) and talk about and answer questions about their own cultures can be a fun and tasty way to learn. It might also help ease culturally based tensions among staff.

Make Information Available to Staff

It is important that clinical staff have easy access to resources with cultural information. There are some excellent books and resources available. A copy of *Culture and Clinical Care*, edited by Lipson and Dibble (2005), belongs at every nursing station. Computers can be bookmarked with links to sites that provide information on cultural issues (see Bibliography and Resources for recommended Web sites). Inexpensive pocket guides (such as my *Cultural Sensitivity: A Pocket Guide for Health Care Professionals*) can be provided for staff members. Information on how to contact an interpreter or cultural resource person should be in clear view at every nursing station.

Show Patients Your Commitment to Cultural Competence

Signs and forms should be printed in the languages of the ethnic groups served. Patients should be surveyed and interviewed regarding how well their cultural and religious needs were met. A category regarding culturally competent care could be added to patient satisfaction surveys. And, most importantly, hospital policies can be modified to accommodate different ethnic and religious groups—for example, regarding visiting hours, dietary practices, and so on.

Conclusion

There is much that can be done to make hospitals more welcoming to patients from a multiplicity of cultures. It is basically a matter of taking individuals and their families into account. All patients, not just those of color. Some of the recommended changes cost money, but most expenses can be recovered in the savings from reduced errors and lawsuits, as well as from increased business once the facility gains a reputation for culturally competent care. Other changes cost little, or can utilize the skills and resources of volunteers. Providing culturally competent care doesn't have to be difficult. And there is much satisfaction to be gained, on everyone's part.

Key Points and Suggestions

- Train bilingual staff to serve as interpreters; post a list on every unit of staff who can provide interpretation services.
- When using telephonic interpreters, use dual receivers/handsets.
- Have signs and forms in multiple languages reflecting the populations served.
- Offer television stations in multiple languages.
- Ask family members to donate books and magazines in their language.
- Serve ethnically appropriate foods and utensils.
- When medically appropriate, allow family members to bring food from home and provide facilities for storage and reheating.
- Offer more modest patient gowns to women.
- Make sure any religious icons on the wall can be removed.
- Allow a place for patients to place religious symbols.
- Extend visiting hours and add visitor chairs.
- Survey and interview patients regarding how well their cultural needs were met. Add a category regarding culturally competent care to patient satisfaction surveys.
- Allow for flexible scheduling in clinics.
- Educate staff on cultural competence.
- Provide on-site continuing education on cultural diversity issues.
- Create a bulletin board in the break room with information about different cultures and health beliefs.
- Motivate staff to become culturally competent.
- Make cultural assessments part of the intake form. This information could be included on the charge sheet to help ensure that the information gets passed on from one shift to the next.
- Require culture-specific nursing interventions as part of nursing care plans.
- Make cultural issues a regular topic for discussion at staff meetings.
- Create a "Cultural Questions Box" for nurses to post questions that could be discussed at staff meetings.
- Make cultural competence policy part of the job description, and thus part of the yearly evaluation.

- Organize potlucks in which each person brings something from his or her own culture, and describes any associated traditions or significance.
- Publicly recognize clinicians who provide culturally competent care. If a nurse's name is specifically mentioned by a patient in the cultural competence category of patient satisfaction surveys, he or she could receive a small reward.
- Have resources easily available for staff to access cultural information.
- Post information at nursing stations on how to contact an interpreter or cultural resource person.

And, finally:

- Be curious about other cultures.
- Don't stereotype!

Appendix 1: Cultural Profiles

It is with some trepidation that I have included cultural profiles for a variety of broad culture areas. It is obvious to all that there are tremendous differences within a single family; it would be ludicrous to assume that every member of a culture would think or act identically. Factors such as religion, class, socioeconomic status, age, gender, education, and time in the United States will often affect their beliefs and behaviors as much as their culture. However, some cultural patterns are common enough to warrant mention. They might serve as useful guideposts for health care providers. It is important to remember, however, that they are merely *generalizations*, meant to be used as starting points, not as something to *stereotype* individuals. They might help health care providers understand behavior in those instances when it deviates from the expected in a culturally consistent direction.

African Americans

Caution: These are broad generalizations and should not be used to stereotype any individuals.

PREJUDICE AND DISCRIMINATION/COMMUNICATION

- Due to a history of slavery and racism, as well as recent studies documenting racial disparities in medical care and the notorious four-decade-long Tuskegee experiment conducted by the U.S. Public Health Service in which African American males with syphilis were left untreated in order to observe the course of the disease, many African Americans may not trust white institutions, including hospitals.
- Realize African Americans may be very sensitive to what they perceive as discrimination, even when it is not intended. If you are late, for example, be sure to explain and apologize.
- Do not use the term "gal" to refer to African American women. It has the same negative connotations as "boy" does for an African American man.
- Address as "Mr." or "Mrs." or by professional title and last name.

RELIGION
- Religion is an important part of the lives of many African Americans. Clergy should be allowed to participate when appropriate. Privacy for prayer is important. Health care practitioners may offer to pray with a patient if all parties involved feel comfortable with it.
- It is customary to visit the sick on Sundays, often straight from church. Quiet time should be allowed for prayer.

FAMILY/GENDER ISSUES
- Family structure may be nuclear, extended, or matriarchal. Close friends may be part of kin support system.
- Father or eldest male may be the spokesperson.
- Egalitarian decision making is practiced outside the household; father may make final decisions within the household, although often it is the woman who is "really" in charge.

TIME ORIENTATION: PRESENT
- Individuals from lower socioeconomic strata may have a present time orientation, which may impede use of preventive medicine and follow-up care. Take special care when prescribing preventive medications (such as those for hypertension) to explain their importance, as well as the need for continuing to take medication (such as antibiotics) even when the symptoms have disappeared.
- Due to time orientation and economic factors, African Americans may put off seeing a physician until conditions are advanced.

EXPRESSION OF PAIN
- Varies widely. African Americans can be equally expected to be loud or stoic.

PREGNANCY AND BIRTH
- Traditionally, only females attend birth, but this may vary.
- New mothers may delay bathing and hair washing until postpartum bleeding stops. Offer sponge bath.

END-OF-LIFE ISSUES
- Blood or organ donation may be rejected with the exception of immediate family's needs for fear it may hasten death of donor.

HEALTH-RELATED PRACTICES
- Rich foods (red) may be thought by some (particularly those in the South) to cause "high" blood, which may be confused with high blood pressure. "High" blood may be treated with clear, white foods to "lower"

blood. Because such foods can include things like pickle juice, which is very high in sodium, this practice should be discussed in detail with the patient. "Low" blood is thought to result from too much vinegar, lemon juice, garlic—and not enough red meat. Be sure to clarify the differences between "low" blood, low blood "count," and low blood pressure.

- There is a rich tradition of herbal remedies in African American culture. Be sure to discuss the use of home or herbal remedies to avoid potential drug interactions.
- Traditionally, African American women in the South would get cravings for red clay dirt when pregnant (pica). Outside of the South, this craving has been replaced by Argo starch. In large amounts, it can cause constipation. In small amounts, it may provide an important comfort measure.
- Because menstruation may be thought to rid the body of dirty and excess blood, any interference with normal menstrual pattern may be feared. With too little flow, the fear is that bad blood may back up in the body; with too much flow, the fear is that it can weaken the body. Keep in mind when discussing birth control methods.
- In addition to "germs," natural causes of disease can include improper diet, exposure to cold/wind; unnatural causes can include God's punishment for sin, voodoo. Treatment should be appropriate to cause.
- For those who believe in voodoo (usually from the South or in rural areas), gastrointestinal (nausea, vomiting, diarrhea, loss of appetite) and unusual behavioral symptoms may be interpreted as signs of voodoo poisoning, which must be treated by a voodoo practitioner (root doctor).

Note: There is wide variation in cultural practices. This material is drawn mainly from the work of Loudell Snow (1977, 1983) and applies largely to lower-class African Americans, especially those in the South. Additional material is from Salamah Locks and Linda Boateng (1996).

Anglo Americans

Refers broadly to those of Northern European descent.

Caution: These are broad generalizations and should not be used to stereotype any individuals.

COMMUNICATION

- Anglo Americans often expect to know details of their condition. Middle- and upper-middle-class Anglo Americans are often well educated about their disease process and treatment options and frequently do a lot of research on the Internet.

- Privacy is important. They may be annoyed with repeated intrusions throughout the day and night while hospitalized.
- Direct eye contact is expected.
- Emotional control is expected.
- Anglo Americans will generally want nurses to provide psychosocial care.

FAMILY/GENDER ISSUES
- Anglo Americans generally have small families. They may not have extended family support system.
- Immediate family refers to spouse, siblings, parents, children.
- Decision making is made by individual for self, or by either parent for child.
- Husbands and wives may have equal authority.
- Independence is valued; self-care will generally be accepted.

TIME ORIENTATION
- Depends on socioeconomic class. Poor people tend to be present oriented; middle- and upper-class individuals tend to be future oriented.

EXPRESSION OF PAIN
- Patients will generally tend to be stoic, although they will want pain medication.

PREGNANCY AND BIRTH
- Prenatal care is generally sought.
- Husband is usually the preferred labor partner.
- Hospital births are generally preferred, although an alternative birthing center within the hospital may be favored.
- No postpartum rituals.
- Breastfeeding is generally practiced for three to six months.

END-OF-LIFE ISSUES
- Patient will generally want to know diagnosis and prognosis.
- Stoicism is valued when someone dies.
- Organ donations and autopsies are acceptable, unless forbidden by religion.
- Cremation or burial acceptable, unless one is preferred by religion.

HEALTH-RELATED PRACTICES
- Anglo Americans generally prefer an aggressive approach to treating illness.
- Western scientific medicine is preferred, although many may also use complementary and alternative medicine. Be sure to inquire about the use of herbal medications.

- Anglo Americans may prefer to be left alone when sick.
- Germs are thought to be the cause of disease; treatment is aimed at destroying germs. Antibiotics are often requested, even for viral illnesses.
- Elderly may fear losing independence or being placed in a nursing home, so they may deny the extent of limitations on completing their activities of daily living.

Asians

Caution: These are broad generalizations and should not be used to stereotype any individuals. Statements are most applicable to the least acculturated individuals.

COMMUNICATION
In order to show respect, patients may:
- agree to what the health care provider says, without having any intention of following through. Make sure the importance of adherence is stressed.
- avoid direct eye contact. Do not assign other meaning to this.
Suggestions for better communication:
- Avoid asking questions that require a "yes" or "no" response. Have the patient demonstrate understanding of any patient teaching.
- Avoid hand gestures; some, such as beckoning with the index finger, are insulting to Filipinos and Koreans.
- Offer things several times; patients may refuse at first in order to be polite.
- Realize that because pronouns don't exist in most Asian languages, they will often confuse "he" and "she."

FAMILY/GENDER ISSUES
- Allow family members to fulfill their familial duty by spending as much time with the patient as possible and by providing nontechnical care.
- Accept that wives may defer to husbands in decision making. Involve the family in decision making.
- Realize that sons may be valued more than daughters.
- Recognize that Asian culture is hierarchical; tremendous respect is often accorded to the elderly.

EXPRESSION OF PAIN
- Patients may not express their pain. Offer pain medication when the condition warrants it, even if patient does not request it. Insist upon giving it when necessary.

PREGNANCY AND BIRTH

- Traditional birth partner may be mother-in-law or other female relative.
- Women are generally stoic while giving birth.
- Traditionally, new mothers avoid cold, bathing, and exercise for one month postpartum ("doing the month"). Respect postpartum prescriptions for rest. Sponge baths may be preferred.
- Because pregnancy is thought to be a "hot" condition in traditional Chinese medicine, birth depletes the body of heat. Restoration of warmth is important. Offer liquids other than ice water, which may be deemed "too cold."
- Parents may avoid naming baby for up to thirty days.

END-OF-LIFE ISSUES

- Family members may wish to shield a terminal diagnosis from the patient. Ask patient upon admission (or before the need arises, if possible) to whom information about his or her condition should be given.

HEALTH-RELATED PRACTICES

- Coining and cupping are traditional medical practices, not forms of abuse, in China, Korea, and Vietnam.
- Fevers are often treated by wrapping in warm blankets and drinking warm liquids.
- Avoid giving ice water, unless requested. Patients may prefer hot liquids, such as tea.
- Use of herbs is common. Be sure to instruct on the use of Western medication.
- Avoid the number 4—it may signify death for Chinese, Japanese, and Koreans.
- Mental illness is highly stigmatized in most Asian countries. Patients with emotional problems are likely to somaticize them and present with physical complaints. Patients may be reluctant to discuss emotional problems with strangers.

Hispanics/Latinos (Primarily Mexicans)

Caution: These are broad generalizations and should not be used to stereotype any individuals. Statements are most applicable to the least acculturated individuals.

COMMUNICATION

- Characterized by *personalismo*: emphasis on personal relationships. Ask about the patient's family and interests before focusing on health issues.

FAMILY/GENDER ISSUES
- Allow family members to express their love and concern by spending as much time with the patient as possible. Allow them to assist patient with activities of daily living if patient is reluctant to do self-care.
- Realize that they may be reluctant to discuss emotional problems outside the family.
- Modesty may be important, especially among older women. Try to keep them covered whenever possible.
- Accept that older, more traditional wives may defer to husbands in decision making, both for their own health and that of their children. Involve the family in decision making.

TIME ORIENTATION: PRESENT
- Many have a present time orientation, which may impede use of preventive medicine and follow-up care.

EXPRESSION OF PAIN
- Patients may tend to be expressive (loud), though varies with audience (males may be more expressive around family members than around health care professionals).

PREGNANCY AND BIRTH
- Pregnancy is seen as a normal condition, so prenatal care may not be sought.
- In labor and delivery, the woman's mother may be the preferred birthing partner.
- Laboring women often yell out "aye yie yie"—best understood as a loud form of controlled breathing. Others will be stoic.
- Traditionally, new mothers avoid cold, bathing, and exercise for six weeks postpartum. Respect postpartum prescriptions for rest. Sponge baths may be preferred.
- Because pregnancy is traditionally thought to be a "hot" condition, birth depletes the body of heat. Restoration of warmth is important. Offer liquids other than ice water, which may be deemed "too cold."

END-OF-LIFE ISSUES
- Because family members may want to withhold a fatal diagnosis from the patient, ask patient upon admission (or before the need arises, if possible) to whom information about his or her condition should be given.

HEALTH-RELATED PRACTICES
- Patients may refuse certain foods or medications that upset hot/cold body balance. Offer alternative foods and liquids.

- Avoid ice water, unless requested.
- Among more traditional women, "fat" is seen as healthy. Many Mexican foods are high in fat and salt. Nutritional counseling may be necessary for diabetics and individuals with high blood pressure.
- Some may believe that complimenting a child without touching the child can cause evil eye. To be safe, touch the child when admiring him or her.
- Ask what herbal remedies, if any, they are using. Most are effective or neutral; however, *azarcón* and *greta* (used to treat *empacho*—stomach pain) contain lead and can be dangerous.

Middle Easterners

Caution: These are broad generalizations and should not be used to stereotype any individuals. Statements are most applicable to the least acculturated individuals.

COMMUNICATION
- Communication should be two-way. You may need to share information about yourself in order for Middle Easterners to share information about themselves.
- Try to avoid direct eye contact with members of the opposite sex to avoid any hint of sexual impropriety.

FAMILY/GENDER ISSUES
- Be patient with "demanding" family members; they may see it as their job to make sure that the patient gets the best care possible. Repetition of demands is often made to show emphasis, as is a loud tone of voice.
- Personal problems are often taken care of within the family; they may not be receptive to counseling.
- It is often appropriate to speak first to the family spokesman.
- Sexual segregation is often extremely important. Assign same-sex caregivers whenever possible, and maintain a woman's modesty at all times.
- Accept the fact that women may defer to husbands for decision making regarding their own and their children's health.
- Accept that the husband may answer questions addressed to his wife. This is not necessarily a sign of spouse abuse.

RELIGION
- Islam is a dominant force in the lives of most, but not all, Middle Easterners.
- Allow Muslims privacy to pray several times a day, facing toward Mecca.
- Many have a fatalistic attitude regarding health: it's all in Allah's hands, so their (health-related) behavior may be of little consequence.

- They may not want to plan for birth or death; it may be seen as challenging the will of Allah.

EXPRESSION OF PAIN
- Muslims often tend to be loud and expressive, especially during childbirth, after someone has died, and when they are in pain.

PREGNANCY AND BIRTH
- Muslims may not make many preparations for birth.
- It is acceptable for women to be very loud and expressive during labor and delivery.
- Male circumcision is common.

END-OF-LIFE ISSUES
- Muslims may be reluctant to agree to DNR or to plan for death.
- Muslims may not allow organ donation or autopsy, since according to Islam, the body should be returned to Allah in the condition in which it was given.

HEALTH-RELATED PRACTICES
- Damp, cold, drafts, and strong emotions may be thought to lead to illness.
- Evil eye (jealousy) may be thought to cause illness or misfortune. Amulets to prevent this may be worn and should not be removed.
- Heavy use of medications is common and thus patient may feel slighted if not given prescription.
- When providing meals, be aware that Muslims may not eat pork.

Native Americans

Caution: These are broad generalizations and should not be used to stereotype any individuals. There are more than 500 different tribes, each with its own culture and variations within each.

COMMUNICATION
- Anecdotes or metaphors may be used; for example, a story about an ill neighbor may be a way of saying the individual is experiencing the same symptoms.
- Long pauses generally indicate that careful consideration is being given to a question. Do not rush patient.
- Direct eye contact may be avoided out of respect and/or concern for soul loss/theft.
- Loudness is often associated with aggressiveness among Navahos and should be avoided.

- Due to history of misuse of signed documents, some may be unwilling to sign informed consent or advanced directives. Some may display hostility toward health care providers due to history of mistreatment of Native Americans by whites.
- Older adults may prefer the term "American Indians" over "Native Americans."

FAMILY/GENDER ISSUES
- Extended family is usually important, and any illness may concern the entire family.
- Decision making varies with kinship structure. Patients will generally make their own decisions. In tribes that are matrilineal (descent reckoned through the female line), women and/or their brothers may make important decisions. Navajo, Hopi, and Zuni tribes are among those that are matrilineal.

TIME ORIENTATION
- Generally flexible, oriented to activities, rather than the clock. "Indian time" may run very late.

EXPRESSION OF PAIN
- Stoicism is often highly valued, and patients may not express their pain, other than by mentioning, "I don't feel so good," or "Something doesn't feel right." If patient reports feeling "uncomfortable" and is not given pain relief, she or he generally won't ask again. Offer pain medication when the condition warrants it, even if patient does not appear to be in pain.

PREGNANCY AND BIRTH
- Female relative may be birth attendant.
- Stoicism often encouraged during labor and delivery.
- Mother and infant may stay inside and rest for twenty days postpartum, or until the umbilical cord falls off, depending upon custom. Parents may want to save umbilical cord, because it may be seen as having spiritual value.

END-OF-LIFE ISSUES
- Names of deceased relatives may be avoided, but relationship term (e.g., brother, father, sister) may be used.
- Members of some tribes may prefer to avoid discussion of terminal prognosis or DNR because negative thoughts are believed to hasten death. Others will use the information to make appropriate preparations.
- Members of some tribes may avoid contact with the dying, while others

will want to be at the bedside twenty-four hours a day. Visitors may display a jovial attitude so as not to demoralize patient. Mourning is done in private, away from the patient.
- After death, wailing and shrieking may occur.
- Some may want to leave a window open for the soul to leave at death; others may orient the patient's body to a cardinal direction before death.

HEALTH-RELATED PRACTICES
- Before cutting or shaving hair, check to see if patient or family wants to keep it. Realize that in some tribes cutting hair is associated with mourning.
- A medicine bag may be worn. Do not treat it casually or remove it without discussing it with the patient. If absolutely necessary to remove it, allow a family member to do so, keep it as close to the patient as possible, and return it as soon as possible.
- Food that is blessed (traditional religion or Christianity) may be thought to be devoid of harm. Nutritional guidance should take this into account. Many traditional foods are high in fat.
- Traditional healers may be combined with use of Western medicine. Allow traditional healers to perform rituals whenever possible. Do not touch or casually admire ritual objects.

Note: the material contained in this profile is adapted from Josea Kramer (1996).

South Asians

Includes Hindus, Sikhs, and Muslims from India, Pakistan, Bangladesh, Sri Lanka, and Nepal. Some may still use the term East Indian interchangeably for South Asian, but the latter is currently the preferred term.

Caution: These are broad generalizations and should not be used to stereotype any individuals. Statements are most applicable to the least acculturated individuals.

COMMUNICATION
- Direct eye contact may be seen as rude or disrespectful, especially among the elderly.
- Silence often indicates acceptance or approval.
- Some patients may not want to sign consents; they consider health care professionals to be the authorities and prefer to have them make the decisions.
- A side-to-side head bob may indicate agreement or uncertainty. An up-and-down nod, which Americans usually interpret as agreement, may indicate disagreement, while acknowledging what the speaker is saying.

- Husbands may answer questions addressed to wife.
- Males should avoid shaking hands with females unless the female offers her hand first.

FAMILY/GENDER ISSUES
- Close female family members will often remain with patient; family members will often take over activities of daily living (such as feeding, grooming, etc.) for patient. Do not insist upon self-care unless medically necessary.
- The father or eldest son usually has decision-making power, but generally family members are consulted before decisions are made.
- Patients may prefer same-sex caregivers due to modesty.

EXPRESSION OF PAIN
- Generally stoic; however, moaning and screaming are acceptable during the birth of the first child.
- Muslim patients may not want narcotics for anything other than severe pain.

PREGNANCY AND BIRTH
- Pregnant Hindu women are often encouraged to eat nuts, raisins, coconuts, and fruits to have a healthy, beautiful baby.
- Dried ginger powder, celery seeds, nuts, and puffed lotus seeds may be given to the new Hindu mother to cleanse her system and restore her strength.
- East Indian women often practice a postpartum lying-in period. It is expected that they feed the baby, but everything else is done for them. Traditionally, female relatives would take over. If none are with them, they may expect nurses to do so.

END-OF-LIFE ISSUES
- Some patients may prefer to have fatal diagnosis given to family member. Family will then decide whether and how much to reveal to the patient. Discuss with patient to whom information should be given. It is best to do this well in advance of need.

HEALTH-RELATED PRACTICES
- Sikhs are enjoined not to cut their hair or shave their beard. Their hair will usually be worn in a turban. Consider this before cutting or shaving any hair in preparation for surgery.
- Hindus will generally not eat meat or fish; some may not eat eggs. Muslims will not eat pork.
- Those who believe in Ayurvedic medicine (Hindus, Sikhs, and some

Muslims) see food in terms of a hot/cold classification, based on qualities inherent in the food rather than on the temperature. "Hot" foods (meat, fish, eggs, yogurt, honey, nuts) will be given for "cold" conditions such as fever or surgery, especially in winter. "Cold" foods (e.g., milk, butter, cheese, fruits, and vegetables) should be eaten in the summer and for "hot" conditions, including pregnancy.

Note: Most of the material contained in this profile is adapted from Rozina Rajwani (1996).

Appendix 2: Selected Religions

Just as culture can have an enormous influence on behavior, so can religion. Although there are differences within the various sects of each religion, and people vary significantly with regard to how closely they adhere to the tenets of their faith, knowledge of religious beliefs and practices may be useful to the clinician. It is important to remember, however, that the information presented in this appendix should be used as *generalizations*, not as something to *stereotype* individuals.

Rachel Spector (2000) was an important source for the information presented in this appendix.

BAHA'I

Autopsy	Acceptable with medical or legal need
Diet	No alcohol or drugs
Euthanasia	No destruction of life
Healing beliefs	Harmony between religion and science
Healing practices	Prayer
Medications	Narcotics with prescriptions
Organ donation	Permitted
Right-to-die issues	Life is unique and precious, so do not destroy
Disposal of the body	Burial preferred; cremation strongly discouraged

BUDDHISM

Autopsy	Matter of individual practice
Diet	Many do not eat meat
Euthanasia	May permit
Healing beliefs	Do not believe in healing through faith
Healing practices	No restrictions
Medications	No restrictions
Organ donation	Considered act of mercy; if hope for recovery, all means taken

Right-to-die issues	With hope, all means encouraged
Spiritual practices	Daily chanting or meditation
Disposal of the body	Burial or cremation, depending upon the wishes of the family. Cremation common.

CHRISTIAN SCIENCE

Autopsy	Not usual; individual or family decide
Diet	No alcohol or tobacco
Euthanasia	Contrary to teachings
Healing beliefs	Accept physical and moral healing
Healing practices	Full-time healing ministers; may use physicians for childbirth and setting broken bones. Healing through prayer
Medications	None
Organ donation	Individual decides
Right-to-die issues	Unlikely to seek medical help to prolong life

HINDUISM

Autopsy	Acceptable
Diet	Most are vegetarian
Euthanasia	Not practiced
Healing beliefs	Some believe in faith healing
Healing practices	Traditional faith healing system
Medications	Acceptable
Organ donation	Acceptable
Disposal of the body	Cremation common
Other practices	Right hand used for eating, left for toileting and hygiene
Right-to-die issues	No restrictions
Spiritual/religious items	Some may wear a thread around wrist or body; do not remove

ISLAM/MUSLIMS

Autopsy	Permitted for medical and legal purposes; otherwise forbidden
Diet	No pork or alcohol; daylight fasting during Ramadan
Disposal of the body	Cremation forbidden; body must be washed by same sex Muslim at death. Burial usually within 24 hours
Euthanasia	Not acceptable
Healing beliefs	Faith healing generally not acceptable
Healing practices	Some use of herbal remedies

Medications	No restrictions
Organ donation	Acceptable
Other practices	Right hand used for eating, left for toileting and hygiene
Right-to-die issues	Attempts to shorten life prohibited
Sabbath	Friday
Spiritual practices	Prayer five times daily, facing Mecca; boys usually circumcised

JEHOVAH'S WITNESSES

Autopsy	Acceptable if required by law
Diet	No tobacco; moderate alcohol allowed
Euthanasia	Forbidden
Healing beliefs	Faith healing forbidden
Healing practices	Reading scriptures can comfort the individual and lead to mental and spiritual healing
Health care issues	No blood or blood products allowed; blood volume expanders okay if not derived from blood; sterilization forbidden
Medications	Accepted except if derived from blood products
Organ donation	Forbidden
Right-to-die issues	Use of extraordinary means an individual's choice

JUDAISM/JEWISH

Autopsy	Permitted if required by law
Diet	Kosher laws for orthodox and some conservative Jews forbid pork, shellfish, and the mixing of meat and dairy products; separate dishes and utensils must be used for meat and dairy
Disposal of the body	Cremation inappropriate; someone should sit with body after death; burial within 24 hours; all body parts including bloody clothing and amputated limbs should be buried with body
Euthanasia	Prohibited
Healing beliefs	Medical care expected
Healing practices	Prayers for the sick
Medications	No restrictions
Organ donation	Complex issue; some practiced
Right-to-die issues	Right to die with dignity. If death is inevitable, no new procedures need to be undertaken, but those ongoing must continue

Religious practices	Boys circumcised on eighth day of life
Sabbath	Sundown Friday to sundown Saturday; Orthodox Jews will avoid all work, including ringing the call button
Spiritual/religious items	Orthodox men may wear prayer shawl, *yarmulka* (skull cap), and *tfillin* (black strings) on arms and forehead while praying

MORMONS (CHURCH OF JESUS CHRIST OF LATTER-DAY SAINTS)

Autopsy	Permitted with consent of next of kin
Baptism	After age eight; not in infancy or at death
Diet	No alcohol, tobacco, coffee, or tea
Disposal of the body	Cremation discouraged; burial common
Euthanasia	Humans must not interfere in God's plan
Healing beliefs	Power of God can bring healing
Healing practices	Anointing with oil, sealing, prayer, laying on of hands
Health care issues	Birth control and abortion forbidden (unless mother's life in danger)
Medications	No restrictions; may use herbal folk remedies
Organ donation	Permitted
Right-to-die issues	If death inevitable, promote a peaceful and dignified death
Spiritual/religious items	"Garment"—a type of underwear that is considered sacred; individuals may not want to remove it

ROMAN CATHOLICISM

Autopsy	Permissible
Disposal of the body	Usually burial, although cremation is now acceptable
Euthanasia	Direct life-ending procedures forbidden
Healing beliefs	Many within religious belief system
Healing practices	Sacrament of sick, candles, laying-on-of-hands
Health care issues	Birth control and abortion forbidden
Medications	May be taken if benefits outweigh risks
Organ donation	Justifiable
Right-to-die issues	Obligated to take ordinary, not extraordinary, means to prolong life
Sabbath	Sunday
Spiritual/religious items	Crucifix, rosary beads
Spiritual practices	Sacrament of the Sick (includes anointing, communion if possible, and blessing by a priest)

SEVENTH-DAY ADVENTISTS

Autopsy	Acceptable
Diet	Vegetarian diet encouraged; alcohol, coffee, tea prohibited
Euthanasia	Not practiced
Healing beliefs	Divine healing
Healing practices	Anointing with oil and prayer
Medications	No restrictions
Organ donation	Acceptable
Right-to-die issues	Follow the ethic of prolonging life
Sabbath	Sundown Friday to sundown Saturday

SIKHISM

Autopsy	Permitted
Diet	Intoxicants, including tobacco, forbidden; many do not eat beef
Euthanasia	Discouraged
Healing practices	Prayer; playing of sacred music
Health care issues	Their bodily hair is not to be cut or shaved; daily washing appreciated; same-sex providers preferred
Medications	No restrictions
Organ donation	Acceptable
Right-to-die issues	Death is a natural process and God's will
Disposal of the body	Cremation preferred
Spiritual/religious items	Male Sikhs are enjoined to carry a dagger and to wear a turban, knee-length pants, and a steel bracelet on the right wrist

UNITARIAN/UNIVERSALIST CHURCH

Autopsy	Recommended
Diet	No restrictions
Euthanasia	Favor non-action; may withdraw therapies if death imminent
Healing beliefs	Faith healing seen as "superstitious"
Healing practices	Use of science to facilitate healing
Medications	No restrictions
Organ donation	Acceptable
Right-to-die issues	Favor the right to die with dignity
Disposal of the body	Cremation common

Appendix 3: Dos and Don'ts of Providing Culturally Competent Care

- Don't stereotype people. Remember that the information given for each culture group is meant to be a broad general guideline, to serve as starting points. Find out whether or not the individual fits the generalization.
- Don't judge a patient's level of pain based upon their expressiveness. Some cultures encourage expressiveness, others encourage stoicism.
- Don't wait to offer pain medication until a patient asks for it; many Asian patients will suffer in silence.
- Don't assume lack of eye contact indicates lack of interest, or guilt, or some other negative point. For Asians, it may be a way of showing respect; for Middle Easterners, a way of maintaining propriety.
- Don't judge people as "pushy" or "cold" based upon how close they stand to you.
- Don't expect that all patients will make their own decisions. In cultures where the family is the primary unit, important decisions may be made by the family. In cultures where males are dominant, the husband may make the final decisions regarding the health care of their wife and children.
- Don't offer ice water as the only liquid for Asians and Hispanics. Many will prefer room temperature or warm liquids.
- Don't confuse traditional health care practices such as coining and cupping with abuse.
- Don't assume that a patient's appetite is based solely on feelings of hunger; some foods prepared by the hospital may violate rules of body balance or religious prohibitions, or may simply be unfamiliar to the patient.
- Don't assume the patient wants to be informed of a fatal diagnosis. Ask the patient upon admission (or before, if possible) to whom he or she would like information about his or her condition to be given. Often family members will want to shield patients from a terminal diagnosis.

DOS

- Do remember to ask the right questions of all your patients: the 4 Cs of Culture (What do you *call* your problem? What do you think *caused* it? What have you done to *cope* with it? What *concerns* you about it? What *concerns* do you have about my recommended treatment?)
- Do try to understand people's values, since they will influence their behavior.
- Do realize that not all patients believe germs caused their disease. Again, ask them what they think caused their illness.
- Do recognize that people with a present time orientation (most poor people, many people from agriculturally based countries) may have difficulty with preventive health care. Make an extra effort to explain the importance of preventive health care, and why it is necessary to continue medication even after the symptoms have disappeared.
- Do try to allow a patient as many visitors as she or he would like to have.
- Do distinguish the degree of self-care necessary for recovery from that which is merely an imposition of the value of independence.
- Do include family members in the patient teaching, if a family member will be caring for a patient at home.
- Do respect a woman's concern for modesty; try to keep her covered.
- Do try to assign same-sex health care providers when possible, especially for Middle Eastern patients.
- Do be sensitive to the fact that most African Americans have been subjected to much racial prejudice and discrimination.
- Do respect patients' religious beliefs; involve clergy in their care when appropriate.
- Do learn about the beliefs and practices of the patient populations you serve.
- Do keep in mind that there is always individual variation within a group.
- Do develop a tolerant accepting attitude about views different from your own.

Appendix 4:
Tips for Working with Interpreters

These guidelines were developed by medical anthropologist M. Jean Gilbert and are included with her gracious permission.

- Brief the interpreter before the encounter if possible; give him/her relevant information about the patient and/or purpose of the conversation.
- When possible, choose an interpreter whose age, gender, background, etc. make it easiest to work with the patient or family.
- Place the interpreter behind the patient or behind you. Never place the interpreter between you and the patient/family.
- When talking, look directly at the patient and speak in first person: "Mrs. Jimenez, I will need to have you go to the lab for a couple of tests."
- Don't tell the interpreter to "Tell Mrs. Jimenez she'll need to go to the lab . . ."
- Ask the interpreter to speak in the first person for you and for the patient instead of saying, "The doctor says . . ." or "Mrs. Jimenez says . . ."
- Don't talk for long without letting the interpreter interpret what you are saying.
- Let the interpreter know that s/he can request clarification from you whenever it's needed.
- Pursue seemingly unconnected issues that the patient raises. These issues may lead to crucial information or uncover difficulties with the interpretation.
- Come back to an issue if you suspect a problem and get a negative response. Use related questions, change the wording and come at it indirectly.
- Learn basic words and sentences in the target language. Asking interpreter about words that have not been translated prompts attention to detail.

- Make sure the interpreter conveys everything the patient says and doesn't abbreviate or paraphrase.

Following these tips keeps you in charge of the encounter and prevents the interpreter from inadvertently taking control. Using first person will seem more natural to the patient and will help you develop and maintain rapport.

Appendix 5:
Summary of Case Studies

Note: Cases demonstrating cultural competence are in italics.

Chapter 1. Basic Concepts

(1) Young Mexican boy presented with symptoms consistent with *susto*.

(2) *African American woman refused an angiogram for acute chest pain because she believes it is punishment for sin and that only God can cure her.*

(3) *Hispanic woman refused pain medication but was in too much pain for physical therapy until culturally sensitive nurse asked her what she had used to cope with the pain before surgery. She had been using herbal teas from a* curandero.

(4) *Culturally competent physician asked her Latino patient the right question and learned he didn't want to take insulin because he feared it caused blindness, because his mother and uncle both went blind after going on insulin.*

(5) Nurse stereotyped a Middle Eastern patient for being loud and later learned that the patient was riddled with cancer.

(6) *Nigerian nurse refrained from stereotyping an African American male patient as drug seeking, due to cultural sensitivity training. It was fortunate he reassessed the patient, because he needed immediate medical intervention.*

(7) Mexican nurse experienced unconscious prejudice regarding a Mexican patient; she assumed she was from a rural area. In fact, she was from the capitol. The patient, in turn, looked down upon the nurse as "provincial" due to the part of town the nurse was from.

(8) Elderly African American man was afraid to have surgery because he didn't trust the white hospital due to historical discrimination against Blacks.

(9) African American woman assumed the physician was being racist when he asked if she wanted her tubes tied after her twelfth pregnancy.

(10) African American woman assumed racism when case manager told her that five-month post-op pain for carpal tunnel release was too long. *Cultural competence restored the situation.*

(11) Nurse used understanding of Hispanic patient's worldview to adjust education on diabetes.

Chapter 2. Communication and Time Orientation

LANGUAGE AND COMMUNICATION

(12) Chinese doctor unfamiliar with the American idiom "cold feet" ordered vascular tests for his patient.

(13) Korean physician didn't understand the idiom "kick the bucket" and responded affirmatively when his patient asked him if that would be the result of his surgery.

(14) English couple were amused when female patient was instructed to slide her fanny up to the middle of the bed. In England, "fanny" is a crude term for a woman's vagina.

(15) Deaf gay male assumed the best when told that his HIV test had come back "positive."

(16) Mexican parents misunderstood the word "puto" when used by a Filipino nurse. They thought she was having sexual relations with a prostitute; she was referring to the rice cake she was having for lunch.

(17) African American man threw a plate of food at a white Canadian nurse when she politely asked, "Do you boys mind if I sit down here?"

(18) Filipino patient and husband said they understood the nurse's discharge instructions when in fact, they didn't, because they wanted to preserve self-esteem.

(19) Chinese woman told her doctor that she would return for a follow-up visit, even though she had no intention of doing so, because to refuse would have been disrespectful.

(20) Hmong patient respectfully agreed with a physician's recommendation to have surgery, even though she had no intentions of undergoing the knife.

(21) Hispanic woman was treated professionally, but without the personal warmth (*personalismo*) valued in Hispanic cultures, so she did not return.

(22) Diabetic Mexican clinic patient on dialysis became more compliant when treated with personalismo.

(23) Culturally competent nurse utilizing personalismo *avoided being named in a lawsuit by a Latino patient's family.*

(24) Hispanic family didn't want to bother the physician with their questions, and told him they had none. Instead, they questioned the nurse.

(25) African American patient didn't respond when nurse called her

by her first name, but did when the nurse gave her the respect of calling her by her last name.

(26) Vietnamese patient avoided a nasogastric tube when an interpreter discovered that her daughter had been bringing her food.

(27) Spanish-speaking woman kept returning to the clinic to treat her abdominal pain. When the staff finally used a professional interpreter rather than the woman's young daughter, it came out that she needed treatment for a sexually transmitted disease.

(28) Gay patient was abandoned when a family member was used to interpret the patient's HIV diagnosis and prognosis.

(29) Mexican home hospice patient didn't want her family to know she was dying. She had an easier time talking to nurse with Hispanic interpreter than when family members were used as interpreters.

(30) Hispanic woman unknowingly signed informed consent for a hysterectomy when her son served as translator. He was embarrassed to talk to his mother about her private sexual parts, and had too much respect for the authority of the nurse to refuse her request to translate.

(31) Arab mother-in-law refused to translate contraception information to her daughter-in-law.

(32) Korean daughter did not pass on information to her father about his condition or instructions given by the nurse because she didn't want to reveal a negative diagnosis and did not feel comfortable telling her father what to do.

(33) Filipino man felt disrespected when staff spoke to his bilingual grandchildren rather than to him.

(34) Adult daughter of a Latino patient was offended when the hospital wanted to use a professional interpreter rather than her.

(35) Mexican patient thought his doctor was crazy when he told him he was going to put a *platano* (banana) in his leg.

(36) Romany (Gypsy) patient's mother-in-law insisted on answering questions put to the patient, probably to ensure she did not give too much information to outsiders.

(37) Navajo woman left long silences when nurse asked her questions while taking a medical history, not because she didn't hear or understand the nurse, but because, in the Navajo style, she was giving thoughtful consideration to her questions.

(38) Middle Eastern man was reluctant to sign informed consent for heart catheterization, believing that since the physician was the one with the expert knowledge, he should take responsibility for making the decision.

(39) Cambodian woman delayed signing consent for a skin graft, probably due to fear stemming from the time of the Khmer Rouge

war, when signed life histories were required from those who were later executed.

(40) Chinese man signed consent for an angiogram out of respect for the physician, who mistook smiling and nodding for understanding, when in fact the patient spoke no English.

(41) Navajo patient avoided making eye contact with nurse while she was giving diabetic health teaching in order to show respect and perhaps to avoid soul loss or theft.

(42) Hmong girl avoided making eye contact with nurse case manager while she was doing health teaching following the birth of the girl's child in order to show respect.

(43) Rabbi ignored the proffered hand of a family member when he was making a hospital visit to a Jewish patient because among ultra Orthodox Jews, it is forbidden to touch the opposite sex unless you are married to the person.

(44) Filipino nurse became angry when a patient beckoned her by motioning with his right index finger because in the Philippines, that gesture is used to call dogs and is thus insulting when used with a person.

(45) Filipino nurse was hurt when she motioned in the Filipino manner for an Anglo aide to come assist her, and the aide simply smiled and waved at her.

TIME ORIENTATION

(46) *Filipino patient was upset when clinic refused to see him after he arrived 30 minutes late. Filipino nurse provided a culturally competent resolution.*

(47) *Mexican woman with kidney failure and diabetes was often late to clinic appointments. Nurse provided a culturally competent resolution.*

(48) Latino patient neglected to adhere to his physician's instructions to take medication for congestive heart failure and hyperkalemia because he stopped experiencing symptoms, and thus had an early, unscheduled return to the hospital.

Chapter 3. Pain

EXPRESSION OF PAIN

(49) Nicaraguan patient recovering from coronary bypass surgery was very expressive of his pain.

(50) Chinese patient recovering from coronary bypass surgery was very stoic.

(51) Mexican woman recovering from femoral bypass surgery complained loudly about pain. Nurse stereotyped her as a loud Mexican patient, but it turned out that she was bleeding internally and in a great deal of pain.

(52) Pakistani doctor didn't understand the significance of a normally stoic Irish woman's complaints about pain prior to surgery, assuming that all women were loud and expressive. Patient died, perhaps due to his lack of cultural competence.

(53) *A culturally competent nurse calmed a dramatic Italian woman with explanations and pain medication.*

(54) A Jewish woman feared that a minor pain in her finger signaled the advent of crippling arthritis, illustrating greater concern for the meaning and signficance of pain than for the pain sensation.

(55) A young Anglo American girl sat stoically through a painful examination, waiting to cry until the physician left the room.

PAIN MEDICATION

(56) Stoic Muslim Nigerian farmer never asked for pain medication following knee surgery, instead offering his pain to Allah.

(57) Filipino patient didn't want to bother the nurse by asking for pain mediation after a shoulder repair.

(58) *An Asian patient didn't request pain medication postoperatively, but his culturally competent nurse noted nonverbal signs of pain and educated him on the importance of pain medication.*

(59) East Indian woman, fearing addiction, stopped taking her medication following a total knee replacement, despite levels of pain that kept her from doing rehab exercises.

(60) Egyptian patient receiving home hospice care for advanced lung cancer preferred injections or IV infusion to oral medication, even though the pills were working.

(61) Hispanic man nearly died of an overdose of pain medication because no one took the time to explain how to take it.

(62) Anglo American woman did not comply with referral to the pain team, despite severe leg pain because she misunderstood the meaning of "pain team"; she felt she had enough pain and did not need more.

(63) Filipino nurse halved the doctor's prescribed dosage of medication for her dying mother because she feared her mother would become addicted to the medication.

Chapter 4. Religion and Spirituality

RELIGIOUS PRACTICES

(64) Buddhist monk from Cambodia became greatly distressed when a female nurse touched his shoulder because it violated the rules of his religion which required sexual segregation.

(65) *Culturally sensitive nurse followed through on a Catholic patient's request for a priest.*

(66) *Christian Scientist with colon cancer allowed doctors to perform a colonoscopy and colostomy, but refused the surgery that would have saved her life because it violated her religious beliefs.*

(67) Spiritual leader of an Indian Orthodox Christian church had to delay open-heart surgery while he underwent a purification ceremony after non-Orthodox Christians performed some medical procedures and a female operated the x-ray machine in the catheterization lab.

(68) Patient called nurse when he saw his roommate on the floor; Muslim patient was on the floor to pray.

(69) Jehovah's Witness's doctor decided to transfuse her and was later sued for assault and battery because he violated her express wish to adhere to her religion's rule against receiving blood.

(70) Jehovah's Witness changed her mind at the last minute and agreed to a blood transfusion.

(71) Jewish father requested the bloody scrubs of the nurse who tried to save his daughter after she was hit by a car because according to Jewish tradition, the individual must be buried whole and the blood was considered part of her body.

(72) *Adult son of Orthodox Jewish man asked to stay with his father's body until it was picked up by the mortuary because according to Jewish custom, the body of the deceased is not to be left unattended.*

(73) Orthodox Jewish man brought his wife to the hospital in labor during the Sabbath, and then could not leave or buy food due to Sabbath laws.

(74) Sikh from India refused to have any of his hair shaved prior to heart catheterization because the Sikh religion forbids cutting or shaving any body hair.

(75) *Culturally competent nurse took the time to explain to Sikh mother and child why she wanted to shave the child to prep him for an appendectomy and allowed the family to make the decision.*

SACRED SYMBOLS

(76) *Culturally competent nurse arranged for Latino patient to wear rosary beads into surgery.*

(77) Italian Catholic woman became upset when her soiled gown was thrown into the laundry without removing her scapular, a spiritual symbol.

(78) *Culturally competent nurse convinced other nurses to allow patients to keep religious statues in the room when Mexican patient explained how important they were to him.*

(79) Buddhist Cambodian woman was disturbed by the crucifix on the wall of her hospital bed.

(80) Mormon woman refused to remove her long underwear because "the garment" signifies adult religious status in the church and is considered sacred; the surgeon refused to operate unless she did.

(81) Culturally competent ICU nurse hung a "soul catcher" over the bed of a Native American.

(82) Cambodian mother became very upset when the nurse first tried to remove the strands of dark brown strings on her infant's wrists, and then inserted an IV line in the infant's scalp. The head is thought to be the seat of life, and holes could allow the child's soul to escape. The strings are thought to "tie in the soul."

(83) Culturally competent nurse prevented nursing assistant from removing a sacred string from Hindu patient's wrist.

SPIRITUAL BELIEFS AND PRACTICES

(84) Filipino woman was upset when the nurse did not respond for several days to her request for a chaplain to bless her daughter who was ill with sepsis and possibly dying.

(85) African American woman complied only with procedures and medications she believed were ordered by God.

(86) Hispanic woman stopped her diabetes medication because a curandera told her that God had cured her. Culturally competent physician handled the situation.

(87) Culturally competent nurse allowed Mexican family to pray together in private before patient had a colonoscopy.

(88) Family of Hmong teenage girl refused to allow her to have surgery when diagnosed with appendicitis for fear that cutting her open would risk having an evil spirit enter her body. Her appendix burst, she became septic and died.

(89) Navajo boy was upset when nurse took his photograph because he believed it would steal his soul.

(90) Mien man refused to have his blood drawn for diabetes test for fear that it would sap his strength and could result in soul loss.

(91) Culturally sensitive nurse took the time to explain to a Cambodian patient the need to draw blood, in case she held traditional beliefs regarding blood loss.

Chapter 5. Activities of Daily Living and the Body

EATING

(92) Culturally sensitive nurse realized it was Ramadan, and apologized to Egyptian Muslim patient for eating in front of her. This opened up communication and led to improved health for patient with diabetes.

(93) Nurses were annoyed at Filipino patient's apparent noncompliance.

Culturally competent nurse learned that the patient was Muslim and following the customs of Ramadan.

(94) A variety of Orthodox Jewish patients refused foods that violated kosher dietary laws.

(95) Hindu man in ER waiting room angrily refused hamburger the nurse had gotten for him because cows are considered sacred and not eaten.

(96) Pakistani woman hospitalized with TB refused many of the foods served to her because they violated rules of "hot" and "cold."

(97) Chinese patient with lung cancer ate only the foods his family brought because, unlike hospital meals, they were consistent with yin/yang (cold/hot) principles. Staff accommodated him.

(98) Mexican woman with diabetes and kidney failure ate only the foods that fit her notion of hot/cold body balance, many of which were bad for her. Situation was handled with cultural competence.

(99) Vietnamese refugee was brought in for observation because she wasn't eating the American-style food she was unused to.

(100) Vietnamese refugee receiving palliative care for cancer would not use dietician's recommended liquid dietary supplement because it was in a taste pleasing to the American palate but not hers. Home health nurse found a substitute more suitable to the Asian palate. (See also case 237 involving the same patient.)

(101) Saudi Arabian patients on dialysis refused to stop eating potassium-rich dates. They believed that Allah determined whether or not they lived or died, not what they ate.

(102) Culturally competent nurse realized that when educating patients about what foods to avoid with certain medications, she needed to consider their typical ethnic diet.

BATHING AND TOILETING

(103) Homeless patient would not bathe because he believed dirt would protect him from illness.

(104) Filipino patient refused to use a bedpan because he did not want to "dirty" his bed and made a mess of the bathroom because he was used to backyard toilets which are rinsed with a bucket of water.

(105) Anglo American woman teaching kindergarten in a Mexican neighborhood didn't realize that students were likely throwing toilet paper on the floor because they assumed the plumbing couldn't handle it.

(106) Arab man would not change colostomy bag, probably because it required two hands and in Arab culture only the left hand is used to clean after going to the bathroom.

HAIR AND BODY

(107) Native American woman took her grandchild out of hospital against medical advice after a nurse cut the child's hair to attach IV lines and would not allow her to keep a medicine bundle on the child's bed.

(108) Nigerian patient was upset because his knee surgery left scars that were too small. How would others know how much he had suffered and thus offered to Allah?

(109) Overweight Anglo nurse was humiliated when her Panamanian boyfriend's family kept telling her how fat she was. They were delighted.

Chapter 6. Family

DECISION MAKING

(110) Latino woman with diabetes would not agree to take insulin without first consulting with her family.

(111) Mexican woman suffering from depression did not want to go on antidepressants without discussing it first with her family.

(112) Twenty-two-year-old Mexican patient refused to sign consent for a kidney biopsy, saying his older brother must make that decision in the absence of his father, who was in Mexico.

ROLE OF THE FAMILY

(113) Nurse handled the 20–30 emotional family members of Hispanic patient with cultural competence by involving them in the patient's care and bending the visiting rules.

(114) Culturally competent labor and delivery nurse found that having family members assist with patient care is often successful in dealing with large numbers of visitors.

(115) Entire Romany (Gypsy) clan took over the hospital when their king was in intensive care.

(116) Anglo American student, injured while in Spain, was attended constantly by friends, even though she wanted to be left alone.

(117) When Lebanese nurse was hospitalized, she realized how important it was to her to have all her family there with her.

(118) Nurse discovered that the Hispanic patient who came to express her complaints was much less angry and more relaxed when treated with cultural competence.

(119) Japanese stroke patient in rehab refused to perform self-care when his family was present because it was their duty to obey and care for him.

(120) Mexican burn patient's wife continued to feed him, even after being told not to because that is how love and concern are demonstrated.

(121) Culturally competent nurse arranged for a demanding Muslim family to have a private room so they could pray together and for the patient to have food that was halal *under Muslim law.*

(122) Culturally competent nurse spoke to Korean patient's adult son to find out if patient knew of his cancer diagnosis.

(123) Pakistani family withheld news of adult son's death for fear that the news would kill their mother.

(124) Adult son of a Korean patient gave the nurse a cash gift upon discharge to show his gratitude and to satisfy a reciprocal obligation.

Chapter 7. Men and Women

SEX ROLES

(125) Anglo public health nurse feared that a fifteen-year-old pregnant Mexican woman, married and living with in-laws, might have been a captive housekeeper and sex slave.

(126) Mexican mother would not sign consent for her ill infant to have a spinal tap in the emergency department, preferring to wait for her husband to make the decision.

(127) Female resident who couldn't get Hispanic mother to sign consent for child's procedure called upon older male physician to speak to child's mother. He got her to agree.

(128) Vietnamese woman who was in motor vehicle accident with her children refused to sign any consents until her husband arrived. Situation resolved when staff called husband on phone and explained everything to him. Wife then agreed to sign consents.

(129) Indian woman would not agree to an epidural, even though she wanted one, because her husband would not allow it. Culturally competent nurse respected the authority structure within the family and spoke with husband; he soon decided she should have the epidural.

(130) Husband of an Indian patient refused to accept discharge instructions from any of the female nurses, only from the male physician.

(131) Iranian couple whose child had cancer became very uncooperative when assigned a female oncologist because they couldn't accept a woman making life-and-death decisions for their son.

(132) Father of a twenty-seven-year-old Saudi Arabian woman refused to allow her to sign consent for a possible hysterectomy prior to

surgery because if she couldn't have children she wouldn't marry and would thus be a burden to her family.

(133) The husband of an Iranian woman who had just given birth would allow no one in the room, answered questions put to her, and told her when to eat and bathe.

GENDER PREFERENCES

(134) Parents of a Chinese boy, dying of liver cancer, ignored their two daughters in favor of spending time with son.

FEMALE PURITY

(135) Husband of Iranian woman with serious heart problems refused to allow a male physician to examine her, thus delaying treatment and endangering her life.

(136) Arab man refused to allow male lab technicians into the room to draw blood from his wife.

(137) *Culturally competent nurse was able to build a trusting relationship with the family of a Lebanese woman.*

(138) When a twelve-year-old Somalian girl was admitted to the hospital with high fever, clinicians discovered she was infibulated.

(139) The vagina of an Egyptian woman in labor was "deformed" due to FGM.

(140) Pregnant Bedouin girl with gunshot wound to pelvis was killed when her father discovered she was pregnant.

(141) Salvadoran receptionist at an imaging center took care to make sure patients getting mammograms were not exposed, reflecting her own concern for the importance of modesty.

(142) *Vietnamese patient was uncomfortable during EKG until culturally sensitive nurse made sure she was completely covered with a blanket.*

(143) Mexican woman refused to be dialyzed when her usual station (which was private) was unavailable because she did not want to be exposed.

(144) *Problems with a "difficult" patient ended when culturally competent charge nurse made sure she was covered with an extra gown and assigned only female nurses to her.*

DOMESTIC VIOLENCE

(145) Iranian woman in traditional garb presented with multiple injuries. Her husband, who accompanied her, refused to allow her to answer questions, instead answering for her. When a male physician's assistant entered the room, he took his wife away.

(146) Mexican woman, beaten by husband, begged emergency department nurse to tell police it was an accident.

Chapter 8. Staff Relations

NURSING: THE ROLE OF THE NURSE

(147) Vietnamese nurse was reluctant to do aspects of the job she never had to do in Vietnam, causing the other nurses to think she was "stuck-up."

(148) Nurse had difficulty advocating for patient with authoritarian Pakistani physician.

(149) When Anglo American nurse questioned an East Indian physician's orders regarding a patient, he became very angry and upset.

(150) When an Anglo nurse refused to follow a Japanese physician's orders regarding patient medication because she thought it would harm the patient, he complained to her supervisor that she should have agreed to do it, and then not followed through.

(151) Iraqi physician was upset when an Anglo nurse questioned his order to discharge their patient.

(152) *The working relationship of an authoritarian Asian physician and an Anglo nurse improved when she applied cultural competence skills.*

(153) Thai nurse was hesitant to question Korean physician when she didn't understand his orders.

(154) Filipino nurse was responsible for the bad outcome of a patient because she did not use critical thinking skills.

CULTURAL INFLUENCES ON NURSING

(155) Nigerian male nurse assistant would not take orders from a female supervisor.

(156) Filipino nurse did not get along with her coworkers. They had very different perceptions of each other's behavior.

(157) Korean charge nurse in ICCU had difficulty doing what the job required because it conflicted with her cultural upbringing: to be passive and avoid conflict.

(158) Filipino nurse with county health department was hurt by the constructive criticism of her Anglo supervisor when she served as translator for an elderly Filipino TB patient who had been violating a county health order to stay in her home.

(159) Filipino aide was insulted when her Anglo supervisor offered to help her out once she had finished her own work. Later, rather than complain directly to her supervisor, she went to her coworkers, who then went to the supervisor.

MEDICINE: THE ROLE OF THE DOCTOR

(160) Anglo patient was angry when a paternalistic Middle Eastern physician would not give her enough information about her condition. In response, he resigned from her case.

LANGUAGE AND COMMUNICATION PROBLEMS

(161) Vietnam veteran, disoriented due to anesthesia, thought he was in prison in a foreign country when he awoke in the recovery room to two nurses speaking in Tagalog.

(162) Russian nurse was uncomfortable refusing food from Filipino nurses during the 40-day period before Easter. When she finally admitted why, it opened the way to more open communication between them.

(163) Chinese nurse's tone of voice did not convey the seriousness of a patient's condition.

(164) Asian nurses, in order to maintain self-esteem, said they knew how to do certain procedures when, in fact, they did not.

(165) Two young Filipino nurses helped an older Filipino nurse to "cheat" on a CEU exam; Anglo American nurse refused to do so.

(166) Anglo nurse had a hostile relationship with her Korean coworker because of the latter's general formality and the fact that she never said "please" or "thank you."

(167) *New Korean nurses hired on a unit were perceived as rude because they did not say "please" or "thank you." When nurse taking cultural competence course explained the reason to the other nurses, morale was greatly improved.*

(168) An American physician, visiting in Japan, was cautioned not to use the phrase "with your permission" when speaking to an audience of faculty members because it is inappropriate for someone of his stature to ask for permission and would diminish the audience's ability to respect anything else he said.

RELIGIOUS CONFLICTS

(169) Nurse who was a Jehovah's Witness refused to hang blood when temporarily transferred to the intensive care unit.

(170) Filipino Catholic nurse was not comfortable circulating on a therapeutic abortion.

(171) Jewish nurse could not take a new position he had applied for because the unit director refused to give him Saturdays off to observe the Sabbath.

Chapter 9. Birth

ANTE PARTUM

(172) Anglo nurse raised her arms above her head, against advice, and had a baby born with the cord wrapped around his neck.

(173) Romany (Gypsy) family was overly concerned about a young woman's bleeding post miscarriage, and wanted her to remain in the hospital as long as possible.

LABOR AND DELIVERY

(174) Filipino woman labored in silence.

(175) African American woman labored loudly.

(176) Cherokee woman labored silently.

(177) Husband of a "difficult" Iranian patient gave her a 3-karat diamond ring following the birth of their son to compensate for the "suffering" she had endured in giving birth.

(178) Orthodox Jewish husband was uncomfortable attending his wife during labor because birth is thought to render women "unclean" and it is thus forbidden for men to touch them.

(179) Arab husband was uncomfortable attending his wife during labor.

(180) Mexican husband was uncomfortable attending his wife during labor.

(181) Mexican father was upset when nurse insisted he join his mother-in-law and sister-in-law in the delivery room.

(182) Elderly Mexican woman had a tattoo on her upper thigh that, due to modesty, neither her husband nor her children had ever seen.

(183) Hmong woman would not consent to a caesarean section during a difficult delivery, perhaps because of fear that souls can leave the body during surgery.

POSTPARTUM

(184) Muslim Arab woman wanted to bury her baby's placenta.

(185) Mexican woman did not want to breastfeed colostrum, thinking it was "bad" milk and not good for the baby.

(186) *Nurse showed cultural sensitivity in respecting Chinese American woman's traditional practices (staying warm and resting) while promoting necessary medical care.*

(187) *Mexican immigrant would not drink ice water, so her culturally sensitive nurse replaced it with warm water, and asked her about other changes she would like to see in her treatment.*

(188) Vietnamese woman did not appear to bond with her infant. It is likely she was trying to avoid attracting attention to the newborn, to protect it from spirits who might want to "steal" the child.

(189) Nurses were upset when woman from India refused to hold her newborn twins except to feed them, consistent with Indian tradition.

(190) Hospital personnel were extremely concerned when a Hindu woman from India did not name her baby immediately after birth. She was waiting the traditional seven days, during which time she would consult an astrologer and allow her husband's sisters the honor of choosing the name.

(191) Middle Eastern couple rejected their newborn baby girl; they had been hoping for a boy to carry on the family name and wealth.

(192) Middle Eastern husband refused to participate in any patient education in baby care techniques; he saw that as the job of women.

BIRTH CONTROL

(193) Hospital required that a Mexican woman get her husband's signed permission before giving her a tubal ligation after delivery.

(194) When told that another pregnancy could prove fatal, a Mexican woman told her physician that she would have to talk to her husband before signing consent to have her tubes tied after delivery.

Chapter 10. End of Life

DYING

(195) Son of elderly Japanese patient asked medical and nursing staff not to let his mother know she had cancer. Patient did not want to know her diagnosis.

(196) Japanese nurse living in the United States for ten years found it difficult to withhold information about her father's condition from him.

(197) *Family of dying Latino man would not leave his bedside for fear that one of the staff might tell their father he was dying. Situation was handled with cultural sensitivity.*

(198) Young physician dealt with situation where family didn't want patient to know he was dying by avoiding the patient.

(199) Physician who believed patients should be told their diagnosis, against the desire of the family, had patients fail to show up for appointments and sometimes never return.

(200) Protective family of Mexican patient wanted hospice care for their dying mother until they learned she would have to sign informed consent for hospice and would learn that she was dying.

(201) *Culturally sensitive physician allowed a* curandera *to perform a ritual healing with a patient.*

(202) Iranian son refused to sign Do Not Resuscitate (DNR) order for his dying mother, perhaps believing that only Allah can decide when someone will die.

(203) African American patient refused to sign an advance directive or DNR because he felt it would be seen by God as giving up or losing faith.

(204) *Culturally competent nurse helped Filipino family decide to change family member's status to DNR and use hospice care.*

(205) Vietnamese man's family refused to remove life support until astrologers deemed the time auspicious.

DEATH

(206) Sephardic family left the room of a dying family member every hour, believing it is too hard for the dying to let go of life in the presence of loved ones.

(207) Relatives of a Romany (Gypsy) king suffering from pneumonia insisted on keeping a lit candle by his bed, despite the presence of an oxygen tent, so at death, his soul would be guided to heaven.

(208) Family of a Romany (Gypsy) king insisted on moving him outside just before he died in order to help free his soul.

(209) Culturally sensitive nurse assisted in preparing the body of a Buddhist patient after his death.

(210) Culturally sensitive nurse had a positive experience helping the family of an elderly male Vietnamese patient who died from a chronic illness.

(211) Family of Arab Muslim began loud wailing when he died, despite the fact that it was 2 A.M. and they were disturbing the other patients. Physician handled the situation with cultural competence.

NUMBERS AND DEATH

(212) Japanese woman became upset when she saw she was being wheeled into operating room 4 for surgery because the number represents "death."

(213) Chinese member of board of directors of hospital serving the Chinese community was upset when put in room 444 due to the association of the number with death.

Chapter 11. Mental Health

MENTAL ILLNESS

(214) Japanese woman was put in a mental hospital by husband for wanting to go to college, and was not released because her culturally appropriate behaviors were seen as signs of psychosis.

(215) Japanese woman tried to kill herself because of shame. Culturally competent nurse created a bond with her and helped the psychiatric treatment team to help her.

(216) Mentally ill Puerto Rican woman's culturally appropriate behaviors confused her diagnosis.

(217) Filipino nurse's visions and symptoms following the sudden death of her aunt and uncle were seen as signs of a nervous breakdown by an Anglo colleague but as normal by a Filipino colleague.

(218) Vietnamese woman visited Student Health Services for a variety of physical complaints, and later attempted suicide.

(219) Korean doctor treated the attempted suicide of a young Korean woman as an "accidental" overdose, rather than follow procedure

for a suicide attempt in order to avoid the stigma of mental illness. The Filipino admitting nurse did not question this obvious misdiagnosis due to respect for the physician.

STRESS AND MENTAL HEALTH

(220) Mexican woman admitted with chest pains would not talk about the fact that her husband had recently left her, even though that was the likely source of her pain, because she was uncomfortable discussing personal problems outside the family.

(221) Mexican woman with depression responded positively to treatment by a curandero *and was more responsive to the therapy prescribed by the psychiatrists as a result.*

(222) Chinese college student felt suicidal over the conflict between the culture of her parents and that of her American friends.

THE SUPERNATURAL

(223) Teenage Mexican boy, hospitalized in a psychiatric unit, seen as psychotic by staff but as having a calling to be a curandero *by his family. Situation was treated with cultural competence.*

(224) Mexican woman in geriatric assessment program believed she was being possessed as punishment for past sins.

(225) Mexican prison inmate appeared to be having a heart attack, believing he had been hexed by a bruja *(witch). Nurse handled the situation with cultural competence.*

Chapter 12. Traditional Medicine

TRADITIONAL OR "FOLK" REMEDIES

(226) Korean man, brought into emergency room unconscious, was covered in red welts. Not understanding that these were caused by the traditional practice of coining, the Emergency Department staff did not discover the cause of his condition until it was too late.

(227) School nurse reported the parents of a Vietnamese girl for child abuse when she discovered red welts on the girl's neck. She didn't realize they were made by coining in an attempt to help her feel better.

(228) A nurse found round red marks all over the upper back of an Armenian man when doing a physical assessment for a myocardial infarction in the critical care unit. They were made by cupping.

(229) Anglo American woman went to acupuncturist who used cupping to treat a cough that antibiotics had failed to cure.

(230) *Japanese patient ignored doctor's instructions for treating his high fever by bundling up and refusing cold liquids and the ice blanket. The nurse acted with cultural competence.*

(231) Mexican woman bundled up in blankets despite her high fever and the efforts of the nurses and refused a rectal temperature.

(232) Mexican mother wrapped her feverish infant in blankets despite the nurses' instructions to cool him down.

(233) African American grandmother became very upset when she saw her grandson put naked into a cool mist tent to reduce his fever.

MEDICATIONS

(234) Home health nurse discovered that a Mexican woman was applying her oral medication as a poultice to the incision site of her cesarean section.

(235) Mexican woman was angry because she got pregnant using birth control pills; she inserted them into her vagina.

(236) A Mexican woman became pregnant while using contraceptive foam; she and her husband applied it to his penis.

(237) Elderly Vietnamese woman did not get the physician's prescription filled for her lung condition because she didn't understand how to fill a prescription. (See also case 100 involving the same patient.)

(238) African American man with congestive heart failure took his medication only when he was short of breath, rather than every day as prescribed.

(239) Hispanic woman gave her infant a potentially dangerous traditional remedy her neighbor obtained from Guatemala.

"FOLK" DISEASES

(240) Medical student observing pediatric visit noticed that Mexican infant's mother changed demeanor when she complimented the child (thus giving the child the evil eye). The mother relaxed when the student touched the child.

(241) *Culturally competent nurse asked mother the meaning of a blue eye amulet worn by an infant at her clinic. It is thought to protect against the evil eye.*

TRADITIONAL HEALERS

(242) *Cherokee woman refused to sign consent for surgery until she saw a medicine man. Situation was resolved with cultural competence.*

(243) *Dying inmate began eating and taking medication again once his culturally competent nurse called in a medicine man to do a ceremony and arranged for him to do a sweat lodge.*

TRADITIONAL MEDICAL SYSTEMS

(244) A Korean man admitted for depression refused to take his medications. The problem was he had been given water or juice with his pills, and this violated hot/cold principles. When they gave him hot tea, he took his medication.

(245) Mexican woman ate nopales to treat her diabetes.

(246) Mexican immigrant recovering from cesarean section was upset because staff would not allow her to give her infant *manzanilla* (chamomile tea) to treat his colic.

(247) Mexican man hospitalized with a stomach problem was upset because the nurse would not allow him to drink the *manzanilla* tea he believed would help.

(248) Young Latino girl died from complications of strep throat two days after presenting in the emergency department. She had been seeing an unlicensed physician who injected her with outdated medications, and this delayed her seeking help from the hospital.

(249) Young Mexican mother treated infant suffering from *caída de la mollera.*

(250) Angry Mexican mother accused home health nurse of giving her child the evil eye when she complimented her.

(251) Nurse spent time trying to convince Mexican patient that Bell's palsy could not have been caused by *susto.*

(252) Mexican patient felt belittled when physician told her there was no such thing as *susto* and it could not have caused her to become ill.

(253) Culturally competent nurse reassured parents of injured Mexican baby that he would not suffer from susto, but they could take the infant to see a curandero if that would make them feel better.

(254) African American woman refused an angiogram for acute chest pain. (An elaboration of case 2)

(255) Family of an African American woman wanted to bring in a voodoo priestess to do a healing ritual for her. Culturally competent nurse came up with a plan to allow the ritual while still adhering to hospital rules.

Bibliography and Resources

Guide to Bibliography and Resources

Books and articles are organized by first by topic and then by ethnicity. The following is a list of topics.

- General Medical Anthropology/Transcultural Health Care
- Communication
- Cultural Competence
- Diet
- Disparities in Health Care
- Domestic Violence
- End-of-Life Care
- Female Genital Cutting and Women's Issues
- Home Health Care
- Interpreters
- Mental Health
- Pain
- Pregnancy and Birth
- Religion and Spirituality
- Staff Relations
- Traditional Medicine
- Values

Journals with a Transcultural Focus

Journal of Transcultural Nursing
Social Science & Medicine
Medical Anthropology Quarterly
Transcultural Psychiatry

Books and Articles

By Topic

GENERAL MEDICAL ANTHROPOLOGY/TRANSCULTURAL HEALTH CARE

Anderson, R. (1996) *Magic, Science, and Health.* New York: Harcourt Brace College.
Andrews, M. M. (1999) How to search for information on transcultural nursing and health subjects: Internet and CD-ROM resources. *Journal of Transcultural Nursing* 10 (1) (January): 69–74.

Andrews, M. M., and J. S. Boyle. (2007) *Transcultural Concepts in Nursing Care.* 5th ed. Philadelphia: Lippincott Williams & Wilkins.

Blackhall, L. J., S. T. Murphy, et al. (1995) Ethnicity and attitudes toward patient autonomy. *JAMA* 274 (10): 820–25.

Chesanow, N. (1998) The versatile doctor's guide to ethnic diversity. *Medical Economics* (September): 135–46.

Culture in Medicine. (2001) Special Issue. *Academic Medicine* 76 (5) (May).

Cross-Cultural Medicine. (1983) Special Issue. *WJM* 139 (6) (December).

Cross-Cultural Medicine—A Decade Later. (1992) Special Issue. *WJM* 157 (3) (September).

Dresser, N. (1996) *Multicultural Manners.* New York: John Wiley and Sons.

Erlen, J. A. (1998) Culture, ethics, and respect: The bottom line is understanding. *Orthopedic Nursing* (November/December): 79–81.

Galanti, G. (2000a) An introduction to cultural differences. *WJM* 172 (5): 335–36.

——. (2000b) Commentary: American health care professionals should respect the traditions of other cultures. *WJM* 173(5): 356.

——. (2001) The challenge of serving and working with diverse populations in American hospitals. *The Diversity Factor* 9 (3): 21–26.

Geiger, J. N., and R. E. Davidhizar, eds. (2007) *Transcultural Nursing: Assessment and Intervention.* 5th ed. St. Louis: C.V. Mosby.

Hahn, R. A. (1995) *Sickness and Healing: An Anthropological Perspective.* New Haven, Conn.: Yale University Press.

Harris, M. (1974) *Cows, Pigs, Wars, and Witches: The Riddles of Culture.* New York: Vintage Books.

Helman, C. G. (2007) *Culture, Health and Illness: An Introduction for Health Professionals.* 5th ed. Boston: Butterworth-Heinemann.

Kavanagh, K. H., and P. H. Kennedy. (1992) *Promoting Cultural Diversity: Strategies for Health Care Professionals.* Newbury Park, Calif.: Sage.

Kleinman, A., L. Eisenberg, and B. Good. (1978) Culture, illness, and care: Clinical lessons from anthropologic and cross-cultural research. *Annals of Internal Medicine* 88: 251–58.

Leininger, M., and M. R. McFarland. (2002) *Transcultural Nursing: Concepts, Theories, Research and Practice.* 3rd ed. New York: McGraw-Hill.

Like, R. C. (1999) Culturally competent managed health care: A family physician's perspective. *Journal of Transcultural Nursing* 10 (4) (October): 288–89.

Lipson, J. G., and S. L. Dibble, eds. (2005) *Culture and Clinical Care.* San Francisco: UCSF Nursing Press.

Loustanau, M., and E. J. Sobo. (1997) *The Cultural Context of Health, Illness, and Medicine.* Westport, Conn.: Bergin and Garvey.

McCullough-Zander K., ed. (2000) *Caring Across Cultures: The Provider's Guide to Cross-Cultural Health.* 2nd ed. Minneapolis: Center for Cross-Cultural Health.

Nakamura, R. M. (1998) *Health in America: A Multicultural Perspective.* Boston: Allyn and Bacon.

Orr, R. D. (1996) Treating patients from other cultures. *American Family Physician* 53 (6) (May): 2004–6.

Payer, L. (1996) *Medicine and Culture: Varieties of Treatment in the United States, England, West Germany, and France.* New York: Holt.

Note: PDF files of the articles from *WJM* are now available through PubMed at http://www.pubmedcentral.nih.gov/tocrender.fcgi?journal=183&action=archive.

Purnell, L., and B. Paulanka, eds. (2003) *Transcultural Health Care: A Culturally Competent Approach.* 2nd ed. Philadelphia: Davis.

Rivera-Andino, J., and L. Lopez. (2000) When culture complicates care. *RN* 63 (7) (July): 47–49.

Spector, R. E. (2003) *Cultural Diversity in Health and Illness.* 6th ed. Upper Saddle River, N.J.: Prentice-Hall.

Stein, H. F. (1990) *American Medicine as Culture.* Boulder, Colo.: Westview Press.

Zoucha, R. (1998) Understanding the significance of culture in emergency care and treatment. *Topics in Emergency Medicine* 20 (4) (December): 40–51.

COMMUNICATION

Betancourt, J. R., J. E. Carrillo, and A. R. Green. (1999) Hypertension in multicultural and minority populations: Linking communication to compliance. *Current Hypertension Reports* 1: 482–88.

Carrese, J. A., and L. A. Rhodes. (2000) Bridging the cultural differences in medical practice: The case of discussing negative information with Navajo patients. *Journal of Internal Medicine* 15: 92–96.

Crowe, K., L. Matheson, and A. Steed. (2000) Informed consent and truth–telling: Cultural directions for healthcare providers. *Journal of Nursing Administration* 30 (3) (March): 148–52.

Flores, G., M. Abreu, I. Schwartz, and M. Hill. (2000) The importance of language and culture in pediatric care: Case studies from the Latino community. *Journal of Pediatrics* 137 (6): 842–48.

Gross, J. (2007) Keeping patients' details private, even from kin. *New York Times*, http://www.nytimes.com/2007/07/03/health/policy/03hipaa.html.

Haffner, L. (1992) Translation is not enough: Interpreting in a medical setting. *WJM* 157 (3): 255–59.

Hall, E. T., and M. R. Hall. (1990) *Understanding Cultural Differences: Germans, French and Americans.* Yarmouth, Minn.: Intercultural Press.

Kuczewski, M., and P. J. McCruden (2001) Informed consent: Does it take a village? The problem of culture and truth telling. *Cambridge Quarterly of Healthcare Ethics* 10 (1) (Winter): 34–46.

Pang, M. C. (1999) Protective truthfulness: The Chinese way of safeguarding patients in informed treatment decisions. *Journal of Medical Ethics* 25 (3) (June): 247–53.

Salimbene, S. (2000) *What Language Does Your Patient Hurt in?™A Practical Guide to Culturally Competent Patient Care.* Amherst, Mass.: Diversity Resources.

Seijo, R., H. Gomez, and J. Freidenberg (1995) Language as a communication barrier in medical care for Hispanic patients. In A. M. Padilla, ed., *Hispanic Psychology: Critical Issues in Theory and Research*, 169–81. Newbury Park, Calif.: Sage.

Torrecillas, L. (1997) Communication of the cancer diagnosis to Mexican patients: Attitudes of physicians and patients. *Annals of the New York Academy of Sciences* 809 (February): 188–96.

CULTURAL COMPETENCE

Betancourt, J. R., A. R. Green, and J. E. Carrillo. (2002) *Cultural Competence in Health Care: Emerging Frameworks and Practical Approaches.* New York: Commonwealth Fund.

Campinha-Bacote, J. (1994) *The Process of Cultural Competence in Health Care: A Culturally Competent Model of Care.* 2nd ed. Wyoming, Ohio: Transcultural C.A.R.E. Associates.

———. (1998) *The Process of Competence in the Delivery of Healthcare Services: A Culturally Competent Model of Care.* Cincinnati: Transcultural C.A.R.E. Associates.

———. (1999) A model and instrument for addressing cultural competence in health care. *Journal of Nursing Education* 38 (5): 203–7.

Chrisman, N. (1991) Culture-sensitive nursing care. In M. Patrick, S. Woods, R. Craven, J. Rokosky, and P. Bruno, eds., *Medical-Surgical Nursing: Pathophysiological Concepts.* 2nd ed., 34–46. New York: J.B. Lippincott.

Chrisman, N. J., and P. A. Zimmer. (2000) Cultural competence in primary care. In P. V. Meredith and N. M. Horan, eds., *Adult Primary Care,* 65–75. Philadelphia: W.B. Saunders.

Flores, G. (2000) Culture and the patient-physician relationship: Achieving cultural competency in health care. *Journal of Pediatrics* 136 (1) (January): 14–23.

Galanti, G. (2007) *Cultural Sensitivity: A Pocket Guide for Health Care Professionals.* Oakbrook Terrace, Ill.: Joint Commission Resources.

Goode, T. D., M. C. Dunne, and S. M. Bronheim. (2006) *The Evidence Base for Cultural and Linguistic Competency in Health Care.* New York: Commonwealth Fund.

Graves D. L., R. C. Like, N. Kelly, and A. Hohensee. (2007) Legislation as intervention: An examination of cultural competence policy in health care. *Journal of Health Care Law and Policy* 10 (2).

Health Resources and Services Administration. (2001) *Cultural Competence Works: Using Cultural Competence to Improve the Quality of Care for Diverse Populations and Add Value to Managed Care Arrangements.* Merrifield, Va.: HRSA Information Center.

Lecca, P. J., I. Quervalu, J. V. Nunes, and H. F. Gonzales. (1998) *Cultural Competency in Health, Social, and Human Services: Directions for the Twenty-First Century.* New York: Garland.

Levin, S. J., R. C. Like, and J. E. Gottlieb. (2000) ETHNIC: A framework for culturally competent clinical practice. In Appendix: Useful clinical interviewing mnemonics. *Patient Care* 34 (9): 188–89.

Mutha, S., C. Allen, and M. Welch. (2002) *Toward Culturally Competent Care: A Toolbox for Teaching Communication Strategies.* San Francisco: Center for the Health Professiona, University of California.

Office of Minority Health. (2001) *National Standards for Culturally and Linguistically Appropriate Services in Health Care: Final Report.* Washington, D.C.: U.S. Department of Health and Human Services. http://www.omhrc.gov/assets/pdf/checked/finalreport.pdf.

Sue, S. (1998) In search of cultural competence in psychotherapy. *American Psychologist* 53: 440–48.

Warda, M. R. (2000) Mexican Americans' perceptions of culturally competent care. *Western Journal of Nursing Research* 22 (2) (March): 203–24.

DIET

Airhihenbuwa, C. O., S. Kumanyika, et al. (1996) Cultural aspects of African American eating patterns. *Ethnicity and Health* 1 (3) (September): 245–60.

Bronner, Y. (1994) Cultural sensitivity and nutrition counseling. *Topics in Clinical Nutrition* 9 (2) (March): 13–19.

Cerrato, P. L. (1996) Customize diets with culture in mind. *Office Nurse* 9 (4) (April): 22–23, 26.

Chaudry, M. M. (1992) Islamic food laws: Philosophical basis and practical implications. *Food Technology* 46 (10) (October): 92.

Counihan, C., and S. Kaplan, eds. (1997) *Food and Culture.* New York: Routledge.

Kilara, A., and K. K. Iya. (1992) Food and dietary habits of the Hindu. *Food Technology* 46 (10) (October): 94–104.

LaFraniere, S. (2007) Nouakchott journal: In Mauritania, seeking to end an overfed ideal. NYTimes.com. July 4 (in World section, Africa). http://www .nytimes.com/2007/07/04/world/africa/04mauritania.html

Lee, S., J. Sobal, et al. (1999) Acculturation and dietary practices among Korean Americans. *Journal of the American Dietetic Association* 99 (9) (September): 1084–89.

Pike, O. A. (1992) The Church of Jesus Christ of Latter-Day Saints: Dietary practices and health. *Food Technology* 46 (10) (October):118–21.

Samolsky, S., K. Dunker, et al. (1990) Feeding the Hispanic hospital patient: Cultural considerations. *Journal of the American Dietetic Association* 90 (12) (December): 1707–10.

Sirota, L. H., J. M. Newman, et al. (1996) Chinese food habit perspectives. *Association for the Study of Food and Society* 1: 31–38.

DISPARITIES IN HEALTH CARE

American College of Cardiology Foundation. (2002) Racial/Ethnic Differences in Cardiac Care: The Weight of the Evidence. Summary Report.

Betancourt, J. R., and O. Ananeh-Firempong II. (2004) Not me! Doctors, decisions, and disparities in health. *Cardiovasc Rev Rep* 25 (3): 105–9. http://www.medscape .com/viewarticle/480602

Hasnain-Wynia, R., D. W. Baker, et al. (2007) Disparities in health care are driven by where minority patients seek care. *Archives of Internal Medicine* 167 (12): 1233–39.

Lillie-Blanton, M., O. E. Rushing, and R. S. Boone. (2002) *Racial/Ethnic Differences in Cardiac Care: The Weight of the Evidence.* Menlo Park, Calif.: Henry J. Kaiser Family Foundation and American College of Cardiology Foundation.

Smedley B. D., A. Y. Stith, and A. R. Nelson, eds. (2003). *Unequal Treatment: Confronting Racial and Ethnic Disparities in Health Care.* Washington, D.C.: National Academy Press.

DOMESTIC VIOLENCE

American Nurses Association. (1998) *Culturally Competent Assessment for Family Violence.* Washington, D.C.: American Nurses Association.

Bui, H. N., and M. Morash. (1999) Domestic violence in the Vietnamese immigrant community: An exploratory study. *Violence Against Women* 5 (7) (July): 769–95.

Campbell, J. C., and D. W. Campbell. (1996) Cultural competence in the care of abused women. *Journal of Nurse Midwifery* 41 (6) (November–December): 457–62.

Chester, B., R. W. Robin, et al. (1994) Grandmother dishonored: Violence against women by male partners in American Indian communities. *Violence and Victims* 9 (3) (Fall): 249–58.

Dasgupta, S. D. (2000) Charting the course: An overview of domestic violence in the South Asian community in the United States. *Journal of Social Distress and the Homeless* 9 (3): 173–85.

Gabler, M., S. E. Stern, et al. (1998) Latin American, Asian, and American cultural differences in perceptions of spousal abuse. *Psychological Reports* 83 (2) (October): 587–92.

Hampton, R. L., and R. J. Gelles. (1994) Violence toward Black women in a nationally representative sample of Black families. *Journal of Comparative Family Studies* 25 (1) (Spring): 105–19.

Horne, S. (1999) Domestic violence in Russia. *American Psychologist* 54 (1) (January): 55–61.

Juckett, G. (2005) Cross-cultural medicine. *American Family Physician* 72 (11): 2267–74.

Kleinman, A., and P. Benson (2006) Anthropology in the clinic: The problem of cultural competency and how to fix it. *PLoS Medicine* 3 (10): e294. doi:10.1371/journal.pmed.0030294.

Korbin, J. E. (1995) Social networks and family violence in cross-cultural perspective. *Nebraska Symposium on Motivation* 42: 107–34.

Kozu, J. (1999) Domestic violence in Japan. *American Psychologist* 54 (1): 50–54.

Krane, J. E. (1996) Violence against women in intimate relations: Insights from cross-cultural analyses. *Transcultural Psychiatric Research Review* 33 (4): 435–65.

Loue, S., and M. Faust. (1999) Intimate partner violence among immigrants. In S. Loue, ed., *Handbook of Immigrant Health*, 521–44. New York: Plenum Press.

Mattson, S., and E. Rodriguez. (1999) Battering in pregnant Latinas. *Issues in Mental Health Nursing* 20 (4) (July–August): 405–22.

Olavarrieta, C. D., and J. Sotelo. (1996) Domestic violence in Mexico. *JAMA* 275 (24): 1937–41.

Rabin, B., E. Markus, et al. (1999) A comparative study of Jewish and Arab battered women presenting in the emergency room of a general hospital. *Social Work in Health Care* 29 (2): 69–84.

Rhee, S. (1997) Domestic violence in the Korean immigrant family. *Journal of Sociology and Social Welfare* 24 (1) (March): 63–77.

Robin, R. W., B. Chester, et al. (1998) Intimate violence in a southwestern American Indian tribal community. *Cultural Diversity and Mental Health* 4 (4): 335–44.

Rodriguez, M. A., H. M. Bauer, et al. (1998) Factors affecting patient-physician communication for abused Latina and Asian immigrant women. *Journal of Family Practice* 47 (4) (October): 309–11.

Wilcox, G. N., and L. J. Armstrong. (1996) Identifying family violence: A community prototype incorporating native Hawaiian values and practices. *Hawaii Medical Journal* 55 (9) (September): 169–70.

END-OF-LIFE CARE

Battaglia, B. (1997a) Cultural views on death and dying, part 1. *Cross Cultural Connection* 3 (1) (July–September): 1–2.

———. (1997b) Cultural views on death and dying, part 2. *Cross Cultural Connection* 3 (2) (October–December): 1–3.

———. (1998) Cultural views on death and dying, part 3. *Cross Cultural Connection* 3 (3) (January–March): 1–4.

Bhungalia, S., and C. Kemp. (2002) (Asian) Indian health beliefs and practices related to the end-of-life. *Journal of Hospice and Palliative Nursing* 4 (1) (January): 54–58.

Blackhall, L. J., G. Frank, et al. (1999) Ethnicity and attitudes towards life sustaining technology. *Social Science and Medicine* 48 (12): 1779–89.

Blackhall, L. J., S. T. Murphy, G. Frank, V. Michel, and S. Azen. (1995) Ethnicity and attitudes toward patient autonomy. *JAMA* 274 (10): 820–25.

Bonura, D., M. Fender, M. Roesler, and D. F. Pacquiao. (2001) Culturally congruent end-of-life care for Jewish patients and their families. *Journal of Transcultural Nursing* 12 (3) (July): 211–20.

Braun, K. L., and R. Nichols. (1997) Death and dying in four Asian American cultures: A descriptive study. *Death Studies* 21 (4) (July/August): 327–59.

Braun, K. L., J. H. Pietsch, et al., eds. (1999) *Cultural Issues in End-of-Life Decision Making.* Thousand Oaks, Calif.: Sage.

Burrs, F. A. (1995) The African American experience: Breaking the barriers to hospices. *Hospice Journal* 10 (2): 15–18.

Crawley, L., P. Marshall, and B. Koeing. (2002) Strategies for culturally effective end-of-life care. *Annals of Internal Medicine* 136 (9) (Supplement, May 7): 673–79.

Crawley, L., R. Payne, et al. (2000) Palliative and end-of-life care in the African American community. *Journal of the American Medical Association* (284): 2518–21.

Danielson, B. L., A. J. LaPree, et al. (1998) Attitudes and beliefs concerning organ donation among Native Americans in the upper Midwest. *Nursing* 8 (3) (September): 153–56.

Davidson, M. N., and P. Devney. (1991) Attitudinal barriers to organ donation among Black Americans. *Transplantation Proceedings* 23: 2531–32.

Dinh, A., C. Kemp, and L. Rasbridge. (2000) Culture and the end of life: Vietnamese health beliefs and practices related to the end of life. *Journal of Hospice and Palliative Nursing* 2 (3) (July–September): 111–17.

Dupree, C. Y. (2000) The attitudes of Black Americans toward advance directives. *Journal of Transcultural Nursing* 11 (1) (January): 12–18.

Eighmy, J. B. (2002) Personal communication, July 30, August 5.

Fetters, M. D. (1998) The family in medical decision making: Japanese perspectives. *Journal of Clinical Ethics* 9 (2): 132–46.

Gelfand, D. E., H. Balcazar, et al. (2001) Mexicans and care for the terminally ill: Family, hospice and the church. *American Journal of Hospice and Palliative Care* 18 (6) (November–December): 391–96.

Green, J. (1992a) Death with dignity: Christianity. *Nursing Times* 88 (3): 26–29.

———. (1992b) Death with dignity: Christian Science. *Nursing Times* 88 (4): 32–33.

———. (1992c) Death with dignity: Jehovah's Witnesses. *Nursing Times* 88 (5): 36–37.

———. (1992d) Death with dignity: The Afro-Caribbean community. *Nursing Times* 88 (8): 50–51.

Haber, D. (1999) Minority access to hospice. *American Journal of Hospice and Palliative Care* 16 (1) (January–February): 386–89.

Hepburn, K., and R. Reed. (1995) Ethical and clinical issues with Native-American elders: End-of-life decision making. *Clinics in Geriatric Medicine* 11 (1) (February): 97–111.

Hern, J. H. E., B. A. Koenig, et al. (1998) The difference that culture can make in end-of-life decision making. *Cambridge Quarterly of Healthcare Ethics* 7 (1) (Winter): 27–40.

Irish, D. P., K. F. Lundquist, and V. J. Nelsen, eds. (1993) *Ethnic Variations in Dying, Death, and Grief.* Washington, D.C.: Taylor and Francis.

Kagawa-Singer, M. (1994) Diverse cultural beliefs and practices about death and dying in the elderly. *Gerontology and Geriatrics Education* 15 (1): 101–16.

Kagawa-Singer, M., and L. J. Blackhall. (2001) Negotiating cross-cultural issues at the end of life. "You've got to go where he lives." *JAMA* 286: 2993–3001.

Kagawa-Singer, M., I. M. Martinson, et al. (1998) Forum focus: A multicultural perspective on death and dying. *Oncology Nursing Forum* 25 (10) (November–December): 1751–63.

Kemp, C. (2001) Culture and the end of life: Hispanic cultures (focus on Mexican-Americans). *Journal of Hospice and Palliative Nursing* 3 (1) (January–March): 29–33.

Kemp, C., and B. Chang (2002) Culture and the end of life: Chinese. *Journal of Hospice and Palliative Nursing* 4 (3) (July): 173–78.

Keovilay, L., L. Rasbridge, et al. (2000) Cambodian and Laotian health beliefs and practices related to the end of life. *Journal of Hospice and Palliative Medicine* 2 (4): 143–51.

Klessig, J. (1992) The effect of values and culture on life-support decisions. *WJM* 157 (3): 316–22.

Koenig, B. (1995) Understanding cultural differences in caring for dying patients. *WJM* 163 (3): 244–49.

Lapine, A., R. Wang-Cheng, M. Goldstein, et al. (2001) When cultures clash: Physician, patient and family wishes in truth disclosure for dying patients. *Journal of Palliative Medicine* 4 (4): 475–80.

Lewis, R. (1990) Death and dying among the American Indians. In J. K. Parry, ed., *Social Work Practice with the Terminally Ill: A Transcultural Perspective*, 23–32. Springfield, Ill.: Charles C. Thomas.

Mouton, C. (2000) Cultural and religious issues for African Americans. In K. Braun, J. H. Pietsch, and P. Blanchette, eds., *Cultural Issues in End-of-Life Decision Making*, 71–82. Thousand Oaks, Calif.: Sage.

Mulhall, A. (1996) The cultural context of death: What nurses need to know. *Nursing Times* 92 (34) (August 21–27): 38–40.

Perkins, H. S., C. M. Geppert, A. Gonzales, et al. (2002) Cross-cultural similarities and differences in attitudes about advance care planning. *Journal of Internal Medicine* 17 (1) (January): 48–57.

Ross, H. M. (1998) Best practice: Jewish tradition in death and dying. *MedSurg Nursing* 7 (5) (October): 275–80.

Sarhill, N., S. LeGrand, R. Islambouli, et al. (2001) The terminally ill Muslim: Death and dying from the Muslim perspective. *American Journal of Hospice and Palliative Care* 18 (4) (July–August): 251–55.

Talamantes, M. A., W. R. Lawler, et al. (1995) Hispanic American elders: Caregiving norms surrounding dying and the use of hospice services. *Hospice Journal* 10 (2): 35–49.

Vawter, D. E., and B. Babbitt. (1997) Hospice care for terminally ill Hmong patients: A good cultural fit? *Minnesota Medicine* 80 (11) (November): 42–44.

Waters, C. M. (2000) End-of-life care directives among African-Americans: Lessons learned: A need for community-centered discussion and education. *Journal of Community Health Nursing* 17 (1): 25–37.

Zimring, S. D. (2001) Multi-cultural issues in advance directives. *Journal of American Medical Directors Association* 2 (5) (September–October): 241–45.

FEMALE GENITAL CUTTING AND WOMEN'S ISSUES

Brooks, G. (1995) *Nine Parts of Desire: The Hidden World of Islamic Women*. New York: Anchor Books.

Burstyn, L. (1995) Female circumcision comes to America. *Atlantic Monthly* (October): 28–35.

Chavez, L. R. H., F. Allan, et al. (1997) The influence of fatalism on self-reported use of papanicolaou smears. *American Journal of Preventive Medicine* 13 (6) (November–December): 418–24.

Hutchinson, M. K., and M. Baqi-Aziz. (1994) Nursing care of the child bearing Muslim family. *Journal of Obstetrics, Gynecologic, and Neonatal Nursing* 23 (9): 767–71.

Kristof, N. D. (1991) Stark data on women: 100 million are missing. *New York Times*, November 5, Science section, C1, C12.

Lightfoot-Klein, H. (1990) *Prisoners of Ritual: An Odyssey into Female Genital Circumcision in Africa.* Binghamton, N.Y.: Haworth Press.

Shaw, E. (1985) Female circumcision. *American Journal of Nursing* 85 (6): 684–87.

HOME HEALTH CARE

Cheng, B. K. (1997) Cultural clash between providers of majority culture and patients of Chinese culture. *Journal of Long-Term Home Health Care* 16: 39–43.

Haddad, L. G., and S. P. Hoeman. (2000) Home healthcare and the Arab-American client. *Home Healthcare Nurse* 18 (3) (March): 189–97.

Narayan, M. C., and K. Rea. (1997) Nursing across cultures: The South Asian client. *Home Healthcare Nurse* 15 (7) (July): 460–69.

Pacquiao, D. F., L. Archeval, et al. (2000) Hispanic client satisfaction with home health care: A study of cultural context of care. In M. L. Kelley and V. M. Fitzsimons, eds., *Understanding Cultural Diversity: Culture, Curriculum, and Community in Nursing,* 229–40. Sudbury, Mass.: Jones and Bartlett.

INTERPRETERS

Kelly, N. (2007) Telephone interpreting in health care settings: Some commonly asked questions. *ATA Chronicle* (June): 18–21.

Kaufert, J. M., and R. W. Putsch. (1997) Communication through interpreters in healthcare: Ethical dilemmas arising from differences in class, culture, language, and power. *Journal of Clinical Ethics* 8 (1) (Spring): 71–87.

MENTAL HEALTH

Arthur, D., H. K. Chan, et al. (1999) Therapeutic communication strategies used by Hong Kong mental health nurses with their Chinese clients. *Journal of Psychiatric and Mental Health Nursing* 6 (1) (February): 29–36.

Barry, D. T., and M. G. Carlos. (2002) Cultural, psychological, and demographic correlates of willingness to use psychological services among East Asian Immigrants. *Journal of Nervous and Mental Disease* 190 (1): 32–39.

Bechtel G. A., R. Davidhizar, and C. M. Tiller. (1998) Patterns of mental health care among Mexican Americans. *Journal of Psychosocial Nursing and Mental Health Services* 36 (11): 20–27.

Behui, K., and D. Bhugra. (1997) Cross-cultural competencies in the psychiatric assessment. *Journal of Hospital Medicine* 57 (10) (May 21–June 3): 492–96.

Campinha-Bacote, J. (1992) Voodoo illness. *Perspectives in Psychiatric Care* 28 (1) (January–March): 11–17.

———. (1994) Cultural competence in psychiatric mental health nursing: A conceptual model. *Mental Health Nursing* 29 (1) (March): 1–8.

———. (1997) *Readings and Resources in Transcultural Health Care and Mental Health.* Cincinnati: Transcultural C.A.R.E. Associates.

Cuellar, I., and F. A. Paniagua, eds. (2000) *Handbook of Multicultural Mental Health.* San Diego: Academic Press.

Erickson, C. D., and N. R. Al-Timimi. (2001) Providing mental health services to Arab Americans: Recommendations and considerations. *Cultural Diversity and Ethnic Minority Psychology* 7 (4) (November): 308–27.

Flaskerud, J. H. (2000) Ethnicity, culture, and neuropsychiatry. *Issues in Mental Health Nursing* 21 (1) (January–February): 5–29.

Gaw, A. C. (2001) *Concise Guide to Cross-Cultural Psychiatry.* Washington, D.C.: American Psychiatric Publishing.

Hammerschlag, C. A. (1988) *The Dancing Healers: A Doctor's Journey of Healing with Native Americans.* San Francisco: Harper and Row.

Hughes, C. C. (1998) The glossary of culture-bound syndromes in DSM-IV: A critique. *Transcultural Psychiatry* 35 (3) (September): 413–21.

Kleinman, A. (1980) *Patients and Healers in the Context of Culture.* Berkeley: University of California Press.

Kung, W. W. (2001) Consideration of cultural factors in working with Chinese American families with a mentally ill patient. *Families in Society* 82 (1): 97–107.

Kuo, C., K. H. Kavanagh, et al. (1994) Chinese perspectives on culture and mental health. *Issues in Mental Health Nursing* 15 (6) (November–December): 551–67.

Lin, K., and F. Cheung. (1999) Mental health issues for Asian Americans. *Psychiatric Services* 50 (6) (June): 774–80.

McGoldrick, M., J. Giordano, and J. K. Pearce, eds. (2005) *Ethnicity and Family Therapy.* 3rd ed. New York: Guilford Press.

Nobles, A. Y., and D. T. Sciarra. (2000) Cultural determinants in the treatment of Arab Americans: A primer for mainstream therapists. *American Journal of Orthopsychiatry* 70 (2) (April): 182–91.

Pang, K. Y. (1998) Symptoms of depression in elderly Korean immigrants: Narration and the healing process. *Culture, Medicine, and Psychiatry* 22 (1) (March): 93–122.

Rodriguez, E. (1999) The heart of the matter: Worldview as a central concept in effective cross-cultural work. *Journal of the California Alliance for the Mentally Ill* 10 (1): 5–7.

Torrey, E. F. (1986) *Witchdoctors and Psychiatrists: The Common Roots of Psychotherapy and Its Future.* New York: Harper and Row.

PAIN

Bates, M. S., L. Rankin-Hill, et al. (1997) The effects of the cultural context of health care on treatment of and response to chronic pain. *Social Science and Medicine* 45 (9) (November): 1433–48.

Davidhizar, R. & J.N. Giger. (2004) A review of the literature on care of clients in pain who are culturally diverse. *International Nursing Review* 51 (1): 47–55.

Galanti, G. (2000) Filipino attitudes toward pain medication. *WJM* 173 (October): 278–79.

Harrison, A. (1991) Arabic pain words. *Pain* 32: 239–50.

Juarez, G., B. Ferrell, et al. (1998) Influence of culture on cancer pain management in Hispanic patients. *Cancer Practice* 6 (5) (September–October): 262–69.

Martinelli, A. M. (1987) Pain and ethnicity. *AORN Journal* 46 (2): 273–81.

Reizian, A., and A. I. Meleis. (1986) Arab-Americans' perceptions of and responses to pain. *Critical Care Nurse* 6 (6): 30–37.

Villarruel, A. M., and B. O. de Montellano. (1992) Culture and pain: A Mesoamerican perspective. *Advances in Nursing Science* 15 (1): 21–32.

Zborowski, M. (1952) Cultural components in response to pain. *Journal of Social Issues* 8: 16–30.

Zola, I. K. (1966) Culture and symptoms: An analysis of patients' presenting complaints. *American Sociological Review* 31: 615–30.

PREGNANCY AND BIRTH

Bodo, K., and N. Gibson. (1999) Childbirth customs in Vietnamese traditions. *Canadian Family Physician* 45 (March): 690–92, 695–97.

Browner, C. H., H. M. Preloran, M. C. Casado, H. N. Bass, and A. P. Walker. (2003) Genetic counseling gone awry: miscommunication between prenatal genetic service providers and Mexican-origin clients. *Social Science and Medicine* 56: 1933–46.

Callister, L. C. (1995) Cultural meanings of childbirth. *Journal of Obstetric, Gynecologic, and Neonatal Nursing* 24 (3): 327–31.

Darabi, K. F., and V. Ortiz. (1987) Childbearing among young Latino women in the U.S. *American Journal of Public Health* 77 (1): 25–28.

Davis, R. E. (2001) The postpartum experience for Southeast Asian women in the United States. *MCN Maternal and Child Nursing* 26 (4) (July–August): 208–13.

DePacheco, M., and M. Hutti. (1998) Cultural beliefs and health care practices of childbearing Puerto Rican American women and Mexican American women: A review of the literature. *Mother Baby Journal* 3 (1) (January): 14–25.

Galanti, G. (2000) Iranian births. *WJM* 173 (1) (July): 67–68.

Han, Y., R. D. Williams, et al. (1999) Breast self examination (BSE) among Korean American women: Knowledge, attitudes, and behaviors. *Journal of Cultural Diversity* 6 (4) (Winter): 115–23.

Higgins, B. (2000) Puerto Rican cultural beliefs: Influence on infant feeding practices in western New York. *Journal of Transcultural Nursing* 11 (1) (January): 19–30.

Hung, P. (2001) Traditional Chinese customs and practices for the postnatal care of Chinese mothers. *Complementary Therapies in Nursing and Midwifery* 7 (4) (November): 202–6.

Jimenez, S. L. (1995) The Hispanic culture, folklore, and perinatal health. *Journal of Perinatal Education* 4 (1): 9–16.

Lefhber, Y., and H. Voorhoeve. (1999) Indigenous first feeding practices in newborn babies. *Midwifery* 15 (2) (June): 97–100.

Mattson, S. (1995) Culturally sensitive perinatal care for Southeast Asians. *Journal of Obstetric, Gynecologic, and Neonatal Nursing* 24 (4) (May): 335–41.

Simpson, E., J. D. Mull, E. Longley, and J. East. (2000) Pica during pregnancy in low-income women born in Mexico. *WJM* 173: 20–24.

RELIGION AND SPIRITUALITY

Beck, S. E., and E. K. Goldberg. (1996) Jewish beliefs, values, and practices: Implications for culturally sensitive nursing care. *Advanced Practice Nursing Quarterly* 2 (2) (Fall): 15–22.

Bonura, D., M. Fender, M. Roesler, and D. F. Pacquiao. (2001) Culturally congruent end-of-life care for Jewish patients and their families. *Journal of Transcultural Nursing* 12 (3) (July): 211–20.

Burgonio-Watson, T. B. (1997) Filipino spirituality: An immigrant's perspective. In M. P. Root, ed., *Filipino Americans*, 324–32. Thousand Oaks, Calif.: Sage.

Falicov, C. J. (1999) Religion and spiritual folk traditions in immigrant families: Therapeutic resources with Latinos. In F. Walsh, ed., *Spiritual Resources in Family Therapy*, 104–20. New York: Guilford Press.

Gallagher, C. (1996) Religious attitudes regarding organ donation. *Journal of Transplant Coordination* 6 (4) (December): 186–90.

Gatrad, A. R. (1994) Muslim customs surrounding death, bereavement, postmortem examinations, and organ transplants. *BMJ* 309 (August 20): 521–23.

Getzel, G. S. (1995) Judaism and death: Practice implications. In J. K. Parry and A. S. Ryan, eds., *A Cross-Cultural Look at Death, Dying, and Religion*, 18–31. Chicago: Nelson-Hall.

Gillman, J. (1999) Religious perspectives on organ donation. *Critical Care Nursing Quarterly* 2 (3) (November): 19–29.

Hunt, L. M., N. H. Arar, and L. L. Akana. (2000) Herbs, prayer, and insulin: Use of medical and alternative treatments by a group of Mexican-American diabetes patients. *Journal of Family Practice* 49: 216–23.

Kapp, M. B. (1993) Living and dying the Jewish way: Secular rights and religious duties. *Death Studies* 17: 267–76.

Katims, I. P. (1999) Buddhist ethics and implications for end-of-life issues. In L. Zhan, ed., *Asian Voices: Asian and Asian-American Health Educators Speak Out,* 106–16. Sudbury, Mass.: Jones and Bartlett.

Mouton, C. (2000) Cultural and religious issues for African Americans. In K. Braun, J. H. Pietsch, and P. Blanchette, eds., *Cultural Issues in End-of-Life Decision Making,* 71–82. Thousand Oaks, Calif.: Sage.

Ross, H. M. (1998) Best practice: Jewish tradition in death and dying. *MedSurg Nursing* 7 (5) (October): 275–80.

Sarhill, N., S. LeGrand, R. Islambouli, et al. (2001) The terminally ill Muslim: Death and dying from the Muslim perspective. *American Journal of Hospice and Palliative Care* 18 (4) (July–August): 251–55.

Stolley, J. M., and J. Koenig. (1997) Religion/spirituality and health among elderly African Americans and Hispanics. *Journal of Psychosocial Nursing and Mental Health Services* 35 (11) (November): 32–38, 45–46.

STAFF RELATIONS

Brislin, R. W. et al. (1986) *Intercultural Interactions: A Practical Guide.* Newbury Park, Calif.: Sage.

Galanti, G. (2006) *65 Tips for Foreign-Born Nurses Working in American Hospitals.* Oakland, Calif.: Support for Nurses. http://supportfornurses.com/toolkit.php

Galanti, G. (2007) *Orienting Foreign-Born Nurses to Work Effectively in American Hospitals: A Training Manual for Health Educators.* Oakland, Calif.: Support for Nurses. http://supportfornurses.com/toolkit.php

Gardenswartz, L., and A. Rowe. (1998) *Managing Diversity in Health Care.* San Francisco: Jossey-Bass.

Thiederman, S. (1991) *Bridging Cultural Barriers for Corporate Success.* Lexington, Mass.: Lexington Books.

TRADITIONAL MEDICINE

Bacardi-Gascon, M. (2007) Lowering effect on postprandial glycemic response of nopales added to Mexican breakfasts, *Diabetes Care* 30 (5) (May): 1264–65, CCINAHL AN: 2009583074.

Baer, R. D., J. Garcia de Alba, et al. (1998) Mexican use of lead in the treatment of empacho: Community, clinic, and longitudinal patterns. *Social Science and Medicine* 47 (9) (November): 1263–66.

Battaglia, B. (1996) Understanding Hispanic folk ailments and illnesses. *Cross Cultural Connection* 2 (2) (October–December): 1–2, 4.

Becerra, R. M., and A. P. Iglehart. (1995) Folk medicine use: Diverse populations in a metropolitan area. *Social Work in Health Care* 21 (4): 37–58.

Beinfield, H., and E. Korngold. (1995) Chinese traditional medicine: An introductory overview. *Alternative Therapies* 1 (1): 44–52.

Centers for Disease Control and Prevention. (1993) Lead poisoning associated with use of traditional ethnic remedies. *California: Morbidity and Mortality Weekly Report* 42: 521–54.

Davis, R. E. (2000) Cultural health care or child abuse? The Southeast Asian practice of cao gio. *Journal of the American Academy of Nurse Practitioners* 12 (3) (March): 89–95.

Engebretson, J. (1994) Folk healing and biomedicine: Culture clash or complementary approach? *Journal of Holistic Nursing* 12 (3) (September): 240–50.

Gordon, S. M. (1994) Hispanic cultural health beliefs and folk remedies. *Journal of Holistic Nursing* 12 (3) (September): 307–22.

Hansen, K. K. (1998) Folk remedies and child abuse: A review with emphasis on *caída de mollera* and its relationship to shaken baby syndrome. *Child Abuse and Neglect* 22 (2) (February): 117–27.

Holden W., J. Joseph, and L. Williamson. (2005) Use of herbal remedies and potential drug interactions in rheumatology outpatients. *Annals of the Rheumatic Diseases* 64: 790.

Hunt, L. M., N. H. Arar, and L. L. Akana. (2000) Herbs, prayer, and insulin: Use of medical and alternative treatments by a group of Mexican American diabetes patients. *Journal of Family Practice* 49: 216–23.

Jenkins, C. N. H., T. Le, et al. (1996) Health care access and preventive care among Vietnamese immigrants: Do traditional beliefs and practices pose barriers? *Social Science and Medicine* 43 (7) (October): 1049–56.

Kaptchuk, T. J. (1983) *The Web That Has No Weaver: Understanding Chinese Medicine.* New York: Congdon and Weed.

Longo, B. (1990) Traditional Southeast Asian medical techniques: What nurses should know. *Nurseweek* (February 5).

Messer, E. (1981) Hot-cold classification: Theoretical and practical implications of a Mexican study. *Social Science and Medicine* 15: 133–45.

Neff, N. (n.d.) Folk Medicine in Hispanics in the Southwestern United States. http://www.rice.edu/projects/HispanicHealth/Courses/mod7/mod7.html, accessed 8/13/07.

Rotblatt, M. and I. Ziment. (2002) *Evidenced-Based Herbal Medicine.* Philadelphia: Hanley and Belfus.

Trotter, R. T. (1997) *Curanderismo: Mexican American Folk Healing.* Athens: University of Georgia Press.

Weldon, M. M., M. S. Smolinski, et al. (2000) Mercury poisoning associated with a Mexican beauty cream. *WJM* 173 (1) (July): 15–18.

Yeatman, G. W. (1980) *Cao gio* (coin rubbing): Vietnamese attitudes toward health care. *JAMA* 244: 2748–49.

Zevin, I. V., N. Altman, and L. V. Zevin. (1997) *A Russian Herbal: Traditional Remedies For Health and Healing.* Rochester, Vt.: Healing Arts Press.

VALUES

Cooper, C. R., H. Baker, et al. (1993) Values and communication of Chinese, Filipino, European, Mexican, and Vietnamese American adolescents and their families and friends. *New Directions for Child Development* 62 (Winter): 73–89.

Kim, B. S. K., P. H. Yang, et al. (2001) Cultural value similarities and differences among Asian American ethnic groups. *Cultural Diversity and Ethnic Minority Psychology* 7 (4) (November): 343–61.

Kluckhohn, C. (1951). Values and value orientations in the theory of action. In T. Parsons and E. Shils, eds., *Toward a General Theory of Action*, 409–14. Cambridge, Mass.: Harvard University Press.

Kluckhohn, F. R. (1953) Dominant and variant value orientations. In P. Brink, ed., *Transcultural Nursing: A Book of Readings*, 63–81. Englewood Cliffs, N.J.: Prentice-Hall.

By Ethnicity

Most of the books and articles focusing on various ethnic groups are listed under their specific topics. The readings listed under ethnic groups are more general or do not fit into any of the topic categories.

AFRICAN AMERICANS

Kaiser Permanente National Diversity Council. (1999) *A Provider's Handbook on Culturally Competent Care: African American.* Oakland, Calif.: Kaiser Permanente National Diversity Council.

Locks, S., and L. Boateng. (1996) Black/African Americans. In J. G. Lipson, S. L. Dibble, and P. A. Minarik, eds. *Culture and Nursing Care: A Pocket Guide,* 37–43. San Francisco: UCSF Nursing Press.

Snow, L. F. (1977) Popular medicine in a Black neighborhood. In E. H. Spicer, ed., *Ethnic Medicine in the Southwest.* Tucson: University of Arizona Press.

———. (1983) Traditional health beliefs and practices among lower class Black Americans. *WJM* 139: 820–28.

———. (1993) *Walkin' over Medicine: Traditional Health Practices in African-American Life.* Boulder, Colo.: Westview Press.

Thomas, S. B., and S. C. Quinn. (1991) The Tuskegee syphilis study, 1932 to 1972: Implications for HIV education and AIDS risk education programs in the Black community. *American Journal of Public Health* 81 (11): 1498–505.

ASIANS

Ahmed, S. M., and J. P. Lemkau. (2000) Cultural issues in the primary care of South Asians. *Journal of Immigrant Health* 2 (2) (April): 89–96.

Barrett, B., K. Shadick, et al. (1998) Hmong/Medicine interactions: Improving cross-cultural health care. *Family Medicine* 30 (3) (March): 179–84.

Chen, Y. (2001) Chinese values, health and nursing. *Journal of Advanced Nursing* 36 (2) (October): 270–73.

Culhane-Pera, K. A., D. E. Vawter, et al., eds. (2003) *Healing by Heart: Clinical and Ethical Case Stories of Hmong Familes and Western Providers.* Nashville, Tenn.: Vanderbilt University Press.

Dasgupta, S. D. (1998) Gender roles and cultural continuity in the Asian Indian immigrant community in the U.S. *Sex Roles: A Journal of Research* 38 (11): 953–75.

Fadiman, A. (1997) *The Spirit Catches You and You Fall Down: A Hmong Child, Her American Doctors, and the Collision of Two Cultures.* New York: Farrar, Straus, and Giroux.

Fetters, M. D. (1998) The family in medical decision making: Japanese perspectives. *Journal of Clinical Ethics* 9 (2): 132–46.

Galanti, G. (2000) Vietnamese family relationships. *WJM* 172 (6): 415–16.

———. (2001) Japanese Americans and Self-Care. *WJM* 174 (3): 208–9.

Johnson, S. K. (2002) Hmong health beliefs and experiences in the Western health care system. *Journal of Transcultural Nursing* 13 (2) (April): 126–32.

Kaiser Permanente National Diversity Council. (1999). *A Provider's Handbook on Culturally Competent Care: Asian and Pacific Island American Population.* Oakland, Calif.: Kaiser Permanente National Diversity Council.

Kristy, S. (1998) Toward understanding Vietnamese attitudes, beliefs and practices regarding blood donation. *Social Sciences in Health: International Journal of Research and Practice* 4 (3) (August): 154–62.

Muecke, M. A. (1983) In search of healers: Southeast Asian refugees in the American health care system. *WJM* 129: 835–40.

Mull, J. D., D. S. Mull, and N. Nguyen. (2001) Vietnamese diabetic patients and their physicians: What ethnography can teach us. *WJM* 175 (November): 307–11.

Ohnuki-Tierney, E. (1984) *Illness and Culture in Contemporary Japan.* New York: Cambridge University Press.

Pourat, N., J. Lubben, et al. (2000) Perceptions of health and use of ambulatory care: Differences between Korean and White elderly. *Journal of Aging and Health* 12 (1) (February): 112–34.

Rajwani, R. J. (1996) South Asians. In J. G. Lipson, S. L. Dibble, and P. A. Minarik, eds., *Culture and Nursing Care: A Pocket Guide*, 264–79. San Francisco: UCSF Nursing Press.

Sharts-Hopko, N. C. (1996) Health and illness concepts for cultural competence with Japanese clients. *Journal of Cultural Diversity* 3 (3) (Fall): 74–79.

Takayama, J. I. (2001) Giving and receiving gifts: One perspective. *WJM* 175: 138–39.

Tsai, J. H. (1999) Meaning of filial piety in the Chinese parent-child relationship: Implications for culturally competent health care. *Journal of Cultural Diversity* 6 (1): 26–34.

GYPSIES (ROM)

Brink, S. (1988) Doctoring Gypsies. *Boston Magazine* 7: 80–86.

Kephart, W. M. (1989) The Gypsies. In E. Angeloni, ed., *Annual Editions: Anthropology 89/90*, 122–37. Guilford, Conn.: Dushkin.

Sutherland, A. (1992) Gypsies and health care. *WJM* 157 (3): 276–80.

HISPANICS/LATINOS

Ailinger, R., and M. Causey. (1995) Health concepts of older Hispanic immigrants. *Western Journal of Nursing Research* 17 (6): 605–13.

Caudle, P. (1993) Providing culturally sensitive health care to Hispanic patients. *Nurse Practitioner* 18 (12): 40–51.

Huff, R. M., and M. V. Kline. (1999) Tips for working with Hispanic populations. In R. M. Huff and M. V. Kline, eds., *Promoting Health in Multicultural Populations: A Handbook for Practitioners*, 189–97. Thousand Oaks, Calif.: Sage.

Kaiser Permanente National Diversity Council. (2001). *A Provider's Handbook on Culturally Competent Care: Latin*. Oakland, Calif.: Kaiser Permanente National Diversity Council.

Mull, D. S., P. F. Agran, et al. (1999) Household poisoning exposure among children of Mexican-born mothers: An ethnographic study. *WJM* 171 (1) (July): 16–19.

Purnell, L. (1999) Panamanians' practices for health promotion and the meaning of respect afforded them by health care providers. *Journal of Transcultural Nursing* 10 (4) (October): 331–39.

Sheppard, H. (1990) Hispanic culture. *Nurseweek* (February 5).

Smart, J. F., and D. W. Smart. (1992) Cultural issues in the rehabilitation of Hispanics. *Journal of Rehabilitation* 63 (4): 9–15.

MIDDLE EASTERNERS

Al-Shahri, M, Z. (2002) Culturally sensitive caring for Saudi patients. *Journal of Transcultural Nursing* 13 (2) (April): 133–38.

Athar, S. (1999) Information for health care providers when dealing with a Muslim patient. *Islamic Medical Association of North America*. www.islam-usa.com/e40.html

Brooks, G. (1995) *Nine Parts of Desire: The Hidden World of Islamic Women*. New York: Anchor Books.

Carlisle, D. (1995) Lifting the veil. *Nursing Times* 9: 22–23.

Fernea, E. W., and R. A. Fernea. (1989) A look behind the veil. In E. Angeloni, ed., *Annual Editions: Anthropology 89/90*, 149–53. Guilford, Conn.: Dushkin.

Ide, Bette A., and T. Sanli. (1992) Health beliefs and behavior of Saudi women. *Women and Health* 19 (1): 97–113.

Kemp, C. (1996) Islamic cultures: Health-care beliefs and practices. *American Journal of Health Behavior* 20 (3): 83–89.

Kulwicki, A. (1996) Health issues among Arab Muslim families. In B. Aswad and B. Belge, eds., *Family and Gender Among American Muslims and Their Descendants*, 187–207. Philadelphia: Temple University Press.

Lawrence, P., and C. Rosmus. (2001) Culturally sensitive care of the Muslim patient. *Journal of Transcultural Nursing* 12 (3): 228–33.

Lipson, J. G., and A. I. Meleis. (1983) Issues in health care of Middle Eastern patients. *WJM* 139: 854–61.

Luna, L. (1989) Transcultural nursing care of Arab Muslims. *Journal of Transcultural Nursing* 1 (1): 22–26.

McKennis, A. T. (1999) Caring for the Islamic patient. *AORN Journal* 69 (6) (June): 1187–96, 1199–206.

Sheikh, A., and A. R. Gatrad, eds. (2000) *Caring for Muslim Patients*. Oxford: Radcliffe Medical Press.

NATIVE AMERICANS

Alvord, L. A., and E. C. Van Pelt. (2000) *The Scalpel and the Silver Bear: The First Navajo Woman Surgeon Combines Western Medicine and Traditional Healing.* New York: Bantam Dell Doubleday.

Bozof, R. P. (1972) Some Navaho attitudes toward available medical care. *American Journal of Public Health* 62: 1620–24.

Coulehan, J. H. (1980) Navaho Indian medicine: Implications for healing. *Journal of Family Practice* 10: 55–61.

Dajer, T. (1989) Medicine man. *Discover* (July): 47–51.

Hammerschlag, C. A. (1988) *The Dancing Healers: A Doctor's Journey of Healing with Native Americans.* San Francisco: Harper and Row.

Kramer, B. J. (1992) Health and aging of urban American Indians. *WJM* 157 (3): 281–85.

Michielutte, R., P. C. Harp, et al. (1994) Cultural issues in the development of cancer control programs for American Indian populations. *Journal of Health Care for the Poor and Underserved* 5 (4): 280–96.

Parker, J. G. (1994) The lived experience of Native Americans with diabetes within a transcultural nursing perspective. *Journal of Transcultural Nursing* 6 (1): 5–11.

Plawecki, H. M., T. R. Sanchez, et al. (1994) Cultural aspects of caring for Navajo Indian clients. *Journal of Holistic Nursing* 12 (3) (September): 291–306.

SOUTH ASIANS

Rajwani, R. J. (1996) South Asians. In J. G. Lipson, S .L. Dibble, and P. A. Minarik, eds., *Culture and Nursing Care: A Pocket Guide*, 264–79. San Francisco: UCSF Nursing Press.

Zachariah, R. (2005) East Indians. In J. G. Lipson and S .L. Dibble, eds., *Culture and Clinical Care*, 146–62. San Francisco: UCSF Nursing Press.

Internet Sites

For an up-to-date list of recommended Websites, go to www.ggalanti.com. From the home page, click on "Related Links" and you will find numerous sites on general and specific topics relevant to culture and health care issues.

Videos, DVDs, and CD-ROMs

For a detailed list of recommended media, go to www.ggalanti.com and click on "Resources."

Index

There are two parts to this index. The first looks at the ethnicity of the various participants by **case number.** The second is a standard index by **page number.**

Case Index by Ethnicity

Again, note that the numbers refer to case numbers, not page numbers. In most cases, the nurses and physicians are Anglo American. They are only identified as such when it was relevant to the case.